Nursing
Research

Third Edition

Jones and Bartlett Nursing Research Titles

Basic Steps in Planning Nursing Research: From Question to Proposal, Fifth Edition, Brink

Grant Application Writer's Handbook, Third Edition, Reif-Lehrer

Institutional Review Board: Management and Function, Amdur

Instruments for Clinical Health-Care Research, Second Edition, Frank-Stromborg

The Methodology of Discourse Analysis, Powers

Nursing Research: A Qualitative Perspective, Third Edition, Munhall

Qualitative Research Proposals and Reports: A Guide, Second Edition, Munhall

Qualitative Inquiry: The Path of Sciencing, Parse

Dorothy Young Brockopp

Marie T. Hastings-Tolsma

FUNDAMENTALS OF
Nursing
Research

Third Edition

JONES AND BARTLETT PUBLISHERS

Sudbury, Massachusetts

BOSTON   TORONTO   LONDON   SINGAPORE

World Headquarters
Jones and Bartlett
Publishers
40 Tall Pine Drive
Sudbury, MA 01776
978-443-5000
info@jbpub.com
www.jbpub.com

Jones and Bartlett
Publishers Canada
2406 Nikanna Road
Mississauga, ON L5C
2W6
CANADA

Jones and Bartlett
Publishers International
Barb House, Barb Mews
London W6 7PA
UK

Library of Congress Cataloging-in-Publication data unavailable at time of printing.

ISBN 0-7637-1567-0

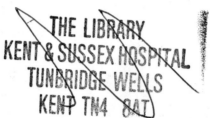

Acquisitions Editor: Penny M. Glynn
Production Manager: Amy Rose
Associate Production Editor: Tara McCormick
Editorial Assistant: Karen Zuck
Production Assistant: Karen C. Ferreira
Marketing Associate: Joy Stark-Vancs
Manufacturing & Inventory Coordinator: Amy Bacus
Composition: Northeast Compositors, Inc.
Text Design: dcdesign
Illustrations: Carolyn H. Kasper/dcdesign
Cover Design: Night & Day Design
Printing and Binding: Malloy, Inc.
Cover Printing: Jaguar Advanced Graphics

This book was typeset in Quark 4.1 on a Macintosh G4. The font families used were Sabon and Futura Condensed.

Printed in the United States of America
06 05 04 03 02   10 9 8 7 6 5 4 3 2 1

DEDICATION

To Gene W. Brockopp
My friend, mentor, and husband,
To whom I owe so much,
With love and appreciation
−dyb

With love and thanks to my mother,
Dorothy M. Owen, RN, PNP, PA
And to my father, William E. Owen, M.D.
−mht

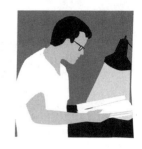

Contents

Preface   xvii
Acknowledgments   xix
Student Introduction   xxi

Unit 1   Evidence-Based Nursing Practice   1

1   *Evolution of a Body of Nursing Knowledge*   3
Introduction   4
Value of Nursing Research   4
Historical Roots   5
   1900-1970: Laying the Groundwork   6
   1970-Present: New World Trends   8
Art and Science of Nursing   8
Development of a Discipline   10
A Unique Body of Nursing Knowledge   10
   Ways of Knowing: Structuring Nursing Knowledge   12
Aim and Purpose of Nursing Research   15
Research Methods   18
Hallmarks of Success   23
   Boundaries for Nursing Study   23
   Scholarly Publications   25
   Resources for Promoting Nursing Research   30

Future of Nursing Research   32

Critical Overview of the Evolution of Nursing
    Knowledge   33

References   35

2   Promoting Evidence-Based Nursing Practice   39

Introduction   40

Research Defined   40

    Problem-Solving Process   40
    Research Process   43

Nursing Research Defined   46

Roles in Nursing Research   49

    The Consumer: A Critical Appraiser of Research   49
    Role as Research Designer and Producer   58
    Role as Replicator   60
    Role as Data Collector   62

Evaluating Research Reports for Use in Practice   64

Categorizing Evidence   64

    Bradford-Hill Guidelines   71

Making Evidence-Based Recommendations   73

Critical Overview of Promoting Evidence-Based Nursing
    Practice   76

References   78

Unit 2   Asking the Research Question   79

3   Initiating a Study   81

Introduction   81

Research Feasibility   82

Purpose of the Investigation   84

Importance of the Study to Nursing   86

Basic Versus Applied Research   88

Kinds of Investigations   92

Conceptual Models   96

Nursing Models   97
Concepts   100
Borrowed Models   102

Theories   105

Propositions   108
Concept-Construct-Variable   111

Scientific Reasoning   116

Deductive   117
Inductive   118

The Problem Statement   120

Specifying the Topic or Concept of Interest   121
Concepts and Their Relationships   125
The Focus of the Study   126

The Population   129

Critical Overview in Initiating a Study   130

References   133

Review of the Literature   137
Introduction   137

Steps in a Review of the Literature   139

The Initial Search   139
The Secondary Search   141

Identifying Publications   144

A Computer Search   145
A Manual Search   148

Keeping a Record   149

Writing the Review of the Literature   151

Critical Overview of the Review of the Literature   154

References   157

5   *Protecting Research Participants   159*
    Introduction   159

    Guidelines for Conducting Research   160
       Professional Guidelines   161
       Federal Guidelines   162

    Research Participants at Risk   164

    Informed Consent   168

    Confidentiality and Anonymity   175

    Participant Withdrawal   181

    Deception   182

    Debriefing   184

    Role of the Research Committee and IRB   185

    Critical Overview of Research Participant Selection and
       Protection   187

    References   190

Unit 3   **Answering the Research Question: Quantitative
         Designs   191**

6   *Measurement   193*
    Introduction   193

    Measuring Variables   194
       The Nominal Level of Measurement   196
       The Ordinal Level of Measurement   198
       The Interval Level of Measurement   201
       The Ratio Level of Measurement   204

    Methods of Measurement   206
       The Instrument   206
       Errors of Measurement   209
       Validity   210
       The Validity of an Instrument   211
       Reliability   215

    Critical Overview of Measurement   219

    References   220

7   *Quantitative Designs in Research   221*
Introduction   221
Experimental Designs   222
 The Experiment   222
 The Quasi-experimental Design   229
Nonexperimental Designs   231
Key Concepts in Quantitative Designs   234
Key Research Concepts   235
 Hypothesis Formation   235
 Identifying Variables   236
 Defining Terms   240
Sample Selection: Choosing Participants   244
 Probability Sampling   244
 Nonprobability Sampling   249
Validity in Relation to the Research Design   251
Critical Overview of Quantitative Designs in
  Research   253
References   255
Bibliography   256

8   *Epidemiologic Research   257*
Introduction   257
Population Health   259
 Causation   261
 Meta-analysis   265
Risk   266
Incidence and Prevalence   268
Rates and Ratios   269
Frequently Used Concepts in Epidemiology   272
 Statistical Estimates: Confidence Intervals   272
 Bias   272
 Confounding Variables   273

Critical Overview of Epidemiology   274

References   275

9   Data Analysis   277

Introduction   277

Basic Concepts in Descriptive Statistics   280

Descriptive Measures   280
The Normal Distribution   289
Correlation   292

Basic Concepts in Inferential Statistics   298

Probability   298
Sampling Error (Standard Error)   300
Null Hypothesis   301
Statistical Significance   303

Inferential Statistical Tests   306

One-Way Analysis of Variance (ANOVA)   309
Factorial Analysis of Variance   312
Analysis of Covariance (ANCOVA)   315
Multivariate Analysis   317
Correlation   319

Inferential Statistical Tests   320

Chi-Square Tests (Nonparametric)   320

Critical Overview of Data Analysis   320

References   322

Unit 4   Answering the Research Question: Qualitative Designs   323

10   Qualitative Designs in Research   325

Introduction   326

Development of Qualitative Research Designs   326

Qualitative Research: Definition and Purpose   327

Qualitative Research Methods   332

Types of Qualitative Inquiry 332
Sources of Data   346
Participant Observation   349
Recording the Data   352
Recording for Bias   354

Critical Overview of Qualitative Research Designs   356

References   358

Bibliography   361

11 Analyzing the Data in Qualitative Research   363

Introduction   364

Analyzing the Data   364

Literature Review   366
   Analyzing the Findings   368

Scientific Adequacy in Qualitative Designs   371

Critical Overview of Analyzing the Data in Qualitative
   Research   373

References   374

Unit 5 Promoting Evidence-Based Practice: Nurse as
Researcher   377

12 Reviewing the Research Findings   379

Introduction   379

Presenting the Findings   380

Interpreting the Results   390

Drawing Conclusions   394

Implications for Nursing   395

Critical Overview of Reviewing the Research Findings   396

References   398

13 Evaluating Research Reports   399

Introduction   399

Aim of Research Evaluation   400

Critique Guidelines   402

Critiquing Process   403

Mapping the Research Report   403
Critique of the Quantitative Research Report   405
Critique of the Qualitative Research Report   411
Basic Consideration in Evaluating Research Reports   419

Format and Preparation of the Research Evaluation   421

Implementing the Research Report Findings in
Practice   422

Critical Overview of the Research Evaluation Process   428

References   429

14 Communicating Study Results   433

Introduction   434

The Research Report   434

Elements of the Research Report   437

Selecting the Target Audience   439

Selecting the Mode of Presentation   442

Written Research Reports   442
Oral Research Reports   443
Tips for Presenting the Research Report   444

Basic Considerations in Facilitating Use of the Research
Report   446

Titling the Research Report   446
Research Abstract   447
References   449
The Investigator's Background and Credentials   450

Critical Overview of Communicating Research   453

References   457

15 *Research and the Entry-Level Professional Nurse* 459

Introduction 459

Guidelines for Participating in Research 460
Expectations of the Profession 460
Societal Expectations 461
Interprofessional Influences 461

Research and the Entry-Level Professional Nurse 463
NLN and ANA Guidelines for Functioning 463

Research Proposal 465

Participating in Grant Applications 468

Promoting Evidence-Based Practice in the Workplace 471

Critical Overview of Research and the Entry-Level Professional Nurse 475

References 477

Appendices 479
Appendix A Elements of Critical Appraisal 481
Appendix B Format for Evaluation of the Quantitative Research Report 493
Appendix C Format for Evaluation of the Qualitative Research Report 499

Glossary 507

Index 521

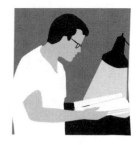

Preface

In the upcoming decade, more than ever before, nurses will be expected to provide evidence-based care for patients. This approach requires us to have a sound working knowledge of research methods, as well as a strong clinical foundation. Although there are a number of different definitions for evidence-based practice, each one assumes the use of systematically derived results in the clinical setting.

The most stringent definition accepts results of randomized controlled trials or quantitative studies as acceptable evidence. Broader views incorporate descriptive studies, qualitative studies, case studies, and expert opinion. Nursing leans toward a broad view that includes clinical expertise, intuition, scientifically derived information, and the ability to comprehend and analyze all facets of a given patient scenario (McPheeters & Lohr, 1999; Titler, Mentes, Rakel, et al., 1999). The Agency for Healthcare Research and Quality (AHRQ) identifies five levels of evidence in a hierarchy of credibility. The most credible evidence is obtained from meta-analysis of available quantitative research on a given phenomenon. The least credible comes from case studies and expert clinical opinion (Stetlet, Brunell, Giuliano, et al., 1998; Stetler, Morsi, Rucki, et al., 1988).

We subscribe to the broad view of evidence-based practice and see quantitative research results as an important but not exclusive component of nursing practice. Our text, therefore, includes qualitative research as an important approach to collecting and analyzing data that can influence care. We also see epidemiology as a method that will be increasingly used as nurses become more influential within our communities. Our goal is for each nurse to understand these structured approaches to generating knowledge at a depth that will enable them to use research findings in a meaningful way.

References

McPheeters, M. & Lohr, K. (1999). Evidence-based practice and nursing: commentary. *Outcomes Management Nursing Practice*. 3(3): 99–101.

Stetler, C., Brunell, J., Giuliano, K., Morsi, D., Prince, L. & Newell-Stokes, V. (1998). Evidence-based practice and the role of nursing leadership. *The Journal of Nursing Administration*. 28(7–8): 45–53.

Stetler, C., Morsi, D., Rucki, S., Broughton, S., Corrigan, B., Fitzgerald, J., Giuliano, K., Havener, P. & Sheridan, E. (1998). Utilization-focused integrative reviews in a nursing service. *Applied Nursing Research*. 11(4): 195–206.

Titler, M., Mentes, J., Rakel, B., Abbott, L. & Baumler, S. (1999). From book to bedside: putting evidence to use in the care of the elderly. *The Joint Commission Journal on Quality Improvement*. 25(10): 545–556.

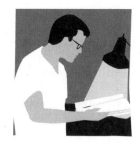

Acknowledgments

We would like to extend our deepest appreciation to those who helped us with our third edition. Penny Glynn, editor at Jones and Bartlett Publishers, was particularly supportive and deserves special mention. Thanks are also extended to Karen Zuck and Tara McCormick. Finally, our warmest thanks to the faculty and students who used the first and second editions and offered valuable comments.

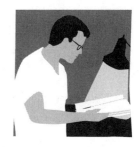

Student Introduction

This text is designed to present the process of nursing research in as clear a manner as possible. To use this text it is important to understand the following elements that help organize the material you will be learning:

- An INTRODUCTION provides an overview of each chapter.
- A WORKING DEFINITION gives a clear description of a concept so that it can be easily understood and readily applied.
- An EXAMPLE provides a practical example of the concept under discussion.
- A PRACTICE suggests an activity that can help the reader understand the concept under discussion.
- A CRITICAL APPRAISAL provides a set of questions on a given topic that can help the reader evaluate a research report.
- A CRITICAL OVERVIEW is an opportunity for the reader to evaluate what has been learned throughout the chapter.

Unit 1

Evidence-Based Nursing Practice

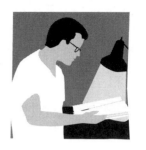

1

Evolution of a Body of Nursing Knowledge

Goals

- *Examine the value of nursing research.*
- *Understand the historical roots of nursing research.*
- *Examine the art and science of nursing.*
- *Describe the development of the discipline of nursing.*
- *Describe ways of knowing in developing nursing knowledge.*
- *Identify hallmarks of success in nursing science.*
- *Describe the future of nursing research.*

Introduction

It is not unusual for the nurse who has not been involved in research before, or whose involvement has been minimal, to feel overwhelmed or frustrated when first encountering the process. Course requirements, job expectations, and personal interest in discovering new knowledge are some of the reasons for examining the research process or initiating a project. Although the research process can be complex and seemingly esoteric, it need not be an activity that elicits feelings of dread, boredom, and helplessness. It can be an exciting process that is much like putting a puzzle together. The evolution of nursing research is particularly exciting and is derived from a rich nursing tradition.

This chapter focuses on the value, need, and use of nursing research. It also addresses how a body of nursing knowledge has evolved—from notable events early in this century to current philosophical thought regarding how nursing care questions can best be answered. This chapter also highlights the hallmarks of nursing's present-day success as a science.

Value of Nursing Research

The primary concern of nurses is to provide high-quality, up-to-date health care to clients. Whether the nurse is practicing in a community setting, acute care facility, long-term care agency, or one of the myriad practice settings, an underlying expectation is that the nurse will provide comprehensive care and will continually seek to incorporate current knowledge into daily practice protocols. Increasing consumer expectations and health care finance constraints make this charge ever challenging. Nurses must challenge themselves to seek better, more cost-effective nursing strategies, while not compromising patients' health care needs.

Nursing research is the key to providing appropriate nursing services. It is the process that allows the multitude of questions that surface in daily nursing practice to be answered. It also provides the data that document the effectiveness and efficacy of nursing care. Patient care based on this information will ensure that the services nurses deliver and the way they deliver those services are based on an ever-growing and refined body of knowledge specific to nursing. The nurse relying on nursing research to guide practice can be reasonably confident that an essential element in competent nursing practice has been met.

Historical Roots

The history of nursing research stems largely from the era of Florence Nightingale. Her classic work, *Notes on Nursing* (1859/1969), stressed the need for careful observation in caring for patients. She believed that through observation, nurses could best determine care for patients. This early emphasis on systematic observation, as opposed to a trial-and-error approach in providing patient care, planted the seeds for the evolution of **nursing science**—a unique body of nursing knowledge.

 WORKING DEFINITION

Nursing Science

Nursing science is the body of knowledge unique to the discipline of nursing. It is the discovery of information that explains, describes, and predicts relationships about the individual and his or her health experience.

Since the turn of the century, it has become increasingly obvious that practice needs to be based on the findings of nursing research. It has not been unusual for the practicing nurse to draw heavily on "experience" in making decisions regarding patient care or to utilize research findings generated from other disciplines. Although many nurses find these approaches helpful in solving patient care problems, there is concern about the need to identify scientific knowledge that has evolved from a nursing frame of reference. Research conducted in nursing has developed in response to key events that formed the groundwork for the development of a body of nursing knowledge (Abdellah & Levine, 1986).

1900–1970: Laying the Groundwork

Significant events that occurred in the early part of this century contributed to the growth of a body of nursing knowledge and the recognition of nursing as a discipline. Prior to this time, and as a result of the organizational efforts of Nightingale, nursing had been viewed as an occupation. Two events that had a fundamental impact on the evolution of nursing and served to shape the direction of research investigations in nursing were the Goldmark Report of 1923 and the Brown Report of 1948.

The Goldmark Report was the result of a comprehensive study conducted to determine the educational preparation necessary for nurses. This study was conducted at a time when nursing education took place within the "training ground" of the hospital. The report recommended that public health nurses receive advanced education and that hospitals provide an opportunity for nursing students to receive formal learning experiences, at a time when they were a source of cheap labor for nursing services. What little nursing research was being conducted at this time focused on the issues of greatest concern to the discipline: nurses' educational needs and the resources necessary to prepare nurses within the structure of higher education. The Goldmark Report encouraged the investigation of issues that would facilitate educational preparation of nurses in a fashion similar to other professionals. This report proved to be a major motivation in the generation of research in nursing.

The Brown Report was the result of intense study of nursing education and service issues. The impact of the report was the generation of research in response to recommendations for analysis of nursing care functions, roles, attitudes, work environment, general welfare, and relationships with clients. Finally, the report led to the development of a system for classifying and accrediting schools of nursing. The dual outcome of the report challenged the nursing community to develop means for appropriate educational preparation, as well as to explore nursing's service realm. Research conducted in response to the report stimulated the development of mechanisms to report research findings (e.g., journals) and the establishment of agencies to support and guide nursing's research endeavors.

Recommendations from the two reports are yet to be fully realized. However, changes in educational requirements from hospital training to college and university preparation and the development of graduate education in nursing were two significant outcomes in the 1950s. These changes were instrumental in socializing nurses to the use of research in discovering knowledge. Other concurrent changes supported the growth of research in nursing. These included the development of a journal to share research findings, *Nursing Research*; the establishment of centers for research; the provision of monies to support research investigations; and the appearance in the literature of the early nursing theory work of Hildegard Peplau.

Since the 1950s, the emphasis of nursing research has noticeably shifted to patient-centered concerns. A review of research publications reveals a growing percentage of studies dealing with practice-related problems, like what to teach new diabetics, how to care for a client with skin alterations, and how to measure those aspects of human behavior that are important in promoting health and preventing illness. This concern with client health contributed to the proliferation of journals dealing with the research process and the reporting of study findings, and of nursing research texts to guide both the designer and the consumer of research.

 PRACTICE

Development of Nursing Science

Review the *Nursing Studies Index* at the library. Identify at least three nursing research investigations for each decade. What is the primary research focus for each decade?

1970–Present: New World Trends

Nursing has reached a new stage of research development. Examination of the direction of research in recent years demonstrates an obvious shift in the focus of research from nursing education and administration (and "nurses studying nurses") to nursing practice problems. Effective practice strategies, expanding on earlier research findings, and building a body of knowledge unique to the profession of nursing are clear research trends.

Art and Science of Nursing

It is generally accepted that nursing is both an art and a science (Peplau, 1988). As members of a practice profession, nurses are concerned with the art of tending to individuals who are experiencing health alterations. Referring to nursing as an art implies the possession of a practical skill acquired by experience or observation (*Webster's II New College Dictionary*, 1995, p. 63). Few nurses would dispute that the way that care is rendered is critical to the healing process. Of equal concern is the recognition that nursing is also a science.

EXAMPLE

Art and Science of Nursing

A nurse working on a maternity unit notes that when she swaddles some newborn infants, they are less fussy and will sleep longer than those infants who are loosely covered with a blanket. The nurse has been teaching the new mothers how to swaddle but wonders why swaddling precipitates this behavior.

This example highlights the skill (art) needed to initiate and teach swaddling to new mothers. The knowledge base (science) for determining which infants to swaddle, the superiority of one swaddling method over another, and the physiological and psychological influences are but a few of the concerns that scientific investigation would clarify.

Acknowledging a distinct body of organized nursing knowledge and the ability of nurses to diagnose and treat health problems are basic to verifying that nursing exists as a science. Studious examination of facts relevant to health promotion and illness prevention is the core of nursing science. This activity is necessary if the nursing care that clients receive (the art) is to be more than care that is based on hunches and trial-and-error methods.

Clients experiencing a health alteration require nursing care that is based on knowledge from scientific investigation. The desire to interact equally with other health professionals and to share scientific findings from research has contributed to the development of nursing science. These professional goals have necessitated the development of strategies effective in the study of areas of interest to nursing.

 PRACTICE

Art versus Science of Nursing

Select a nursing technique from the following list and discuss whether the technique is art or science.

catheter care	inserting a nasogastic tube
backrub	care of pressure sores
bedbath	taking a blood pressure
starting an intravenous infusion	making an occupied bed

Nurses need to be concerned with how an investigation contributes to both the refinement of the art of nursing and the development of nursing science. Although every study may not directly contribute to the art and science of nursing, the potential to do so should be made clear.

CRITICAL APPRAISAL

Art and Science of Nursing

Does the researcher describe how the study relates to the development of the art and science of nursing?

Development of a Discipline

Development of a discipline is marked, in part, by the growth of knowledge that is useful in solving problems encountered in practice (Donaldson & Crowley, 1978; Riegel et al., 1992). This process, which can be slow, is influenced by several factors. Educational preparation of nurses, the ability to conduct and communicate new knowledge discovered through research, and the way in which the knowledge is used by practitioners are some of the key aspects.

Nursing has made impressive strides in the enunciation of knowledge appropriate to providing improved patient care. Examination of research produced in past decades demonstrates monumental advances in developing new knowledge (Gortner, 1983). Most nurses would now agree that nursing is a distinct discipline, with its own concerns for how best to proceed in solving problems unique to their own focus of inquiry.

A Unique Body of Nursing Knowledge

It is difficult to understand exactly what is meant by a *unique body of nursing knowledge*. Knowledge is continually changing and expanding. The knowledge that is valued by a discipline is always being altered by new discoveries and findings from research. The speed with which professionals are able to generate and absorb new findings is central to determining how that discipline's body of knowledge emerges.

It is probably misleading to describe the knowledge as "unique" to nursing. In fact, no single discipline holds ownership on knowledge. After knowledge is discovered, it may be useful to many disciplines (McMurrey, 1982). For example, a physicist may make an important discovery regarding energy transformation. This knowledge is part of the growing body of knowledge in physics and is thus unique to that discipline. However, it is not reserved for use by physicists. It may be useful in other fields of study, like nursing, engineering, biology, and medicine. After knowledge reaches the public domain, the public has the right to use that information.

Reference to a unique body of knowledge is appropriate when describing a discipline that has determined that its focus of inquiry, or purpose, is unique. Nursing has the unique focus of knowing, experiencing, and understanding patients and their experience of health. No other discipline purports to be concerned with the whole person and with how health is lived (Rogers, 1980).

 WORKING DEFINITION

A Unique Body of Nursing Knowledge

A unique body of nursing knowledge represents the knowing, experiencing, and understanding of the phenomena related to providing nursing care to patients.

The evolution and emergence of a unique body of organized knowledge is nursing science (Carper, 1978; Jacobs & Huether, 1978; Woods & Cantanzaro, 1988). Those individuals who have primary responsibility for the structure of nursing knowledge are referred to as *nurse scientists*. These doctorally prepared individuals are the researchers who design and expand the tree of nursing knowledge.

For the practitioner of nursing there is a growing understanding of the utility of nursing science. An expanding body of nursing knowledge serves as a reservoir that can verify role performance and intervention strategies. Continued attention to the development of relevant research means the development of unique knowledge that the practitioner can use in solving patient care problems.

Ways of Knowing: Structuring Nursing Knowledge

New knowledge can be gained in a variety of ways (Kaplan, 1964). Intuition, a problem-solving approach using logical reasoning, experience, and scientific inquiry are all **ways of acquiring new knowledge** that could be useful in nursing practice. **Scientific inquiry**, however, is of primary concern to nursing as a science.

 WORKING DEFINITION

Ways of Knowing

Ways of knowing are the variety of modes available to find new knowledge. They include intuition, problem solving, practical experience, and scientific inquiry.

Nursing is interested in explaining the relationships among the individual, the environment, and the experience of health. As in other disciplines, theories are posited to help explain what can be expected. The study of how well a given theory explains a particular phenomenon is the concern of research. Those conducting nursing research are seeking new knowledge in an attempt to answer a particular health care question or solve a problem that has emerged, based on a proposed theory.

 EXAMPLE

Theory-Based Research

Martha Rogers' nursing model was used to design a national study comparing power and spirituality in people who had and had not survived a life-threatening illness. *Power* was described as actively taking part in the process of change; *spiri-*

tuality was described as choosing to actualize potential reflected in certain "identifiable values in regard to self, others, nature, life, and whatever one considers to be the Ultimate." According to Rogers, the idea that people are "subjected to negative influences with pathological outcomes overlook their 'unity with nature' and 'evolutionary becoming.'" Polio survivors ($n = 172$), selected as an exemplar population, showed greater spirituality ($p = .001$) and the same power as people who have not had polio or any similar or life-threatening illness ($n = 80$). The findings of growth through adversity may have implications for people who survive other critical illnesses (Smith, 1992).

The use of scientific inquiry to gain new knowledge in nursing means that research methods are used to systematically observe events, behavior, or objects. Scientific inquiry specifies an approach to inquiry that seeks to systematically collect empirical evidence. The collection of data gathered through the five senses had been traditionally defined as empirical evidence. This view, however, stems largely from the sixteenth-century philosophical work of René Descartes, who wrote of the need to separate mind and body. The influence of this notion has been far-reaching and important in the development of new knowledge about specific diseases and in the rapid growth of the natural sciences.

 WORKING DEFINITION

Scientific Inquiry

Scientific inquiry is the process of critically analyzing the data that are systematically gathered about a particular phenomenon.

What is not widely acknowledged is the massive influence Descartes' work had on the human sciences, including nursing. As medicine grew to understand more about specific disease entities, medical specialties proliferated. Orthopedics, internal medicine, psychiatry, cardiovascular medicine, obstetrics, and rheumatology are some of the specialty areas in medicine. The trend toward specialization is equally obvious in nursing practice areas (e.g., obstetrical, psychiatric, or orthopedic nursing). The concern is that this approach to gaining new knowledge is limited to the "observable parts" such as a fractured hip, gangrenous limb, or infected wound. In light of nursing's commitment to caring for the whole person, concern has been expressed that scientific inquiry based only on data gained through the five senses is too limiting for nursing (Reeder, 1984).

Research is a process of systematically examining and explaining the observables. Research seeks to generate an *answer* to the problem, as well as suggesting additional *questions* in need of further inquiry. Scientists use the research process not only to answer a particular research question, but also to generate further questions for scientific inquiry. This dual purpose of research seems contradictory, a paradox. Ludeman (1979) has described this paradox, with the search for understanding as the questioning side and the attempt to predict knowledge as the answering side, and has identified a need to develop comfort with both values (see Figure 1.1).

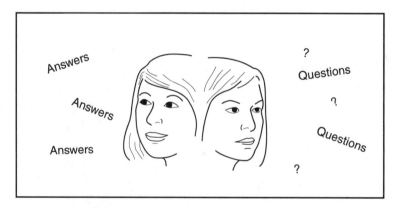

FIGURE 1.1 The paradox of nursing research

WORKING DEFINITION

Paradox of Nursing Research

The paradox of nursing research is the dual nature of research—the attempt to answer a question and at the same time generate further questions for study.

EXAMPLE

Paradox of Nursing Research

A nurse researcher conducts an investigation to determine attachment behaviors of maternal grandmothers who attend the birth of a grandchild. The investigation is developed to answer the following research question: What is the maternal grandmother's level of attachment to a grandchild when she has attended the birth?

The findings of the research investigation not only answered the research question, but also suggested several questions in need of further study. For example, how does a grandmother's own birthing experience(s) influence the willingness to attend the birth of a grandchild? Or, how does intergenerational family functioning relate to the development of attachment behaviors?

Aim and Purpose of Nursing Research

The importance of a body of nursing knowledge is self-evident. A stock of knowledge specific to the understanding of nursing practice would clearly further understanding of patient care problems. The development of nursing science through research is the nursing profession's responsibility to society (Peplau, 1987). The clear demarcation of knowledge about the patient and the experience of health is the aim of nursing research.

WORKING DEFINITION

Aim of Nursing Research

The aim of nursing research is the identification and understanding of knowledge relevant to the client and the experience of health.

The purpose of nursing research, the *raison d'etre*, is nursing practice (Jacox, 1986). Thus, the nurse researcher needs to address how the investigation is relevant to practice (see Figure 1.2). The application may not be immediate, but the potential for clinical benefit is an area of concern.

WORKING DEFINITION

Purpose of Nursing Research

The purpose of nursing research is to develop a unique body of nursing knowledge for the eventual improvement of the nursing care that clients receive.

It is easy to identify problems that merit further study for the benefit of clients. Research investigation could contribute to countless savings in time, energy, discomfort, and finances. The prevention of urinary tract infections, skin breakdown, and anxiety are only a few of the areas that would benefit clients through additional study.

Clinical research priorities have been established in nursing. In the 1970s, primary areas in need of research were determined (*Delphi Survey of Clinical Research Priorities,* 1974). A survey of selected nurses revealed 150 significant nursing research concerns. These items were classified into three areas: patient welfare, the nursing profession, and nursing responsibility. This effort to detail the direction that future nursing research should take has been instrumental in guiding the design of research. In 1985, the American Nurses Association Cabinet on Nursing Research (1985) identified priorities that help focus research efforts, and the National Center for Nurs-

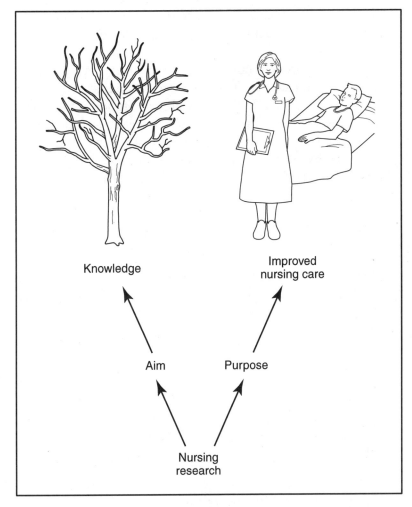

Knowledge

Improved
nursing care

Aim   Purpose

Nursing
research

FIGURE 1.2 The aim and purpose of nursing research

ing Research (Hinshaw, 1987) put forth a policy statement. More recently and in follow-up to these works, Hinshaw (2000) identified five major research priorities from nine articles published from 1994 to 1999. The reports reviewed were by American professional organizations or leading researchers. The top five nursing research priorities identified were: quality of care outcomes and their measurement, impact/effectiveness of nursing interventions, symptom assessment and management, healthcare delivery systems, and health promotion/risk reduction.

Similarly, many nursing organizations have developed research priorities relative to regional needs and concerns. These varied research priorities play an important role in fostering research activity in high-priority areas, as well as serving as a guide for funding agencies and organizations. Research priorities by these groups are usually updated and revised at periodic intervals.

 PRACTICE

Development of Nursing Knowledge

Identify a nursing research study that would contribute to understanding patients and their health experience.

 CRITICAL APPRAISAL

Development of a Discipline

- Does the discovered knowledge seek to contribute to understanding the patient and the health experience?

- Does the researcher answer a research question, as well as generate new questions for nursing study?

- Is the investigation consistent with the purpose and aim of nursing research?

Research Methods

The application of the research process through an appropriate method of inquiry enables nurse researchers to generate scientific knowledge needed by nursing. The way the knowledge is developed, how it is linked with other research findings, and an understandable form of presentation are important if the consumer is to have confidence in the research.

The way in which new knowledge in nursing is developed is an issue of frequent controversy and confusion. Growing criticism has been expressed about the selection of modes of inquiry that seem to be inconsistent with nursing concerns. It is generally accepted that the health care nursing delivers is conducted in a humanistic and holistic fashion. These notions are discussed in the works of many nursing theorists and appear to be a basic assumption in the nursing literature. Nursing is concerned with more than the disease or ailment afflicting the individual.

Because nursing's orientation is toward holistic care, the way new knowledge is gathered, or the mode of inquiry, needs to be carefully selected. For example, a nurse researcher is interested in examining the impact of dislocation on elderly people who are moved from their own homes into an extended care facility. The experiential aspect (i.e., how the elderly feel about the move) could be one key aspect for study. If the researcher were to limit the study to only the data that are "observable" through the five senses, significant data might never be known about dislocation effects on the elderly.

Traditional science methods advocate complete objectivity and concern for gathering data that are verifiable, or repeatable by another researcher under similar conditions. Traditional scientific inquiry is sometimes referred to as quantitative research because of the emphasis on "objective" observation by the researcher, as well as concern with the ability to generalize the findings to other populations. This view of science has been regarded by some critics as a scientific approach that disregards nursing's concern with the individual's holistic nature. It has raised a host of philosophical questions about the value of multiple modes of inquiry.

The decision regarding what is an acceptable method of conducting scientific inquiry is an issue that is being debated by nursing scholars. Should scientific inquiry in nursing be concerned with discovering knowledge that has immediate application (e.g., methods of pain reduction), or should effort be focused on discovering abstract knowledge that clarifies the domain of nursing (e.g., the meaning of health, or the historical evolution of holistic health care)?

 WORKING DEFINITION

Quantitative Research

Quantitative research is an approach to structuring knowledge by determining how much of a given behavior, characteristic, or phenomenon is present. Quantitative research methods are particularly concerned with objectivity and the ability to generalize the findings to others.

 EXAMPLE

Quantitative Research

A nurse working on a surgical unit is interested in studying the effectiveness of two different treatments in preventing atelectasis (blocking of the bronchial tubes in the lung with mucous and other respiratory secretions) in patients after abdominal surgery. The nurse divides patients into two treatment groups, then measures temperature, pulse, and quality of respirations to ascertain the effectiveness of each of the two treatments.

In this study the nurse is concerned with gathering data that quantify the amount: pulse rate, temperature, and depth and rate of respirations. Controlling the situation and manipulating the treatment given are two key concepts in quantitative research investigations.

Nursing concerns do not always fit well with older world views of how to do science. Although some research problems in nursing can be solved using traditional methodologies, many nursing problems require new and different methodologies to uncover the desired knowledge. Gortner (1983) and

Silva and Rothbart (1984) argue for the selection of scientific methods that fit the problem being studied, and Wolfer (1993) insists that different methods are required for fundamentally different phenomena (p. 145). These would include forms of scientific inquiry that are both **quantitative** (determining the *amount* of something) and **qualitative** (determining the *meaning* of a particular experience).

 WORKING DEFINITION

Qualitative Research

Qualitative research is an approach to structuring knowledge that utilizes methods of inquiry that emphasize subjectivity and the meaning of the experience to the individual.

 EXAMPLE

Qualitative Research

A nurse works at an inner-city health facility that provides care for a growing number of Hispanic mothers who are undocumented citizens and their infants. The nurse is interested in describing the experience of being an undocumented citizen and in need of health care for a sick baby. The nurse finds Hispanic mothers who attend the clinic and are willing to participate, and proceeds to discover what the experience is like for them. The information shared by the mothers is coded, analyzed, and categorized.

In this study the nurse is concerned with capturing the human experience of needing health care for a sick child when the mother is a Hispanic undocumented citizen. The nurse researcher's ability to understand the experience from the Hispanic mother's perspective is paramount to the qualitative focus of the study.

Carper (1978) describes a convenient way of viewing the kind of knowledge necessary in nursing. These knowledge areas include scientific, or empirical, knowledge; ethical knowledge, or knowledge of the values of nurses and nursing; esthetic knowledge, or knowledge of the art of nursing; and personal knowledge of the therapeutic use of self (p. 22). It is helpful to use these areas as a framework for thinking about structuring knowledge in nursing. The development of nursing knowledge in each of these four areas will require multiple modes of inquiry to establish a useful body of knowledge (Fawcett, 1984) and knowledge in all four areas is needed to advance evidence-based nursing practice (Fawcett, Watson, Neuman, Walker, & Fitzpatrick, 2001).

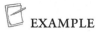 EXAMPLE

Structuring Knowledge in Nursing

- *Scientific knowledge:* Development of nursing knowledge that is factual in nature and is used to describe, explain, and predict. It includes both quantitative and qualitative methods. For example, what is the effect of viewing violent television programming on the development of motor skills in toddlers?

- *Ethical knowledge:* Development of knowledge that describes the values of nurses, as well as ways to analyze and solve ethical dilemmas—for example, an analysis of the advocacy role in nursing.

- *Esthetic knowledge:* Development of knowledge that focuses on the art of nursing. For example, what is the lived experience of incorporating a Down's syndrome child into the family unit?

- Knowledge of therapeutic use of self: Development of knowledge that is concerned with the nurse's ability to use the self therapeutically, to interact in an authentic fashion with patients—for example, an investigation of the enactment of empathy behaviors by senior nursing students working with drug-addicted pregnant women.

CRITICAL APPRAISAL

Structuring Knowledge in Nursing

- Does the researcher link the study to other related studies?

- Is the way the researcher discovers new knowledge appropriate to nursing concern?

- Does the research support the development of scientific, ethical, esthetic, or personal knowledge?

Hallmarks of Success

Nursing is largely considered to be a young profession and discipline. The achievements that have been accomplished in building a body of nursing knowledge are impressive. Three areas are of particular significance in marking research success: clarification of the boundaries for appropriate study in nursing, establishment of scholarly publications, and the growth of professional research organizations.

Boundaries for Nursing Study

Fawcett (1984) has noted that one of the most impressive hallmarks of success in nursing research has been the delineation of the boundaries for study. This means that through the development of nursing conceptual systems and theories, the parameters of concern have been set. All of the published nursing models and theories demonstrate a consensus that the main concepts for study in nursing are **person, environment, health,** and **nursing**

23

(p. 2). The broad boundaries for what nursing research should study have been identified and essentially agreed on by nurses.

WORKING DEFINITION

Boundaries for Nursing Study

Boundaries for nursing study have been identified as the body of knowledge formed by the interrelationship of the concepts of individual (person), environment, health, and nursing.

EXAMPLE

Boundaries for Nursing Study

A group of home health care nurses initiate a research project to examine the impact of nursing support on client adjustment to a disfiguring surgery. This study would fall within the boundaries for nursing study because the nurses have identified a theoretical framework for the study that addresses the project's concern with disfigured patients (*persons*) in their home (*environment*), their adjustment to the disfigurement (*health*), and the impact of *nursing*.

PRACTICE

Boundaries for Nursing Study

Identify a client care problem noted in nursing practice. Describe how an investigation of that problem could be related to nursing's four key concepts. Sketch out the interrelationship of the concepts in the study.

CRITICAL APPRAISAL

Boundaries for Nursing Study

- Does the researcher identify how the four major concepts for nursing study (person, environment, health, and nursing) articulate with the project under investigation?

- Does the research project focus on studying an area of concern to nursing?

Scholarly Publications

Publications that are used to disseminate scholarly work within a discipline are crucial to the growth of its members. It is generally believed that the average practitioner in any discipline is using knowledge in everyday practice that is about ten years old. In other words, there appears to be a ten-year gap between publication of research findings and the widespread knowledge and use of those findings in practice.

WORKING DEFINITION

Scholarly Publications

Scholarly publications are the documents that serve to communicate to other professionals the methods and achievements produced through academic study and research investigation.

Research utilization in nursing reflects a similar knowledge gap. For example, Ketefian (1975) studied a sample of 87 nurses to ascertain their knowledge of the correct placement time for taking oral temperatures. This function is virtually uniform across specialty areas, and it could be assumed that nurses would be equally concerned with this knowledge. Ketefian noted that three separate studies exploring the correct placement time for oral temperatures had been widely published in scholarly nursing journals in the preceding decade.

25

Despite this fact, only *one* nurse correctly reported the information. The other research participants were either unaware that the research existed or were unable to make sense of the reported findings.

Similarly, Kirchhoff (1982) surveyed intensive care nurses regarding their knowledge of widely published findings that supported the discontinuation of restricting ice water and rectal temperature measurements in coronary care patients. Despite the available literature refuting the practices, approximately three-quarters of the nurses still reported restricting ice water and approximately two-thirds still restricted rectal temperature measurements. Coyle and Sokop (1990) provided further support for poor utilization of research findings in practice when they replicated a study done by Brett in 1987. They randomly surveyed hospital nurses in North Carolina to determine whether those in practice had adopted nursing innovations from 14 different studies. There was widely varying knowledge of the findings from the various studies, demonstrating a continued gap between knowledge and practice.

Scholarly journals are one key means of communicating the vital aspects of a study to nurses. Since 1952 nursing has accumulated an impressive core of journals that are designed to report the findings from research investigations. Some of the primary nursing research journals published in the United States include *Advances in Nursing Science (ANS)*, *Applied Nursing Research (ANR)*, *Nursing Research (NR)*, *Research in Nursing and Health (RINAH)*, and *Western Journal of Nursing Research (WJNR)*.

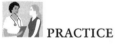

PRACTICE

Scholarly Research Publications

Obtain one issue of each of the following: *ANS*, *ANR*, *NR*, *RINAH*, and *WJNR*. Select one research study from each journal and evaluate the article for readability and for how clearly the implications for practice are discussed.

Each of the major research journal publications attempts to provide a forum for the scholarly presentation and discussion of scientific investigations related to the development of nursing and the improvement of health care.

The journals devoted primarily to research proceedings sometimes seem abstruse and difficult to comprehend for the general practicing nurse. Editors and researchers continue to be concerned with the problem of how to best disseminate research findings in the journal medium. Increased emphasis has been placed on the need to publish research reports that discuss the project in clear terms and explicitly state the implications for practice.

It is interesting to note that many of the general and specialty journals in nursing have addressed the need to report research activities and findings. Over the past few years, many journals have developed strategies for disseminating research findings of interest to the subscribers of that particular journal. For example, some specialty journals now identify "research briefs" that summarize key points from a particular study, retain a researcher to address methodological concerns of importance to nurses conducting research within a given specialty setting, or publish full research studies that have been developed so that the general practicing nurse can more easily understand the full implications of the research. If a research report is difficult to follow, its obscurity should not be confused with scholarliness or quality.

Growing emphasis on the presentation of research findings in an interesting and understandable manner has contributed to the proliferation of research reports appearing in nursing journals. Use of specialty journals to disseminate practice-related research findings to nurses working in that area is an effective means of spurring the implementation of research findings in a clinical specialty.

Although the journals identified as "research journals" are important and noteworthy, excellent research can be found in many of the general and specialty nursing journals. For example, the consumer of nursing research can find a wealth of relevant scientific knowledge in the specialty nursing journals *Oncology Nursing Forum* or *American Journal of Maternal Child Nursing*. For the designer of a research project, reporting the research outcomes in a nursing specialty journal can facilitate the growth and utilization of knowledge in that area of practice.

PRACTICE

Scholarly Research Publications

Obtain a copy of a specialty journal that reports a full research project, as well as a copy of a research journal. Note the differences in readability and ease of application to clinical situations.

Swanson, McCloskey, and Bodensteiner (1991) present an excellent listing of administrative, educational, general practice, and specialty nursing journals. This compilation identifies the circulation, issue frequency, information for prospective authors, length of time from submission to publication, and whether the journal is refereed.

A refereed journal submits manuscripts to a blind review process by a panel of experts who are knowledgeable in that content or practice area. For example, if a nurse researcher were to submit the findings from a research project to *Nursing Research* for possible publication, the editor would initiate the review process established for that journal. This would include the following major activities: an initial screening by the journal editor to determine whether the manuscript is consistent with the goals, purpose, and aims of the journal; selection of individuals from the journal's review board who are knowledgeable about the research topic or methodology; and the determination of whether the reviewed project is amenable to the journal's expectations and needs.

WORKING DEFINITION

Refereed Journal

A refereed journal is a journal that submits manuscripts to a review process using a panel of experts to determine the quality of the work.

Whether or not a journal is refereed should be noted when evaluating any research report appearing in the nursing literature. Although publication of a research report in a refereed journal does not guarantee quality or relevance to nursing, it does suggest that it has merit beyond what is claimed by the researcher. Being aware that a journal submits work to a scholarly critiquing process fosters the development, execution, and reporting of project findings that are of the highest quality. Knowing that a journal is refereed does not ensure quality, but it is a factor that should be considered when deciding whether to subscribe to a particular journal.

 PRACTICE

Refereed Journals

Select a nursing journal that publishes full research studies. Determine whether the journal is refereed and, if referred, note the number of review board members and their credentials.

Regular scrutiny of both the general and specialty literature is important for the practicing nurse. As illustrated in the discussion of the Ketefian investigation, large gaps appear to exist between the identification and utilization of new knowledge. The practicing nurse can keep current with the rapid expansion of knowledge generated by research through regular review of one research journal (e.g., *Research in Nursing and Health*), a specialty journal (e.g., *Journal of Gerontological Nursing*), and a general practice journal (e.g., *American Journal of Nursing*). Regular perusal of these (or equivalent) publications is essential to ensure the professional nurse's competence in practice.

Keeping abreast of current nursing knowledge is difficult for many nurses who may not have been socialized to the research process. Consistent effort to read research reports, education to become familiar with the research process, contact with skilled nurse researchers who are able to act as mentors in conducting research, and participation in research activities in the practice setting will eventually provide those unfamiliar or unskilled in research with the tools necessary to utilize research findings in practice.

CRITICAL APPRAISAL

Refereed Journals

Does the research report appear in a journal that is refereed?

Resources for Promoting Nursing Research

Nursing research organizations have multiplied in response to the need for support of research activities. These support and resource organizations can be divided into two categories: research centers established to guide and promote research activities, and organizations that serve to develop and support a network of researchers.

Research centers established to promote and guide research have received earnest attention in recent years. The American Nurses Association (ANA) has been a significant force in providing a relatively comprehensive and accessible research center. In 1983 the first Center for Nursing Research evolved. It is charged with initiating a research program that supports established research policy, and securing and administering funding for projects. Housed in Washington, D.C., the Center for Nursing Research includes the American Nurses Foundation (ANF), an agency designated by the ANA to provide financial support for research and to disseminate findings.

The center also encompasses the American Academy of Nursing (AAN). The AAN is the ANA's means of recognizing outstanding scholars who have made a significant contribution to the development of nursing research and theory. Individuals who are nominated for membership to the academy are voted on for membership by those who have already been admitted to the AAN. Those who have been selected are designated by the use of "F.A.A.N." (Fellow of the American Academy of Nursing) after their names.

The National Center for Nursing Research (NCNR) was established by Congress in 1985. Now the National Institute for Nursing Research (NINR), its purpose is to conduct a program of grants and awards to support nursing research and training, to promote health, and to further the prevention and mitigation of the effects of disease (Merritt, 1986). The creation of the NINR in 1993 is significant in the recognition and continued growth of nursing science.

Many colleges and universities have also developed research centers to address the development of nursing knowledge on a local or regional level. These centers are an important complement to the national centers that have been described.

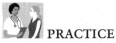 PRACTICE

Promoting Nursing Research

Contact a nurse who has conducted research at a health or academic facility and inquire what mechanisms exist for the support and promotion of nursing research.

Finally, organizations exist that serve to support networking of nurse researchers and the scholarly progression of nursing. One such highly respected organization is Sigma Theta Tau International, the honor society for nursing. Accepting eligible members from accredited baccalaureate and higher degree programs, Sigma Theta Tau seeks to foster scholarship in nursing. A few of the accomplishments of the organization include the development of a national research fund to support the work of nurse researchers, monies raised through local chapters for research efforts, regional research conferences, the publication of the scholarly journal *Journal of Nursing Scholarship*, and the establishment of a National Center for Nursing Scholarship.

The National Center for Nursing Scholarship, located in Indianapolis, Indiana, is the central headquarters for the compilation of knowledge crucial to the evolution of nursing science. A key facet of knowledge building in nursing is a well thought-out plan for the support and execution of research.

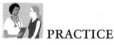 PRACTICE

Promoting Nursing Research

Contact a local Sigma Theta Tau chapter and arrange to attend a general membership meeting or a research conference.

Future of Nursing Research

Nursing is developing as an art and a science at an unparalleled rate. This explosion in nursing knowledge has also made it clear that multiple means of developing new knowledge are absolutely necessary. A major challenge in attempting to answer the myriad questions faced by nurses is to continue to develop a philosophy of nursing science that is consistent with the values of the discipline (Phillips, 1988; Riegel et al., 1992). This will mean that new research methods—different ways of answering questions influencing nursing practice—will emerge.

If current trends are any indication, future nursing research activity will continue to demonstrate a proclivity toward clinical research that aims to answer questions of a pressing, everyday nature. This emphasis will mean examining nursing therapeutics and evaluating client outcomes. The philosophical basis from which these projects are developed will need to be carefully examined so that projects can be designed to use or contribute to the further refinement of nursing theory. Finally, replicating studies to determine the usefulness of the findings with other clients in varying situations will be crucial to the establishment of a repertoire of scientifically based nursing therapeutics.

To date, the evolution of nursing science has gone hand in hand with nurses who are increasingly well prepared to participate in research activity at all levels. The importance of well-prepared, astute practitioners of nursing, who are proactive in ensuring nursing's role in the health care system, is vital to the continued evolution of a nursing science that best serves the patient in need of health care services.

Critical Overview of the Evolution of Nursing Knowledge

The future of nursing science is both exciting and promising. Research activities to build a body of nursing knowledge have proliferated in a relatively short period of time. Ongoing support of nursing research is noteworthy. Continued attention to scholarly growth of nursing knowledge will give greater clarity to the meaning of the health experience.

Use of the research process is fundamental to the development of nursing knowledge. When the process is based on methods appropriate to nursing and findings are related to other scientific work, the knowledge tree that is formed is even more meaningful. Each piece of knowledge that is uncovered links with another, and the mosaic of nursing science becomes increasingly intricate.

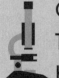

CRITICAL OVERVIEW
THE EVOLUTION OF NURSING
KNOWLEDGE

Excerpt A

A family health nurse working at a neighborhood health center assesses family sleep/rest patterns and notes that it is not uncommon for parents to let their toddler and preschool children sleep with them. The nurse is curious about the impact of this behavior on the children.

Some of the literature suggests that children who sleep with their parents experience higher levels of separation anxiety but have fewer fears of abandonment and of the unknown. The nurse wants to gather evidence to support the advice parents should be given regarding this sleep pattern.

Activity 1

- Suggest an investigation that is quantitative in nature, and one that would be qualitative.

- Would the knowledge generated from the proposed quantitative study be knowledge that was scientific, ethical, esthetic, or personal? And the qualitative study?

- Identify one refereed specialty journal and one refereed general nursing journal in which it would be appropriate to publish the project's findings.

Activity 2

Identify some of the resources that the nurse could use to support the study financially.

Excerpt B

A student nurse is doing a clinical rotation in the emergency room (ER) of a large inner-city children's hospital. The student notes that young children who come to the ER and have an invasive procedure performed frequently exhibit emotional outbursts, withdrawal behavior, or abusive activity. No planned strategy for interacting with these children is utilized by the nursing staff.

The student talks with some of the senior nursing staff about how they deal with these children. Based on their suggestions, the student nurse reviews the pediatric nursing literature and finds several articles on use of play therapy in the acute care setting.

A protocol is developed by the student nurse for use by the ER staff. Included in the protocol are suggestions for use of hand puppets, face masks, dolls, and medical equipment. Guidelines are also suggested for parental participation.

Activity 1

- Discuss how the protocol developed by the student nurse contributes to nursing as an art and a science.

Activity 2

- Has the protocol for using play therapy been derived from intuition, problem solving, practical experience, or scientific inquiry?

References

Abdellah, F. & Levine, E. (1986). *Better patient care through nursing research* (3rd Edition). New York: Macmillan.

American Nurses Association Cabinet on Nursing Research. (1985). *Directions for nursing research: Toward the twenty-first century*. Kansas City, MO: American Nurses Association.

Brett, J. L. L. (1987). Use of nursing practice research findings. *Nursing Research*, 36:344–349.

Carper, B. A. (1978). Fundamental patterns of knowing in nursing. *Advances in Nursing Science*, 1(1):13–23.

Coyle, L. A. & Sokop, A. G. (1990). Innovation adoption behavior among nurses. *Nursing Research*, 39:176–180.

Delphi survey of clinical nursing research priorities. (1974). Boulder, CO: Western Interstate Commission for Higher Education (WICHE).

Donaldson, S. K. & Crowley, D. M. (1978). The discipline of nursing. *Nursing Outlook*, 26(2):113–120.

Fawcett, J. (1984). Hallmarks of success in nursing research. *Advances in Nursing Science*, 7(1):1–11.

Fawcett, J., Watson, J., Neuman, B., Walker, P. H. & Fitzpatrick, J. J. (2001). On nursing theories and evidence. *Journal of Nursing Scholarship*, 33(2):115–119.

Gortner, S. R. (1983). The history and philosophy of nursing science and research. *Advances in Nursing Science*, 5(2):1–8.

Hinshaw, A. (1987). *National Center for Nursing Research Priorities*. Washington, DC: National Institutes of Health.

Hinshaw, A. S. (2000). Nursing knowledge for the 21st century: Opportunities and challenges. *Journal of Nursing Scholarship*, 32(2):117–123.

Jacobs, M. K. & Huether, S. E. (1978). Nursing science: The theory-practice link. *Advances in Nursing Science*, 1(1):63–73.

Jacox, A. (1986). The coming of age of nursing research. *Nursing Outlook*, 34(6):276–281.

Kaplan, A. (1964). *The conduct of inquiry*. New York: Thomas Y. Crowell.

Ketefian, S. (1975). Application of selected nursing research findings into nursing practice: A pilot study. *Nursing Research*, 24(2):89–92.

Kirchhoff, K. T. (1982). A diffusion survey of coronary precautions. *Nursing Research*, 31:196–201.

Ludeman, R. (1979). The paradoxical nature of nursing research. *Image: The Journal of Nursing Scholarship*, 11(1):2–8.

McMurrey, P. H. (1982). Toward a unique knowledge base in nursing. *Image: The Journal of Nursing Scholarship*, 14(1):12–15.

Merritt, D. H. (1986). The National Center for Nursing Research. *Image: The Journal of Nursing Scholarship*, 18(3):84–85.

Nightingale, F. (1859/1969). *Notes on Nursing*. New York: Dover.

Peplau, H. E. (1987). Nursing science: A historical perspective. In R. R. Parse (Ed.), *Nursing science: Major paradigms, theories, and critiques* (pp. 13–29). Philadelphia: W. B. Saunders.

Peplau, H. E. (1988). The art and science of nursing: Similarities, differences, and relations. *Nursing Science Quarterly*, 1(1):8–15.

Phillips, J. R. (1988). Research blenders. *Nursing Science Quarterly*, 1:4–5.

Reeder, F. (1984). Philosophical issues in the Rogerian science of unitary human beings. *Advances in Nursing Science*, 6(2):14–23.

Riegel, B., Omery, A., Calvillo, E., Elsayed, N. G., Lee, P., Shuler, P. & Siegal, B. E. (1992). Moving beyond: A generative philosophy of science. *Image: The Journal of Nursing Scholarship*, 24(2):115–120.

Rogers, M. E. (1980). Nursing: A science of unitary man. In J. P. Riehl & C. Roy (Eds.). *Conceptual models for nursing practice* (pp. 329–337). New York: Appleton-Century-Crofts.

Silva, M. C. & Rothbart, D. (1984). An analysis of changing trends in philosophies of science on nursing theory development and testing. *Advances in Nursing Science*, 2(6):1–13.

Smith, D. W. (1992). *A study of power and spirituality in polio survivors using the nursing model of Martha E. Rogers*. Unpublished Ph.D. dissertation. New York University. UMI, 9222966.

Swanson, E., McCloskey, J. C. & Bodensteiner, A. (1991). Publishing opportunities for nurses: A comparison of 92 U.S. journals. *Image: The Journal of Nursing Scholarship*, 23(1):33–38.

Webster's II New College Dictionary (1995). Boston: Houghton Mifflin Co.

Wolfer, J. (1993). Aspects of reality and ways of knowing in nursing: In search of an integrating paradigm. *Image: The Journal of Nursing Scholarship*, 25(2):141–146.

Woods, N. R. & Cantanzaro, M. (1988). *Nursing research: Theory and practice*. St. Louis: C.V. Mosby.

2

Promoting Evidence-Based Nursing Practice

Goals

- *Describe critical inquiry processes in nursing.*
- *Examine the basic components of the research process.*
- *Differentiate roles in nursing research.*
- *Detail strategies for evaluating research reports to support evidence-based nursing practice.*
- *Describe strategies for making evidence-based practice recommendations.*

Introduction

The goal of patient care is to provide quality nursing services that are effective in promoting health and wellness and alleviating the discomforts of the illness. When efficacious nursing care is given, cost and time can be reduced, ineffective interventions can be eliminated, and outcomes can be validated. In a time of shrinking resources and patients with increasingly acute health care needs, it is important for evidence-based nursing practice to be utilized. To use research-based interventions in practice, nurses need to learn how to evaluate research reports, describe the level of evidence that exists on a particular topic, and identify the strength of the association for the research evidence that does exist.

Research Defined

In the provision of nursing care, the nurse is constantly challenged by questions related to client care. Is one method of applying a heat lamp more effective than another? What is the effect of exposing newborn infants to bright lights in the nursery? What are the differences in maternal outcome depending on birthing positions (i.e., squatting, side-lying, semi-Fowler's, supine, and sitting)? What relaxation techniques are most effective in reducing anxiety for individuals with Type A personality? Under what conditions is the use of elastic stockings effective in decreasing the incidence of thrombi formation? These are only a few of the questions that the nurse may have wondered about (see Figure 2.1).

The use of research can be a valuable vehicle for helping to determine the best way to solve patient care problems. The research process involves the use of discrete steps that are similar but not identical to those of the problem-solving process.

Problem-Solving Process

Most nurses have utilized the problem-solving process in attempting to solve a patient care problem that has surfaced.

40

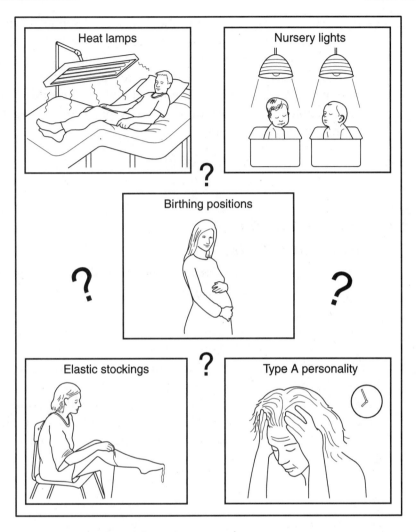

FIGURE 2.1 Questions relating to patient care

Typically, the nurse must make a determination about how to act in a new or novel situation. The nurse generally examines past experiences with similar problems and extrapolates relevant facts to be applied to the current situation.

Knowledge that cannot be derived from experience is generally "problem-solved." For example, a community health nurse makes home visits to new parents who are part of the

41

early discharge program at the local hospital. While visiting one new family, the nurse discovers that the family has been giving the newborn baby lemon juice to "purify the blood after birth." Discussion with the family reveals a cultural basis for this practice. Concern for the infant's welfare requires the nurse to explore other solutions. This is problem solving to meet an immediate problem.

WORKING DEFINITION

Problem-Solving Process

The problem-solving process is the practical determination of a solution to an immediate problem.

Problems that surface in everyday nursing practice often cannot wait for a research investigation to provide the best answer. Nurses find themselves in a position of needing to make an immediate decision about how to solve the problem. The process of problem solving involves identifying the problem, specifying all options available to solve the problem, implementing the best alternative, and evaluating for effectiveness.

EXAMPLE

Problem-Solving Process

A school nurse is working with elementary school children in a rural area where head lice have reached epidemic proportions. The nurse, who is particularly concerned with the incidence of reinfestation of many of the children, notes that the parents are not fully carrying out the prescribed treatment.

The nurse has identified reinfestation as the problem requiring an immediate, practical solution. The nurse lists all the possible solutions that would be appropriate to prevent lice reinfestation. The nurse decides that the best solution would be to bar the infested child from school until the parents have signed a form verifying that treatment has been completed and the nurse has inspected each child. The nurse would evaluate the effectiveness of this particular course of action by noting whether the incidence of reinfestation significantly decreases.

 PRACTICE

Problem-Solving Process

Identify a patient care problem recently encountered in practice. List all the possible alternatives that could be used to solve the problem, identify the best alternative, and suggest how the effectiveness of the action could be evaluated.

Research Process

Course requirements frequently identify the need to conduct research on a particular topic. For many students, the term *research* conjures up an image of long hours in the library, poring over the literature on a given topic. This general view of research as the careful study of information is held by many nurses who have not been exposed to a formal research course. Although researching a particular topic is important in developing a broader understanding of what is already known, it is only one component of a process that is essential in generating nursing knowledge.

In the scientific sense, the term 'research" is used to denote an active process of identifying a research problem needing a solution, and then systematically gathering, examining, and interpreting knowledge about how to best solve that problem. Research in the scientific sense is more than a literature study of a particular topic or problem. Rather, it is making an effort to review what is already known about a particular problem (literature review), then skillfully proposing solutions through systematic study of patients experiencing that problem.

WORKING DEFINITION

Research Process

The research process is the examination and analysis of systematically gathered facts about a particular problem. The aim of the research process is the discovery or validation of knowledge.

The research process is used in all disciplines as the method for finding solutions to problems or questions. Use of this process allows scientists from different disciplines to he able to communicate with each other in an understandable, common manner. Table 2.1 identifies the major components of the research process.

 TABLE 2.1   Major Components of the Research Process

Research problem identification:

• Clearly state the research problem.

• Review the literature to support the need for the problem to be studied.

• Develop a conceptual framework.

Addressing the research problem:

• Select an appropriate method to study the problem.

• Conduct systematic observation to determine accuracy of possible solution.

• Analyze and interpret the findings.

• Communicate the findings to other scientists and professionals.

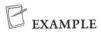 EXAMPLE

Research Process

Research Problem Identification

A researcher has been working with full-time mothers attending a support group. The researcher notes that the participants express feelings of frustration with their role and exhibit signs of low self-esteem. The following research problem is identified: What is the relationship between self-esteem and level of frustration in full-time mothers? The researcher reviews the literature and develops the following hypothesis: Mothers with lower self-esteem will demonstrate higher levels of frustration.

Addressing the Research Problem

Using a descriptive design, the researcher studies 100 mothers. The mothers are asked to complete two paper-and-pencil tests to determine levels of frustration and self-esteem. Using appropriate statistical tests, the researcher determines that the research hypothesis is supported by the findings.

 PRACTICE

Research Process

Identify a topic of interest to nursing practice. Clearly specify the research problem and describe in broad terms how it might be addressed.

 CRITICAL APPRAISAL

Research Process

Has a researchable problem relevant to nursing been identified?

Nursing Research Defined

The discipline of nursing is as concerned as other sciences are with the use of the research process to generate new knowledge. It is accepted as the means through which nursing science evolves (Abdellah, 1969; Chinn & Kramer, 1991). The term **nursing research** refers to the application of scientific inquiry to phenomena of concern to nursing. The systematic investigation of patients and their health experience is the primary concern of nursing (Schlotfetdt, 1977). Nursing research seeks to find new knowledge that can eventually be applied in providing nursing care to patients. It includes both qualitative and quantitative methodologies.

WORKING DEFINITION

Nursing Research

Nursing research is the application of scientific inquiry to the phenomena of concern to nursing: clients (individual/family/community) and their health experience.

In contrast to nursing research, "research *in* nursing" refers to research that is conducted outside the realm of patients and their experience of health (Notter, 1968). Research in nursing has frequently been viewed as nurses studying nurses (see Figure 2.2). For example, a study investigating management styles of clinical nursing supervisors would be considered research *in* nursing because it does not focus directly on the patient and the health experience.

Research in nursing is no less valuable than nursing research. In fact, many nursing leaders consider the differences to be so fine that no distinction need be made. However, there has been disagreement within the profession about what constitutes a legitimate subject for nursing investigation. Some nurses are concerned that for nursing to develop fully as a science, research effort must be directed primarily to the study of practice-related phenomena and not the profession of nursing itself (Gortner, 1975). It is undoubtedly true that concentrated

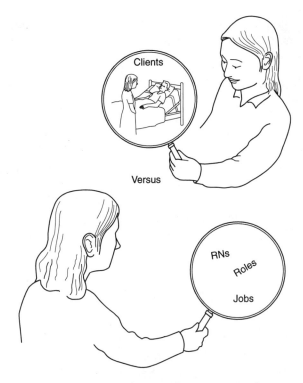

FIGURE 2.2 Focus of nursing research

energy needs to be focused on expanding the knowledge base for nursing practice. The discipline of nursing critically needs inquiry from a nursing perspective (Donaldson & Crowley, 1978). However, studies that help clarify how nursing resources can best be developed, distributed, and evaluated can only serve to support the development of scientific nursing scholars who have the capacity to conduct increasingly refined investigations.

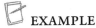 EXAMPLE

Nursing Research versus Research in Nursing
Projects that are *nursing research:*

- An exploratory study of mothering for the elderly primigravida

- Development of a nursometric (nursing measurement) instrument for use in quantifying diversity of pattern in healthy adults

- Disengagement behaviors of elderly retired parents toward their adult children

Projects that are *research in nursing:*

- Perceived role discrepancy for adult nurse practitioners

- Performance attributes of A.D., B.S., and diploma nurses

- Administrative styles of nurse leaders

EXAMPLE

Nursing Research

A nurse works with adolescents at an eating disorder clinic. Interested in studying the phenomenon of self-help in bulimic clients, the nurse develops the following problem for study: Is group or individual counseling more effective for bulimic adolescents in initiating self-help behaviors?

The nurse could draw on experience to decide which type of counseling would be more effective. However, using research methodology to study bulimic adolescents in both group and individual counseling situations would be preferable. A research approach would increase the likelihood of accuracy and would provide data to support the development of a particular treatment approach effective in supporting self-help behavior.

PRACTICE

Nursing Research

From the following list of research projects, identify those that are *nursing research* and those that are *research in nursing.*

- Nursing attitudes and values in health care policy formation and administration

- An exploratory nursing study of the development of the role of grandparent

- A nursing investigation of the ethical dilemma of placebo administration for pain relief

- A nursing investigation of the lived experience of fear in patients facing treatment of cancer

- A study of the impact of the nurse's attitude toward breast-feeding on length of breast-feeding in first-time mothers

CRITICAL APPRAISAL

Nursing Research

Does the investigation examine a problem that is related to phenomena of nursing concern?

Roles in Nursing Research

Participation in nursing research can involve multiple roles. These roles include that of research consumer, collaborator in the design and production of a research project, replicator of research, and data collector (Mallick, 1983). These roles can be conducted with others, such as with a multidisciplinary group of health professionals, or can be done individually.

The Consumer: A Critical Appraiser of Research

The role of research consumer encompasses the critical appraisal of a research study. The appraisal determines the significance of the research problem, the merits of the design, and the appropriateness of implementing the findings in nursing practice. Developing the skills to critically analyze a research piece is not easy and evolves over time with knowledge of the research process, growing clinical nursing skills, and repeated practice in research appraisal.

One important means of developing the research consumer role is for the nurse to read research reports consistently and thoroughly. This activity contributes to the nurse's competence and helps to ensure that the practitioner is informed of current scientific findings. Reading a research report initially requires a great deal of effort. Perseverance in reading research reports will eventually assist the nurse in making a knowledgeable determination about the report with greater ease.

 WORKING DEFINITION

Research Consumer

The research consumer determines the quality and merit of a given research report through systematic review and critique.

Most individuals are consumers of research. Each day we are confronted with the findings from research investigations and suggestions for improving our lifestyles as a result. To be a research consumer from the vantage point of a professional nurse, however, means that criteria are used to determine quality and merit of the study in question *before* the findings are implemented in practice.

The development of an ability to discriminate "good" research from "questionable or poor" research involves the systematic analysis of all phases of the investigation. Only after careful inquiry into the study's design and method has been conducted should the nurse make a determination regarding whether the findings are worthy of initiating a change in clinical practice.

The ultimate goal of nursing research is to improve nursing practice (Polit & Hungler, 1995; Woods & Catanzaro, 1988). Changes in nursing practice can be very costly, and conversely, cost-effective. To recommend a change in practice, the nurse needs to feel confident that the findings of the study are accurate and will make an improvement in nursing service to patients. Changes are sometimes initiated on the basis of one well-conducted research investigation. In other situations, it may be important to find several studies that support the proposed change.

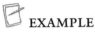 EXAMPLE

Consumer of Research

A nurse working on an oncology unit is concerned with the excessive nausea and vomiting experienced by clients on a new chemotherapeutic agent. None of the conventional methods of dealing with nausea and vomiting provide significant relief, so the nurse conducts a review of the research literature to ascertain new treatments that might be of use.

The nurse locates one small-scale study ($n = 22$) of research participants who were given a new treatment for relief of nausea and vomiting after chemotherapy. Critique of the research report reveals a well-conducted investigation, despite the small sample size. Although the nurse would like to find other studies supporting the study findings, the problem is of sufficient concern to warrant implementation of the treatment.

 PRACTICE

Consumer of Research

Following are four problems that have been noted in clinical practice. Select one problem and review the current research literature to ascertain the extent of research relevant to the problem. For each research study found, identify the sample size and show how the researcher(s) studied the problem.

- Fall prevention during institutionalization

- Treatment of skin breakdown in the elderly

- Available support for breast-feeding mothers

- Impact of limited visitation on clients in the critical care unit

To act as a knowledgeable consumer of nursing research, the nurse needs to develop a systematic approach to the review and evaluation of the major components of a research investigation. The research review and research critique are two critical aspects of developing skills as a research consumer.

Research Review versus Research Critique Two critical, but different, activities associated with being a consumer of nursing research are the *research review* and the *research critique*. A **research review** is the process of summarizing the overall points and features of a given research report. The purpose of the review is to become familiar with the major features of the research report.

WORKING DEFINITION

Research Review

A research review is the summarization of the key points and characteristics of a research report.

Conducting a research review is generally the first step in developing the role of research consumer. A review involves pointing out the major features of the study without making a judgment regarding the merit and quality (Leininger, 1968). Learning to do the research review is a valuable activity that will help the nurse who is new to the research process become familiar with both the components of a research report and research terminology.

PRACTICE

Research Review

Select a research report from a nursing journal and write a summary of the major aspects of the investigation, using the following structure:

Journal citation	
Problem statement	
Review of the literature	
Hypotheses (if any)	
Method of studying the research problem	
Instruments used	
Data analysis	
Findings or summary	

The **research critique** is similar to the research review in that both summarize the study's main components. It is different, however, in that the research critique involves the deliberative process of making a judgment about the worth of the study (see Figure 2.3). In conducting the research critique, the nurse

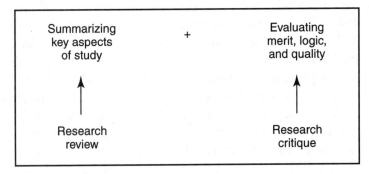

FIGURE 2.3 The research review and the research critique

53

would summarize the main features of the study while also making comments about the positive and negative aspects of the study. The purpose of the critique is to help the researcher in conducting further study in the area of investigation, as well as to assist other consumers in making a judgment about the worth of the findings.

WORKING DEFINITION

Research Critique

The research critique is the process of summarizing the key aspects of a research report, then determining the quality and merit of the study on the basis of predetermined criteria.

In making positive and negative judgments about a research piece, it is important to remember that it is the study that is being reviewed, not the researchers themselves. All research investigations have weaknesses and strengths. Conducting research involves making compromises based on financial, institutional, and time restrictions, to name a few. In conducting a critique of a given research piece, the nurse must determine the overall merit of the study, based on the identified strengths and weaknesses of each component.

The nurse needs to structure the criticism of the study in such a way that thoughtful, constructive feedback is provided (Leininger, 1968). There is no value in writing a critique that is destructive and attempts to lower the researcher's self-esteem. Sensitivity to the efforts of the researcher should be kept in mind at all times.

The process of conducting a research critique is the critical appraisal of a study's credibility (Duffy, 1985). Theoretically, each section of the research process is equally important. In practice, however, a research report may emphasize some areas of the process to a greater extent than other areas. All components of the research process need to be appraised because overlooking some elements may contribute to a less-than-thorough critique.

EXAMPLE

Research Critique

The research critique examines each element of the research process. A research project may emphasize some elements over others.

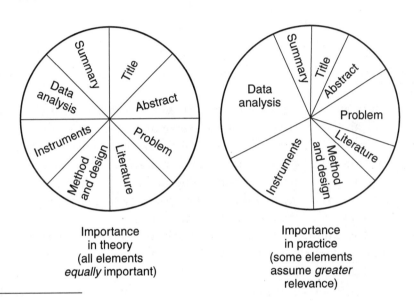

Importance
in theory
(all elements
equally important)

Importance
in practice
(some elements
assume *greater*
relevance)

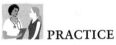

PRACTICE

Research Critique

Select a research report and determine the emphasis placed on each of the major research process elements by completing the circle graph.

55

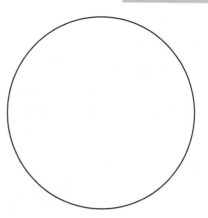

- Title
- Abstract
- Problem
- Review of literature
- Methodology and design
- Instruments
- Data analysis
- Discussion and summary

Framework for Evaluating Research Reports Initiating a research critique involves the systematic coverage of the study using specified criteria. The criteria are guidelines recognized as crucial in carrying out "good research," which assist the research consumer in maintaining objectivity while evaluating the research report. Table 2.2 provides key points to be considered in reviewing a research investigation.

The findings of the research critique should be written as concisely as possible. Unless the investigation is unusually complicated or lengthy, the report probably need not be longer than three or four pages. The paper should address all parts of the report equally, with strengths and weaknesses outlined where appropriate. The research appraiser should attempt to highlight the strengths first, followed by a sensitively worded, honest discussion of the weaknesses. Where possible, the evaluator should make suggestions for how the study could be improved.

Finally, it is helpful to have a colleague read the critique before final presentation. Unnecessarily harsh language, over-criticism, and unclear points can often be detected by an individual removed from the task at hand.

Table 2.2　The Research Critique

Purpose of the investigation:

- Is the purpose clear?
- Is the problem relevant to nursing?

Problem under study:

- Is the problem stated clearly?
- Are hypotheses stated clearly?
- Is the problem placed in the context of a theoretical framework?

Literature review:

- Is it relevant to the stated problem?
- Is it logically presented?
- Is the review comprehensive?

Research design/methods/instruments:

- Is the design identified and described?
- Are data-collection measures clearly described?

Research sample:

- Is the sample representative of the population under study?
- How were research participants selected?
- Was informed consent obtained?

Analysis of the data:

- Were appropriate statistical tests employed?
- Are the meanings of the statistical tests discussed?

(continued)

Table 2.2   (continued)

Findings/summary of study:

- Does the researcher discuss how the research problem was answered?
- Do the data support the researcher's interpretation?
- Are findings clearly and logically organized?
- Are implications for education, practice, and research given?
- Are limitations of the study noted?
- Are recommendations for further research made?

CRITICAL APPRAISAL

Consumer of Research

- Can the consumer systematically appraise the research report?
- Are judgments made regarding the strengths and weaknesses of the report?

Role as Research Designer and Producer

Designing and producing research is the process of identifying a problem requiring study, and then designing a project that will answer the question under investigation. Designing and producing research requires original, creative, and pragmatic skills in determining an appropriate and relevant problem for nursing study.

WORKING DEFINITION

Research Designer and Producer

The process of designing and producing research involves the identification of a relevant problem for nursing study, as well as a clear plan for carrying out a relevant research design.

Designing and producing research is a complex activity. The nurse researcher prepared at the graduate level is viewed as having full responsibility for producing nursing knowledge. It is not unusual however, for the entry-level nurse to be asked to participate in the design and production of a study. Involvement at this level is likely to be most satisfying when carried out with a more experienced researcher.

It is important that the professional nurse fully understand how a research report should be designed and produced. This knowledge is crucial to the development of the research consumer role. The capacity to understand fully how research is designed and produced is a skill that evolves over time and is sharpened with experience. All nurses should possess basic skills in examining the design and production of nursing research and should actively suggest problems in need of study. Active participation by the professional nurse in identifying areas in need of research will contribute to the generation of research that is relevant and supportive of practice-related problems.

 EXAMPLE

Designer and Producer of Research

A nurse working on a surgical unit notes that clients awaiting a biopsy after finding a mass in the breast experience near-panic-level anxiety. The nurse is interested in studying the impact of a progressive relaxation protocol on these women.

The nurse designs a study based on the identified problem. The protocol is carried out with individuals willing to participate in the study.

 PRACTICE

Designer and Producer of Research

Identify a problem in need of nursing study. Outline the major steps to be used in designing a study to solve the problem.

CRITICAL APPRAISAL

Designer and Producer of Research

- Has a problem relevant to nursing been identified?
- Has a plan for studying the problem been clearly identified and executed?

Role as Replicator

The process of duplicating a research investigation that has already been conducted is referred to as replicating a study. **Replication** may involve repeating a study under the same conditions with similar research participants as were used in the initial investigation. Replication studies may also involve the use of a different sample, setting, and timing, but are otherwise virtually the same. Repeating the study under different conditions makes the research more generalizable (Shelley, 1984) and establishes further the validity of the findings.

WORKING DEFINITION

Replicator of Research

Replicating research involves repeating a research investigation that has been conducted previously.

The role of research replicator has been largely undervalued. The importance of replicating all studies cannot be stressed enough. It is often difficult to justify the use of research findings from one singular study. To find similar study results under different conditions and with different populations provides additional support for the generalizability of the findings. When findings are not supported, suggestions can be made for additional study or changes in the research design. Meeting with the original nurse investigator to discuss various aspects of the original study can be enormously helpful for the nurse attempting to replicate another researcher's work.

EXAMPLE

Replicator of Research

A nurse working on a maternity unit reads a research report describing the use of therapeutic touch promoting relaxation and inducing sleep in postcholecystectomy patients. The nurse is interested in duplicating the study using a group of mothers who have had a cesarean section.

The nurse should consider replicability with every nursing research report that is examined. Whether the study appears in a published source or is presented orally, the nurse can use these diverse sources in identifying reports in need of replication. Knowing that a piece of research has been replicated suggests improved credibility and may give the practitioner increased confidence that the findings merit application or additional replication (Hailer, 1986).

PRACTICE

Replicator of Research

Review current issues of a nursing research journal. Identify a research study that would be suitable for replication in the practice setting. Identify the components that need to remain the same to duplicate the study.

CRITICAL APPRAISAL

Replicator of Research

- Does the researcher virtually duplicate a study that has already been completed?

- Does the replicator of the research make suggestions for improving generalizability?

61

Role as Data Collector

It is not unusual for the nurse working in a clinical setting to be asked to participate in a research project as a **data collector**. Participating in research as a data collector usually means that the nurse assists in carrying out the implementation phase of a research study designed by another researcher. For example, a physician may be conducting research to determine which of two treatments for an orthopedic condition is more effective. Similarly, a nurse investigator may be studying a new procedure designed to reduce the incidence of phantom pain after lower-limb amputation. The nurse may be asked by the nurse researcher or a researcher from another health-related discipline to participate in carrying out the research protocol.

 WORKING DEFINITION

Data Collector in Research

Acting as a data collector in a research project involves participation in gathering data relevant to the problem under investigation.

Participating as a data collector in a research project that has already been designed is an important aspect of developing the research role. This activity can be invaluable in developing knowledge about the research process. Additionally, the nurse working in the clinical setting generally has close and consistent contact with a client and is in a unique position to act as participant on the research team. Changes in client behavior, problems in carrying out the treatment protocol, and concern for client welfare are all readily noted by the nurse who has prolonged and consistent interaction with a client serving as a research participant. The nurse can serve as client/subject advocate and contribute to the integrity of the study while serving as a data collector.

Serving as a data collector for a study that has been designed by a researcher from nursing or some other discipline requires that the nurse who is collecting data be given information about the study. Questions regarding the nature of the study, potential harm to the research participant, and debriefing procedures should all be fully answered prior to agreeing to participate.

 EXAMPLE

Data Collector in Research

A nurse working at a visiting nurse agency is asked by a nurse researcher to participate in a project. The researcher is interested in evaluating the adjustment of parents to their children who have tracheostomies. The researcher informs the nurse about the full nature of the study, what participation would mean, and the impact of participation on these families.

 PRACTICE

Data Collector in Research

Identify a nursing research study being conducted in a health care agency. Describe the role a data collector would assume if participating.

 CRITICAL APPRAISAL

Data Collector in Research

Does the researcher inform the data collector about the full nature of the project, including the impact of participation for research participants?

Evaluating Research Reports for Use in Practice

To effectively carry out research roles and to promote evidence-based practice, the nurse must learn the skill of critiquing research reports to determine the quality of the work. To do so, specific criteria can be used to analyze the major aspects of a report. Evaluating research reports is a skill that develops over time and with growing knowledge of how research is conducted, as well as with growing clinical expertise. Research findings should be evaluated within the context of actual or potential usefulness in practice. The nurse's acumen regarding practice in a particular specialty will sharpen this skill.

The criteria for evaluating reports can be set according to the type of report that is being conducted, quantitative or qualitative. Table 2.3 details the components used to evaluate a quantitative report, and Table 2.4 details those used to evaluate a qualitative report.

By using evaluation criteria when critiquing the quantitative or qualitative report, a consistent review of the most important aspects of the study can be undertaken. The process allows the reviewer to make a judgment about the strength of each study and to use the findings based on the merit of the report. The ability to critique a report is a critical skill to learn as a professional nurse and is fundamental to review of a group of reports. Skillful examination of a group of reports related to a particular topic allow for appropriate categorization of evidence for sound practice recommendations.

Categorizing Evidence

One of the initial steps needed in developing recommendations for practice that are evidence-based is to systematically review what research has been done. This involves conducting a thorough review of the literature to identify the relevant literature on the topic of interest. Specific criteria are usually used to determine whether a particular research report will be

◈ TABLE 2.3   Evaluation Criteria for Evaluating Quantitative Research Reports

Component	Description
Title	Name of the report. Clearly identifies what the research study was about.
Abstract	A brief summary of the research report, including the problem, how the study was done, the number of participants, and the major findings. Found at the beginning of the research report.
Author Credentials	The education, experience, and background of the researcher(s). Supports the authors' ability to do the research.
Style/Organization	Layout of the research report. Report should be clearly and succinctly detailed. Style should be consistent with requirements of the journal or book.
Purpose of the Study	The reason the study was done, in a clearly stated manner.
Problem	The problem(s) under study, clearly stated as either a statement or an interrogative.
Hypothesis	The hypothesis (or hypotheses) stating what the researcher expects the answer to the problem will be. They should be clearly identified.
Theoretical Framework	The researcher's thoughts regarding how the problem and the proposed answer could be explained. The theoretical framework may be another's work or may be developed specifically for the study.
Literature Review	A specific section identified in the report that summarizes the available knowledge about the topic under study.

(continued)

65

◈ TABLE 2.3 (continued)

Component	Description
Research Design/ Methods	The blueprint for conducting the study, which details the specific process that will be used to conduct the study.
Data Collection Measures	A description of the manner in which each of the concepts under study were measured.
Sample	The participants in the study, who represent the larger population or group. This can be people, animals, bacteria, or the like. Should include a discussion of how the ethical rights of participants were protected.
Analysis of the Data	A clearly presented section that details how the data that was collected were analyzed. This would include the statistical tests that were utilized.
Findings/Summary	A description of the results of the statistical analyses. Major findings are detailed.
Implications of Findings	A discussion of what the findings mean in relation to the problem under study, with suggestions for use of the findings in practice.

included in the systematic review. For example, a clinical nurse specialist working in the surgical intensive care unit wonders about the impact of the unit lighting on biorhythms and healing. The nurse decides to collect and evaluate all available research reports in English on the topic of ambient lighting and healing times in surgical patients.

The reports that are selected for review are then evaluated and a determination is made regarding how much evidence is really present and whether there is causation. To facilitate the process of categorizing the information, the reports are typically grouped by study type (see Table 2.5). Note that the lower the number, the better the evidence.

◈ TABLE 2.4   Evaluation Criteria for Evaluating Qualitative Research Reports

Component	Description
Title	Name of the report. Clearly identifies what the research study was about.
Abstract	A brief summary of the research report, including the problem, how the study was done, the number of participants, and the major findings. Found at the beginning of the research report.
Author Credentials	The education, experience, and background of the researcher(s). Supports the authors' ability to do the research.
Style/Organization	Layout of the research report. Report should be clearly and succinctly detailed. Style should be consistent with requirements of the journal or book.
Purpose of the Study	The reason the study was done, in a clearly stated manner.
Problem	The problem(s) under study, clearly stated as either a statement or an interrogative.
Sample	A clear statement of participants selected to be in the study and why they were chosen. Discussion of how the ethical rights of participants were protected.
Measures for Collecting Data	A description of how the researcher gathered the data to be analyzed. This might include interviews, written reports, diaries, artwork, and so on.
Data Collection Procedures: Method	The process used to collect the data.
Data Collection Procedures: Time/Length of Study	The time framework during which the study was conducted. A rationale for the length of the study should have been presented.

(continued)

67

◈ TABLE 2.4 (continued)

Component	Description
Data Collection Procedures: Nature/Number of Settings/Participants	A discussion of the number of participants who actually participated in the study and where and how that participation occurred.
Data Collection Procedures: Participant Involvement	Detail about how the individuals were involved in the phenomenon under study.
Data Collection Procedures: Researcher's Feelings	Discussion about how the researcher felt about his or her involvement and their relation to the phenomenon under study.
Data Collection Procedures: Researcher–Participant Relationship	A statement regarding the researcher's relationship to the participants in the study.
Data Collection Procedures: Checking for Bias	The researcher states what biases might be in process and how those potential or actual biases were dealt with in the study.
Data Collection Procedures: Organizing, Categorizing, Summarizing	A section in the report that describes how the data, once gathered, was organized for analysis. Categories are clearly described, along with a rationale for the selection of those categories. The entire process is summarized.
Scientific Adequacy: Credibility, Transferability, Dependability, Confirmability	The researcher discusses how findings were verified and by whom. Threats to credible findings are identified. Findings appear credible.

(continued)

◈ TABLE 2.4 (continued)

Component	Description
Results of Data Gathered	Succinct description of what the researcher found on data analysis.
Implications of Findings	Discussion of what the findings mean for further research and practice.
Suggestions for Use of Findings	The researcher suggests how the findings could be used.

It needs to be noted that descriptive studies, case reports, and opinions of respected authorities do not represent scientific evidence. These types of reports can be very helpful in clinical decision making but are not at the same level as controlled studies. The information from uncontrolled studies and opinion cannot be used to make a causal inference. Sometimes clinicians have no choice but to use uncontrolled studies and expert opinion because there may be no other evidence available. However, when controlled study findings are accessible, their weight would be of paramount importance.

WORKING DEFINITION

Categorizing Evidence

Categorizing evidence involves locating the available research on a topic of interest and using specific criteria for review of the reports. The reports are then critiqued using specific criteria. After all the reports are evaluated, the researcher makes a decision regarding the extent to which the findings support causation.

◈ TABLE 2.5   Levels of Evidence in the Evaluation of Research Reports

Evidence Level	Type of studies evidence derives from
I	Evidence is obtained from at least one properly randomized control trial.
II-1	Evidence is obtained from well-designed controlled trials without randomization.
II-2	Evidence is obtained from well-designed cohort and case-control studies. Cohort studies focus on specific subpopulations (e.g., first-time mothers) from which different samples are examined at different times. Case-control studies compare a case (e.g., prostate cancer) with a control (a man without prostate cancer, but otherwise matched).
II-3	Evidence obtained from cross-sectional studies (observations at different points in time to infer trends), studies with external control groups, or ecological studies (observational studies that look at aggregate or group data, e.g., breast feeding rates and infant mortality). Also, this category contains dramatic results obtained in uncontrolled experiments, such as the introduction of antibiotics in the 1940s.
III	Evidence derived from the report of expert committee, which itself used a scientific approach to arrive at a scientific opinion. The distinction that is made here is that some review committees publish a consensus opinion that is based on nothing more than the opinion of the committee members. This approach is not consistent with the scientific method. Other scientific review groups use a systematic process to review the literature, so the way the report was generated needs to be determined.

EXAMPLE

Categorizing Evidence

A nurse working on a community primary prevention program is interested in the use of aspirin and the incidence of colon cancer. She selects three randomized control trials, each having 40 of more study subjects, all in English and on the topic of use of aspirin and colon cancer. After reviewing each report, she determines that the findings from the combined studies provide Level I evidence.

PRACTICE

Categorizing Evidence

Find two research reports that examine the use of ginkgo biloba and mental alertness in adults. Evaluate the reports and suggest the level of evidence the findings provide. Provide a rationale for your suggestion.

CRITICAL APPRAISAL

Categorizing Evidence

- Are the reports that are reviewed clearly identified?
- Are the criteria for selecting and evaluating the reports described?
- Is the level of evidence (I through III) identified and a rationale provided?

Bradford-Hill Guidelines

Sir Austin Bradford-Hill (1971) developed nine criteria that can be used to evaluate consistency across research reports.

Evaluating each report using these same criteria fosters continuity in the evaluation process and permits the determination of the level of evidence and the strength of the association.

The nine Bradford-Hill criteria are the *strength of the association, confounding variables and bias, temporality, biologic gradient, specificity, consistency, biologic plausibility, studies appropriately done (having clear comparison group, blinding, description of the study methods used, analysis consistent with study design),* and *freedom from bias and confounding variables.* Systematic evaluation of each study using the Bradford-Hill criteria help in making a determination about the consistency of findings across studies. The ultimate goal is to determine the existence of a cause-and-effect relationship.

Researchers evaluate the scientific evidence to first determine if a statistically significant association exists between a particular exposure (e.g., environmental pollutants) and the presence or absence of a particular outcome (e.g., asthma). If there is an association, then the extent to which bias and other factors relate to the findings is detailed. One way that researchers can determine if bias and confounding variables contributed to the association is to do a meta-analysis. A meta-analysis analyzes several previously conducted studies. The purpose is to see if the presence of the incidence of asthma, for example, is truly due to increased exposure to environmental pollutants or if the studies had flaws. Failure to control for bias and other confounding variables could make it look like there is an increased incidence of asthma when exposed to environmental pollutants when the asthma might be due to some other factor. An alternative approach to doing a meta-analysis is to analyze the relevant studies using the Bradford-Hill criteria.

More information about Bradford-Hill criteria and meta-analysis can be found in Chapter 8.

 WORKING DEFINITION

Bradford-Hill Guidelines

Bradford-Hill criteria are nine specific criteria that are used to evaluate studies for the existence of a cause-and-effect relationship. Consistent use of the criteria aids in the determination that the increased relative risk is not likely the result of bias or other factors.

EXAMPLE

Bradford-Hill Guidelines

Concerned that perineal lacerations are caused by a failure to have women keep their feet flat on the bed during birth, the nurse locates two small observational studies that both conclude that there is a significant association. The studies are evaluated using the nine criteria and the nurse determines that the studies were poorly conducted and no cause-and-effect relationship can be suggested.

CRITICAL APPRAISAL

Bradford-Hill Guidelines

Are the criteria specified in the guidelines clearly stated in the review of the research reports?

Making Evidence-Based Recommendations

After the relevant research on a particular topic has been selected and reviewed, the researcher needs to rank the resulting evidence. The ranking is a way to describe the evidence to support a cause-and-effect interpretation of the association. Table 2.6 details the A through E rankings.

The A and B rankings indicate that there have been some well-done studies, preferably by different investigators, where there is consistency of findings. There would be an A level of certainty with an increasing number of studies and the consistency of findings is pretty uniformly similar. Generally, there needs to be findings from several studies and not a single observational or case study report. However, there may be exceptions to this. For example, reports of patients taking

◈ TABLE 2.6   Ranking Evidence in Making Evidence-Based Recommendations

Ranking	Required Evidence
A	There is good evidence to support a cause-and-effect interpretation of the association.
B	There is fair evidence to support a cause-and-effect interpretation of the association.
C	There is insufficient evidence to support or reject a cause-and-effect interpretation of the association.
C1	The available evidence is conflicting and the conflict unresolvable.
C2	There is no evidence or data.
C3	The interpretation of the existing evidence leads one to two or more reasonably close alternative explanations, each of which has biologic plausibility.
D	There is fair evidence against a cause-and-effect interpretation of the association.
E	There is good evidence against a cause-and-effect interpretation of the association.

diethylstilbesterol during pregnancy to prevent recurrent loss and the subsequent development of uterine abnormalities and an unusual vaginal cancer in the offspring, provided causal information.

Level D and E evidence means that the evidence that is available supports the notion that there is no cause-and-effect association. For example, a clinician might be interested in making a determination about whether Hormone Replacement Therapy (HRT) causes uterine cancer. In reviewing the available research reports, the clinician would look to see the risk associated. If there were no evidence that there is an association between HRT and uterine cancer, Level D and E evidence would exist.

WORKING DEFINITION

Evidence-Based Recommendations

Evidence-based recommendations come from a critical review of a group of studies to make a determination about what the overall findings are related to a particular topic. Quality of the research and consistency of findings are key.

EXAMPLE

Evidence-Based Recommendations

A nurse reviews the available literature regarding the use of oral contraceptives and the development of ovarian cancer. She locates five large retrospective studies that are well done. All show a substantial reduction in the development of ovarian cancer that increases with length of time that oral contraceptives are used. The nurse makes a determination that the strength of the association is at a B level.

PRACTICE

Evidence-Based Recommendations

You have conducted a review of the literature on use of a popular herb during pregnancy and the incidence of spontaneous abortion. You find several case reports that detail pregnancy loss when used in the first trimester but no reports can be located that show loss during the second and third trimesters. Identify the strength of the association that you think would be most appropriate and the reason why.

CRITICAL APPRAISAL

Evidence-Based Recommendations

- Are relevant studies identified for analysis?

- At what level are the studies done?

- What is the strength of association when relevant study findings are considered all together?

Critical Overview of Promoting Evidence-Based Nursing Practice

Evidence-based nursing practice requires that the nurse first identify the available research related to a particular topic. Each report must then be evaluated regarding how the study was conducted. When the critique of each report is completed, a determination must be made about what the research demonstrates. The reviewer must decide the level of evidence that the studies provide and, finally, how strong the evidence is when considered all together. When this process is complete, recommendations to promote evidence-based practice can be initiated.

Working to promote evidence-based practice promotes quality care that has been demonstrated to be effective. Delivering care that is based on solid research findings facilitates cost containment in health care and quality services. It is the responsibility of the nurse to provide care that is consistent with current research findings and to promote that care in the work environment.

CRITICAL OVERVIEW EVIDENCE-BASED NURSING PRACTICE

A nurse working in the newborn nursery is interested in how pain is managed during the circumcision procedure. She has heard comments that "babies can't feel pain," as well as comments about the use of pain medications with the newborn being unsafe. The nurse decides to research the subject so that recommendations for evidence-based nursing practice can be made.

Activity 1

Locate three research reports on the topic of the use of pain medication prior to circumcision in the newborn. Critique each report summarizing the strengths and weaknesses of each study.

Activity 2

Based on the research critiques on pain medication used prior to circumcision in the newborn, identify the level of evidence and the strength of the evidence.

Activity 3

Describe specific recommendations for pain medication use prior to circumcision based on the research you have critiqued and the level of evidence and strength of the research found.

References

Abdellah, F. G. (1969). The nature of nursing science. *Nursing Research*, *18*(5):390–394.

Bradford-Hill, A. (1971). *Principles of Medical Statistics* (9th Edition). New York: Oxford University Press, pp. 309–323.

Chinn, P. L. & Kramer, M. K. (1991). *Theory and nursing: A systematic approach* (3rd Edition), St. Louis: Mosby Year Book.

Donaldson, S. K. & Crowley, D. M. (1978). The discipline of nursing. *Nursing Outlook*, *26*(2):113–120.

Duffy, M. E. (1985). A research appraisal checklist for evaluating nursing research reports. *Nursing and Health Care*, *6*(10):538–547.

Gortner, S. R. (1983). The history and philosophy of nursing science and research. *Advances in Nursing Science*, *5*(2):1–8.

Haller, K. B. (1986). The value of replication research. *American Journal of Maternal/Child Nursing*, *11*(5):364.

Leininger, M. M. (1968). The research critique: Nature, function and art. *Nursing Research*, *17*(4):444–449.

Mallick, M. J. (1983). A constant comparative method for teaching research critiquing to baccalaureate nursing students. *Image: The Journal of Nursing Scholarship*, *15*(4):120–123.

Notter, L. E. (1968). The nature of science and nursing (editorial). *Nursing Research*, *17*(6):483.

Polit, D. F. & Hungler, B. P. (1995). *Nursing research: Principles and methods* (5th Edition). Philadelphia: J. B. Lippincott.

Schlotfeldt, R. M. (1977). Nursing research: Reflection of values. *Nursing Research*, *26*(1):4–8.

Shelley, S. I. (1984). *Research methods in nursing and health*. Boston: Little, Brown.

Woods, N. F. & Catanzaro, M. (1988). *Nursing research: Theory and practice*. St. Louis: C. V. Mosby.

Unit 2
Asking the Research Question

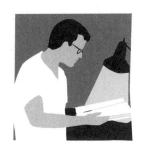

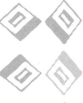

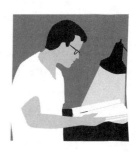

3

Initiating a Study

Goals

- *Describe the process of selecting a research topic.*
- *Describe the purpose of conceptual models and theories in relation to the research process.*
- *Analyze the components of conceptual models and theories.*
- *Describe the processes of reasoning, identifying the topic of interest, and formulating a problem statement.*

Introduction

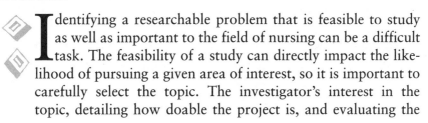

Identifying a researchable problem that is feasible to study as well as important to the field of nursing can be a difficult task. The feasibility of a study can directly impact the likelihood of pursuing a given area of interest, so it is important to carefully select the topic. The investigator's interest in the topic, detailing how doable the project is, and evaluating the investigator's expertise and capability to conduct the study are central to successful execution.

Part of ultimately determining the importance of a study to nursing is identifying the conceptual framework that gives structure to the topic, problem for study, and findings. The framework for study of a particular phenomenon needs to be identified early in the research process so that direction is given for a relevant literature review and concept selection. The ultimate problem for study flows from the early and succinct articulation of a conceptual framework. Failure to clearly detail the conceptual framework early in the research project will result in a study that is disconnected from a meaningful frame of reference or that fails to relate to other important research findings.

The investigator's commitment to a particular area, the need in a particular institution or locality, and priorities set by the National Center for Nursing Research are examples of priority setting strategies. Because research requires perseverance and hard work, the investigator's commitment to the work is one of the most important considerations in relation to successfully completing a project.

This chapter addresses topic selection, feasibility, expertise required to conduct the study, and a study's relevance and importance to nursing. A clearly directed nursing investigation is one that begins with the careful examination of how these elements of the research process fit together.

Research Feasibility

The feasibility of conducting a study refers to the ease with which the particular study can be completed. Questions related to feasibility include the following:

- Can a sufficient number of research participants be located?
- Will participants willingly and honestly respond to the questionnaire or interview?

- Will available resources (money, people, equipment) be sufficient to complete the research?
- Are the questionnaires/interviews appropriate for the desired collection of information?

Some investigations are called *feasibility studies*, and their primary purpose is to find out whether a major study on a given topic is actually possible (feasible). These studies may also be referred to as *pilot studies* or *small-scale administration studies*. Major funding sources (federal, institutional, foundations, etc.) may require that a feasibility study be conducted prior to supporting a major research project. The rationale for examining feasibility is that even the best research design formulated by experienced researchers can encounter problems. The results of a small feasibility study can help the researcher to identify problems in the design and modify the major investigation accordingly.

WORKING DEFINITION

Feasibility

Feasibility refers to the ease (or conversely the difficulty) of completing a study.

EXAMPLE

Feasibility

Before conducting a study of 300 nurses to examine the effectiveness of small group interactions on nurses' negative attitudes toward specific groups of patients in pain, a feasibility study was planned. Investigators were concerned that their measures might not be appropriate and wondered about the timing and content of the group interaction. Five nurses experienced the small group process and the data was collected on them and their patients. As a result, one nurse attitude measure was changed, the length of the group process was modified, and several patient measures were added.

PRACTICE

Feasibility

Select an area of research interest and formulate appropriate feasibility questions related to study participants, measures, and resources.

CRITICAL APPRAISAL

Feasibility

If there are problems with the findings of the study, are they due to misunderstandings regarding the feasibility of the research?

Purpose of the Investigation

• The **purpose** of the investigation reflects the need for the findings of a given research project. Need can be thought of as responding to a desire for knowledge that is not immediately applicable (basic research) or knowledge that facilitates actions within a given field of endeavor (applied research). The identification of the specific purpose of the study clarifies the intent of the investigator and frames the results in a practical manner (Wilson, 1987). The nurse who studies the career attitudes of associate's degree- versus baccalaureate-prepared nurses may do so in order to modify the educational preparation these groups receive or may do so in order to seek higher paying jobs for the more career-oriented group. Funding agencies are particularly interested in the purpose of a given study. If the purpose of a study does not agree with the particular philosophy of a funding agency, funds will not be awarded to the investigator. For example, some funding agencies will award monies only to those investigations whose findings have immediate applicability.

WORKING DEFINITION

Purpose of the study

The purpose of a study describes why the study has been designed. The purpose reflects the intent of the investigator and the use of the knowledge derived.

EXAMPLE

Purpose of the Study

Two faculty members design a study to correlate the board scores of the five preceding classes with students' clinical grades. The purpose of the study is to provide the coordinators of the clinical courses with useful information regarding the relationship between clinical performance and success on the boards.

In the example above, the purpose of the study is to provide educators with data that may influence their structuring of clinical courses. Other possible purposes of this study include developing a rationale for the increase or decrease of clinical experiences within a curriculum, providing information to the state board of examiners as to the relevance of their examination to clinical performance, or developing a rationale for appeals of failing grades on the professional licensure examination.

Although the results of the study may be used at some future date in myriad ways, including those listed in the preceding paragraph, the specifying of the investigator's purpose is instrumental in obtaining funds as well as other kinds of support necessary to conduct a study. In addition, the specification of the purpose of the study assists the investigator in clarifying the direction of the research study.

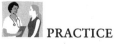

PRACTICE

Purpose of the Study

Identify an area for study and list three different purposes for conducting the research.

CRITICAL APPRAISAL

Purpose of the Study

- Does the purpose describe why the study was designed?
- Does the purpose reflect how results will be used?
- Is the purpose *clearly* specified?

Importance of the Study to Nursing

At the national level, priorities for nursing research are set by the National Institute for Nursing Research (NINR). Research priorities are set in relation to the health care needs of the country. For example, the management of pain and the care of individuals at the end of their lives have been priorities on several occasions. Unfortunately, our health care system has not provided optimal care for many patients who are dying and for patients who experience moderate to severe pain. Funding decisions are influenced by these priorities.

At the local level, the importance of a specific area of research may be dictated by the needs of a particular institution or group of patients. Nurses working in acute care institutions or community agencies are often in an ideal situation to identify patient care problems that should be investigated. In these instances, funding of studies is frequently an issue. Vendors and/or the agencies themselves may be willing to provide a moderate level of support for such things as a research assistant to collect data and costs for input and analysis of data.

Priorities shift in nursing research based on changing health needs and challenges. Problems regarding best practices for patient care have been most heavily studied. However, the long-standing emphasis on clinically focused research in nursing has limited the attention given to some other areas of research, such as educational research. As nursing experiences a workforce shortage, as well as other problems in the discipline, attention to research about the profession may be of growing import. For example, attention to models of nursing education and strategies to grow a new pool of nurse educators are two aspects that will need research study. A historical difficulty in accessing funding for educational research has resulted in little knowledge growth in this area, and targeted priorities to investigate these problems will be required.

 WORKING DEFINITION

Importance of the Study to Nursing

The importance of a study to nursing is related to national priorities, local needs, and researcher interest. In terms of funding, clinical studies are more likely to receive support than educational projects.

 EXAMPLE

Importance of the Study to Nursing

A doctoral student in nursing has spent 10 years as a hospice nurse. Her research interests are related to the quality of the lives of individuals who are within months of dying. She discovers that NINR has identified end-of-life care as an important priority and that the Oncology Nursing Society (ONS) is very interested in the same area. She receives funding from ONS to conduct a pilot study and then a grant from NINR to complete her dissertation.

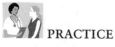

PRACTICE

Importance of the Study to Nursing

Access the NINR database and identify the priorities for nursing research for the year.

CRITICAL APPRAISAL

Importance of the Study to Nursing

- In review of a databased article, is the area under study related to national or professional priorities?

- Is a clear benefit to nursing theoretically or practically apparent?

Basic Versus Applied Research

The term **basic research** refers to those studies that are designed to seek knowledge for its own sake. When investigators examine the characteristics of a human cell, they do so to develop a better understanding of that specific structure. Although information gained may be useful at some later date in the development of a particular treatment or drug, the purpose of the study is to advance knowledge in a given area (Oyster, Hanten, & Llorens, 1987, p. 4).

Nursing has not, for the most part, been involved in basic research. Such topics as "Can death be viewed as a part of a developmental continuum rather than an end to be resisted?" or "What characteristics of parenting are typical of females in contrast to males?" might add to our knowledge regarding human behavior but do not suggest an immediate application.

WORKING DEFINITION

Basic Research

Basic research is research that seeks to gain knowledge for its own sake and does not therefore specify an application of the findings.

Basic research is conducted in order to understand the relationships among phenomena (LoBiondo-Wood & Haber, 1997). This kind of research describes these relationships and permits scientists to make predictions about the phenomena under study. Basic research is not aimed toward the solution of problems or the facilitation of decision making. The results of basic research tend to influence the way individuals think about behaviors and situations.

EXAMPLE

Basic Research

A group of nurse investigators decide to examine the meaning of parenting during adolescence.

In the example above, the researcher is interested in examining value systems without any immediate concern or interest in how the findings might be applied to modify a given situation. The findings of the study would simply add to the body of knowledge regarding value systems and how they relate to particular professions.

PRACTICE

Basic Research

Identify three possible areas for conducting basic research that are related to nursing.

89

CRITICAL APPRAISAL

Basic Research

Is the research designed to make predictions about the phenomena under study, with no attention given to direct application?

The term **applied research** refers to those studies that have as their purpose an identified practical use or application. A problem is investigated, and some resolution is sought by way of the research findings (Poolit & Hungler, 1995). Problems that nurses investigate include clinical/patient care difficulties, educational concerns, and administrative issues. In each case, the investigator hopes to contribute to some modification of present practices.

Applied research is conducted to solve problems, make decisions, develop something new, or evaluate something of interest (Abdellah & Levine, 1986). An example of solving a problem related to nursing practice would be an investigation into the reaction of siblings to a child's death. Using research to assist with decision making suggests that a choice among alternatives must be made. For example, nurse researchers might examine the patient care implications of primary care versus team nursing. An evaluation of a technique of interest might involve an experiment to test the effectiveness of therapeutic touch (Figure 3.1).

WORKING DEFINITION

Applied Research

Applied research is research that is designed to produce findings that can be used to remediate or modify a given situation.

Research can also play a role in the development of a new approach to the provision of nursing care. If a group of nurses wished to implement a new method of communicating patient data to other members of the health care team, they could

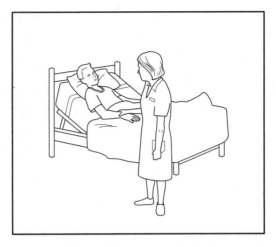

FIGURE 3.1 The efficacy of therapeutic touch. This nurse is practicing therapeutic touch (Krieger, 1979) as part of a research study on the efficacy of this approach.

design a study or a series of studies to assist in the design and implementation of this new approach. Similarly, a new approach to nursing practice can be evaluated by designing a study to assess the outcomes of the particular approach.

Evaluation research in some research texts is viewed as an additional category; that is, there are three major divisions within research: basic, applied, and evaluation (McMillan & Schumacher, 1984). Other authors include evaluation research within the "applied" category (Abdellah & Levine, 1986; LoBiondo-Wood & Haber, 1997).

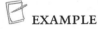 EXAMPLE

Applied Research

Two nurse investigators wish to examine the difference between two interventions designed to prevent the formation of decubitus ulcers.

In the preceding example, the researchers clearly wish to determine which approach to the prevention of decubitus ulcers is more effective. The investigators would probably recommend the use of one treatment over the other depending on the findings of the study. In this instance they choose to focus on the acquisition of knowledge that will have an immediate application.

PRACTICE

Applied Research

Identify three possible areas for conducting applied research that are related to nursing.

CRITICAL APPRAISAL

Applied Research

Is the research designed to have an immediate impact on nursing care?

Kinds of Investigations

Even at the stage of selecting a topic to research, it is probably helpful to have some understanding of what kinds of investigations are possible for a given area of interest. The conduct of research implies a systematic approach to seeking knowledge, and there are various ways to accomplish this task systematically. Decisions as to how to proceed may be made on the basis of appropriateness to a given topic or the proposed use of the information acquired.

There are three important considerations when examining the kinds of investigations available: (1) the type of information desired, (2) the present knowledge base in the topic area, and (3) the proposed use of the information derived from conducting the study. The depth of knowledge available in a given area may dictate the level of research possible. The proposed use of the information derived may dictate the choice of a method of study.

The type of information desired refers to the goal of the study. Does the investigator wish to simply describe "what is" in relation to the topic area, or to explain the relationship between two or more occurrences? The investigator who designs a study to examine the psychosocial needs of a particular population may be interested in simply describing what exists. When investigators design a study to explain why the diagnosis of cancer brings with it intense feelings of helplessness, they want to explain a relationship.

The present knowledge base in a given area may dictate how nurse researchers begin their investigation. For example, a nurse may discover that several patients suffering from a particular condition are responding to care in an unusual manner. The nurse may then examine the literature and find little or nothing written about the particular phenomenon. The next step might be to design a study that would describe similar patients who have the same condition to discover if in fact the observed occurrence happens in most or all instances. The results of the study would demonstrate as much as possible the reality related to the observed phenomenon.

Given that an extensive knowledge base exists in relation to a given topic area, a nurse researcher may choose to use existing information as a basis for a study. Investigators, for example, who believe that a strong sense of personal control has a positive effect on a patient's general health status can go to the psychological literature and find both clinical opinion (articles written by clinical experts) and empirical evidence (results of research) to support their premise. They might then design a study to evaluate an intervention aimed at increasing the personal control of patients.

The proposed use of the information acquired through a research project may dictate the method used to conduct the study. For example, when a powerful drug is being tested for possible use in a patient population, the most stringent method possible for the testing of the drug is recommended. The issue of ensuring that the results obtained will apply to any member of the patient population is of utmost importance. In this case, a highly controlled experiment would be the research method of choice. In many instances, however, particularly in nursing science, important topic areas do not lend themselves to the experimental approach. The study of interventions designed to decrease the number of suicides in the population is one example where the experimental approach is not applicable.

WORKING DEFINITION

Kinds of Investigations

The kinds of investigations used refers to (1) the type of information desired, (2) the present knowledge base in the topic area, and (3) the proposed use of information derived from conducting the study.

EXAMPLE

Kinds of Investigations

A nursing official within the government wishes to determine the value of educating and employing nurse practitioners within the health care system. The proposed use of the results is to modify funding to those programs that train practitioners in the direction of the findings. A quantitative method of investigation is chosen.

The study in the above example seeks to explain the difference between care provided by a nurse practitioner and a variety of other health care professionals. The investigator is not merely interested in describing what exists, but wants to be able to predict that care provided by this particular health care professional either will make a difference (either positive or negative) or, perhaps, will be the same as care provided by others.

There is some background information in the literature on the nature of the activities performed by nurse practitioners. Although there are opposing opinions as to the ability of any investigator to design a study that could accurately provide the information desired from this project, there is sufficient background material to warrant the design of an experiment.

The most stringent method of investigation has been chosen in this example. The outcome of the proposed research—that is, the use of the findings—can affect in a major way the future of the profession of nursing. The effects would be felt on a national level, and both the educational system and the health care system would be affected.

Other kinds of investigation allow the researcher to explain phenomena. A historical approach, in which the researcher carefully and thoroughly examines all past documents that relate to the topic in question, can provide data that will explain relationships. In addition, the investigator may choose an approach that is similar to an experiment but with fewer controls. Although the information derived from these studies can be of considerable value, the applicability of the findings is different.

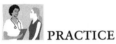 PRACTICE

Kinds of Investigations

Identify three topic areas that would lend themselves to describing "what is" and three topic areas in which relationships could be explained.

 CRITICAL APPRAISAL

Kinds of Investigations

- What kind of information is presented: Descriptive? Explanatory? Predictive?

- What is the knowledge base in the particular area?

- What is the proposed use for the findings of the investigation?

Conceptual Models

An important consideration when designing a study is the decision regarding the conceptual framework or theoretical foundation of the research.

A **conceptual model** is a framework for communicating a particular perception of the world. A conceptual model represents ideas or notions that have been put together in a unique way to describe a particular area of concern. It may be likened to experiencing the world by "looking through someone else's glasses" or "walking in someone else's shoes." Because each person has different perspectives and life experiences, wearing another's shoes changes the experience of events. Similarly, conceptual models put specific ideas or notions into a meaningful framework for viewing the world. One's world view as perceived within one conceptual model may differ greatly from that perceived within another conceptual model. Specifically, conceptual models assist individuals in organizing their thinking in order to select a focus of study and in interpreting the findings (Morse, 1992).

WORKING DEFINITION

Conceptual Models

A conceptual model provides organization for thinking, observing, and interpreting what is seen, gives direction to the search for identifying a question to ask about the phenomenon, and points out solutions to problems.

All disciplines or fields of study, such as psychology, sociology, and physics, specify boundaries for the areas that are examined within each particular field. Psychology is largely concerned with the study of individual human behavior and interaction; sociology examines the behaviors of groups of individuals; and physics is concerned with the study of the laws of physical matter. Nursing, as a distinct discipline, has been concerned historically with four key concepts: humans, environment, nursing, and health. Nursing is concerned with the interaction between humans and the environment in relation to health (Marriner-Tomey & Alligood, 1997; Meleis, 1991). More than a dozen nurses have designed conceptual models that link the key concepts of the discipline in unique ways. Some examples are Orem's (1985) self-care model, King's (1989) open systems model, Roy's (Roy & Andrews, 1989; 1998) adaptation model, and Rogers' (1970, 1980, 1990) developmental life process model.

Nursing Models

Nursing conceptual models not only are helpful in that they provide a direction for study, but they also provide an understanding of the world in terms of nursing's major concerns, namely humans, environment, nursing, and health (Fawcett, 2000; Fitzpatrick & Whall, 1996; Nursing Theories Conference Group, 1996). Although many nurse researchers have successfully used models that do not reflect these four concepts, the advantage of using a nursing model is that the researcher views the study from a nursing point of view from its inception. Within the nursing framework, each nursing model defines and relates the four major concepts in a unique manner. Thus, viewing the world through Roy's glasses as opposed to Orem's gives the researcher quite a different understanding of nursing and its concerns. In essence, a nursing conceptual model frames the way in which nursing's concerns will be viewed and the direction that a research project will take. Figures 3.2 and 3.3 depict how two different nursing models view the four key concepts and their interrelationship.

In addition to describing relationships between key concepts, the nursing model provides definitions of the key concepts that make sense within the specific framework. Concepts such as adaptation, development, self-care, and many others are defined by the designer of the given model. These concepts can be defined differently by different individuals, and it is therefore important to understand the particular definition

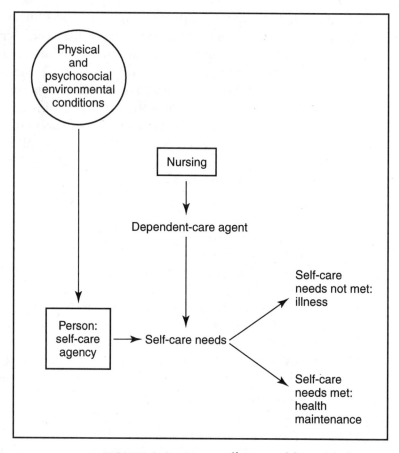

FIGURE 3.2 Orem's self-care model

used within a specific model. Figure 3.4 depicts the concept of adaptation as Roy defines it in her model.

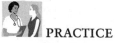

PRACTICE

Nursing Models

Select one of the following nursing models and identify the major key concepts as they are used in the model. Diagram the interrelationships between those concepts.

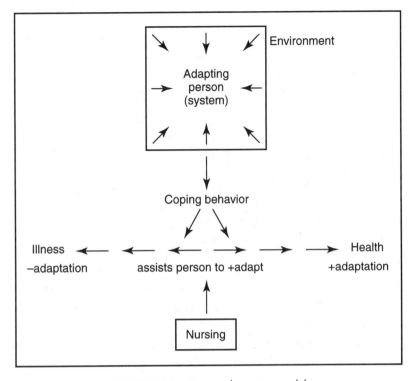

FIGURE 3.3 Roy's adaptation model

- King's (1989) open systems model
- Rogers's (1970, 1980, 1990) developmental life process model
- Neuman's (1994) systems model
- Johnson's (1980) behavioral systems model
- Peplau's (1952) interpersonal relations model

CRITICAL APPRAISAL

Conceptual Models

- Is a clear conceptual model (framework) described in the study?

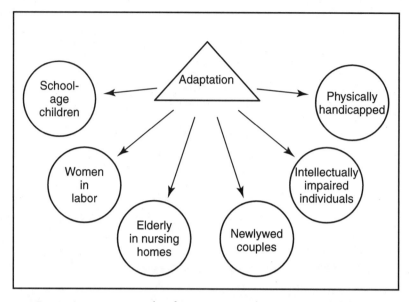

FIGURE 3.4 Concept identification. Roy's adaptation model defines the concept of adaptation as a process of responding positively to environmental changes; this concept can be applied to all living organisms (Roy & Andrews, 1998).

- Are the major concepts of the model identified and defined?
- Are the relationships among concepts within the model described?
- Is the conceptual model relevant to nursing research?
- Does the conceptual model presented make logical sense?

Concepts

The directions that a conceptual model provides to the nurse researcher are general and somewhat vague. This situation arises in part from the fact that the **concepts** themselves are abstract entities and not directly observable in the real world (Chinn & Jacobs, 1998). For example, most individuals speak of having "energy," and their family and friends seem to understand the reference. Yet someone who was asked to observe energy might experience some confusion. Energy is obviously an abstract concept and can be defined in a variety of ways. Each conceptual model has a set of abstract concepts that require definition to understand their meaning. When all of the concepts in a particular model are defined and related to one another, they help to give meaning to how the world is experienced within that framework. Models do not apply only to one particular event, group of individuals, or situation (see Figure 3.5). Rather, models help to structure the way any situation, event, or group of individuals could be viewed.

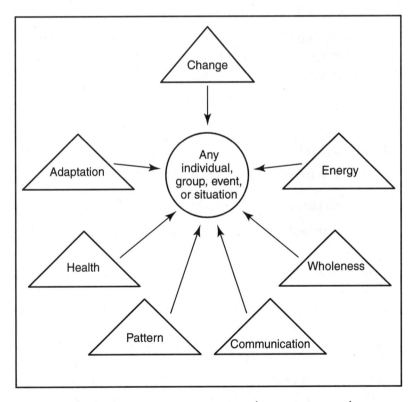

FIGURE 3.5 Common concepts used in nursing research

WORKING DEFINITION

Concepts

Concepts are imaginary, abstract pictures or mental images formed from real-world observations of things, objects, or events that an individual has experienced.

PRACTICE

Concept Selection in Nursing Research

Using a nursing model, complete the following:

• Select and define one concept from the model.

• Describe how the concept could (or could not) apply to the following: children, adults, families, groups other than families, communities.

CRITICAL APPRAISAL

Concept Selection in Nursing Research

• Are the concepts under study clearly identified and defined?

• Are relationships among the concepts under study described?

Borrowed Models

The use of a given nursing model has distinct advantages in conducting research that is relevant to nursing. Nurse researchers can, however, select conceptual frameworks that have been developed within other disciplines. This practice is referred to as using a **borrowed model**. For example, the sociologist Talcott Parsons (1951) developed a conceptual model (framework) that attempts to organize the individual's experience of the sick role. In order for nurse researchers to use Parsons' framework, they would have to explain the relationship between Parsons' model and the major concepts of nursing—that is, humans, environment, health, and nursing.

WORKING DEFINITION

Borrowed Models

Borrowed models are conceptual models taken from scientific disciplines outside of nursing that are thought to provide a better explanation of what we see in nursing and a more relevant explanation of how the world operates.

Nurse researchers have often selected Maslow's (1970) model of human motivation as a framework for examining questions pertinent to nursing. This model, taken from psychology, can help nurse researchers to explain how humans are motivated to reach their full potential. If a study is designed to examine an aspect of human motivation as it relates to nursing and Maslow's model is selected as the framework, the researcher would first identify the major concepts of the model. In the next step, the nurse researcher would relate the key concepts of Maslow's model to the four major concepts of nursing: environment, nursing, human beings, and health. These initial steps are an important part of the development of the study's conceptual framework and are crucial when borrowing a model from another discipline.

The identification of the major concepts in Maslow's model would be a first step in using the model as a framework for a nursing study. For example, according to Maslow, *individuals* strive to satisfy their needs by moving up the hierarchy from physiological to self-actualization needs; motivation to satisfy needs is affected by *environmental* situations and events; nursing attempts to assist humans in their movement to satisfy needs, and ultimately to reach full integration, or *health* (see Figure 3.6). Thus, this brief explanation provides the investigator with a rationale for borrowing from another discipline a model that appears to explain or fit a question under study

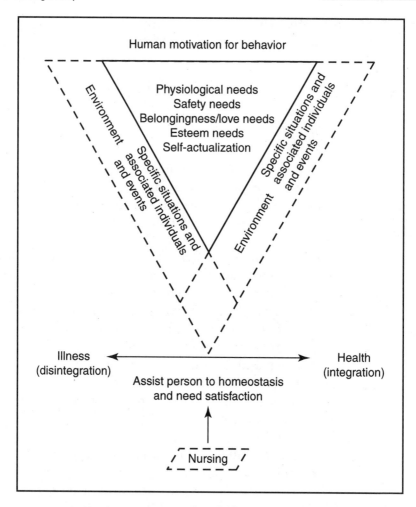

Human motivation for behavior

Environment

Specific situations and associated individuals and events

Physiological needs
Safety needs
Belongingness/love needs
Esteem needs
Self-actualization

Specific situations and associated individuals and events

Environment

Illness
(disintegration)

Health
(integration)

Assist person to homeostasis
and need satisfaction

Nursing

FIGURE 3.6 A borrowed model for use in nursing research
(Maslow, 1970).

better than a given nursing model. The fit between the model
and nursing is obvious.

The consumer of research should evaluate the investigator's
use of a conceptual model in terms of its logical adequacy. The
consumer needs to ask: Does the use of the model make logical
sense for viewing nursing concerns? Is it logical to understand
the world from the perspective of the selected model?

Borrowing conceptual models (frameworks) is generally viewed as an acceptable practice within nursing, as long as the relevance to nursing is clarified. Borrowed models, as well as models developed by nurses within their own discipline, are varied and numerous. At this time, consensus does not exist in regard to a *preferred* nursing model. Unlike many other professions, nursing is considered a young science and does not yet have one dominant, universally accepted model. The continued generation of research within nursing may eventually lead the profession to adopt one or two theoretical positions. At present, however, there are many options, a situation that frequently leads to some confusion and frustration.

CRITICAL APPRAISAL

Borrowed Models

- Does the selected model best explain the phenomena under study?

- Are the major concepts of the model identified and defined?

- Is the model discussed as it relates to nursing's four key concepts (human, environment, health, and nursing)?

Theories

Theories are similar to conceptual models in that they are also composed of interrelated concepts. Theories, however, unlike conceptual models, contain more specific information. In order to understand a basic difference between a conceptual model and a theory, imagine a family visiting an architect who is in the process of building their house. If the family were to visit a building site where the frame had already been erected, they would become immediately aware of the general layout of the house. For example, they would be able to tell whether the house would be a one-story or a two-story dwelling. They would also be able to discern where the doors and rooms would be located. They would not be able to tell what the kitchen would look like when completed, however, nor would they be able to envision where decorative items would eventually be placed.

If the architect were to show the family the detailed plans for the house, their mental image of the house would be quite different. Similarly, when an individual uses a conceptual model, a frame is provided with few specific details. The specificity of the architect's plans can be likened to a theory in that more detailed information is provided.

WORKING DEFINITION

Theories

A theory is composed of specific concepts and propositions that attempt to account for a particular notion that is observed in the real world. Theory assumes that a particular conceptual model is utilized. The purpose of using theory is to describe a notion, to explain an idea, or to predict what might be observed.

EXAMPLE

Theories

- Describe an idea: Identifying factors that influence feelings of loneliness in the elderly.

- Explain an idea: Identifying how pain is experienced during acute stress.

- Predict what might be observed: Stating what social supports affect coping behaviors.

In each of the above examples, the relationship between what is hypothesized and real-life events is apparent. A definitive piece of reality is suggested in a very concrete manner—much less obscure than the information presented by a conceptual model. Each example assists in forming a different type of relationship between concepts that, once tested, become useful to nursing. Thus, when a particular theory is proposed to explain a nursing concern, it is tested for accuracy. As portions of theory are tested and found to be accurate representations of the world, the researcher moves closer to "objective" reality.

 PRACTICE

Theories

From the following examples identify whether the theory describes, explains, or predicts a relationship:

- The extent of support systems and attitudinal factors that affect success in nursing.

- Factors influencing feelings of isolation among institutionalized individuals.

- Describing the grieving experience.

- Identifying and describing characteristics of burnout.

- Feelings of loneliness and sleep-wake patterns.

- Support systems that affect paternal-fetal attachments.

 CRITICAL APPRAISAL

Evaluating the Use of Theory

- Does the theory clearly describe a notion, explain an idea, or predict what might be observed?

- Is the purpose for using selected theories stated?

- Is the theory useful to nursing practice, education, and research?

107

Propositions

The statements within a theory are attempts to link the concepts together so that a prediction, explanation, or description of something can be provided. The statements that interrelate concepts are the result of previous knowledge and research and are assumed to be true and accurate. For example, as participation in decision making increases, satisfaction increases. As a result of previous study, this observation is largely assumed to be true. There are two types of statements that can form **propositions**. These statements are termed **axioms** and **theorems** (see Figure 3.7). Figure 3.8 shows how a proposition could be developed.

WORKING DEFINITION

Propositions

Propositions are statements that suggest a specific relationship between two or more concepts. A proposition may take the form of an axiom or a theorem.

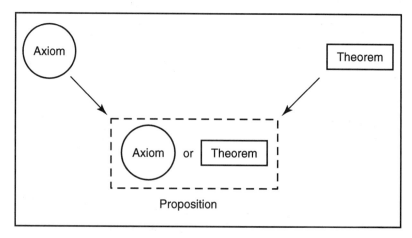

FIGURE 3.7 Forms that a proposition may take

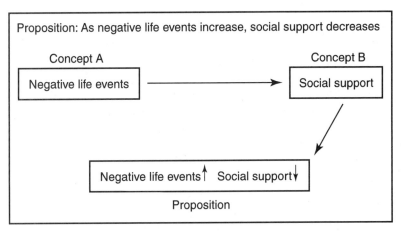

FIGURE 3.8 Developing a proposition

PRACTICE

Propositions

From the following statements, identify those that are propositions:

- Fear is innate in humans.

- As anxiety increases, learning decreases.

- Love produces affectional behavior.

- As control increases, feelings of power decrease.

- Nurses frequently feel frustration.

WORKING DEFINITION

Axiom

An axiom is a statement that links the concepts of a theory. The links or relationships between concepts are assumed to be true.

109

WORKING DEFINITION

Theorem

A theorem is a statement that designates a relationship between concepts that are deduced from relationships already formed by axioms.

It is the previously assumed or designated relationships among concepts (axioms) that form the underpinnings of theory and ultimately a research study. The investigator proposes new relationships that have not heretofore been established in the form of theorems (see Figure 3.9). The investigator must have a clear awareness of those relationships that have been established, the evidence that permits the designation of given relationships, and those relationships that have not been tested. Consumers of research must be able to identify clearly the same kind of information when they read a research report.

PRACTICE

Deducing Theorems from Axioms

Following are two sets of axioms. Deduce a theorem from each set.

- As depression increases, isolation increases.

- As isolation increases, feelings of helplessness increase.

Axiom: As fear increases, tension increases.

Axiom: As tension increases, stress increases.

Deduced theorem: As fear increases, stress increases.

FIGURE 3.9 Deducing theorems from axioms

110

- As pain increases, muscle tension increases.
- As muscle tension increases, irritability increases.

CRITICAL APPRAISAL

Propositions

- Are the propositions in the theory clearly identifiable?
- Does the researcher state the relevance of the propositions?
- Is the theorem to be tested clearly stated?

Concept-Construct-Variable

Unlike the concepts within a conceptual model, the concepts within a theory are specific and may relate to only a very select group of individuals, situations, or events. Figure 3.10 illustrates how the composition of the conceptual model provides a framework for examining a phenomenon of interest but does

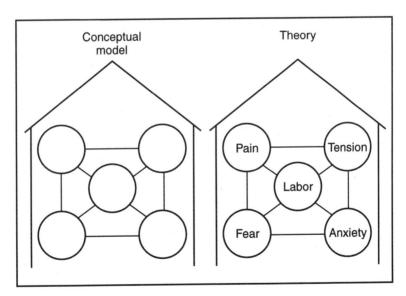

FIGURE 3.10 Interrelationships among concepts in a model and a theory

111

so in a general, abstract manner. The concepts within a theory are clearly delineated and must be defined very specifically. The clear identification of how the concepts interrelate determines how the theory is supported.

Concepts within a theory must be clearer and more concrete than those of a conceptual model because a theory seeks to produce knowledge about a very narrow, specific problem. Because a theory tends to deal with "special interests," the concepts found in theory tend to be concepts that can be tied to a particular individual, group, event, or situation. For example, in using a theory of boredom in young adults, it is easy to think of many individuals, situations, or events where the theory might not apply. For example, very small children, people of a particular culture, or individuals during certain periods of their lives may not experience boredom in the same fashion.

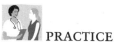 PRACTICE

Concept Specificity

Select one of the following concepts and identify the individuals, groups, events, or situations for which the concept may not apply:

- Stress
- Loneliness
- Disengagement

- Grief
- Hostility
- Sadness

- Pain
- Bonding
- Love

Concepts are not defined or clarified in everyday usage. Understanding the general intent of the speaker is usually sufficient. For example, clients may describe themselves as being sad, and, given a knowledge of their particular situation, that description may be sufficient. If the concept of *sad* were to be studied in any depth, however, *sad* would have to be specified and clarified.

A concrete example of the need to specify the meaning of concepts can be found in Figure 3.11. The concept depicted is

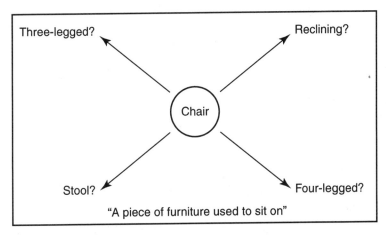

FIGURE 3.11 Concept specificity

chair. Although each person holds a specific notion of this concept, all individuals may not share the same definition. Greater specificity in relation to the concept *chair* would be required if the concept were under examination.

When a concept is clarified so that it is potentially observable and in a form that is open to measurement, it is considered a **construct**. To formulate a construct, the researcher must take a concept that is relatively fuzzy and unclear and list all of the aspects of that concept that could be seen in the real world. Although the concept itself is not directly observable, the construct that is formulated from the concept narrows the meaning for study.

WORKING DEFINITION

Construct

A construct reflects the specific, potentially observable characteristics of a concept and thus facilitates testing of the idea.

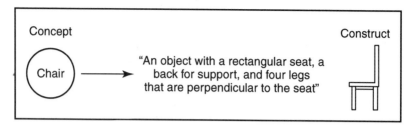

FIGURE 3.12 Construct

Figure 3.12 depicts how the concept *chair* is specified as a construct by identifying its measurable aspects.

Making a concept potentially observable, and thus a construct, does not mean that all individuals who read the translation of the concept would understand exactly what to measure, observe, control, or look for in the real world. **Variables** are the final pieces that ensure continuity in observing real-world phenomena in a precise fashion.

WORKING DEFINITION

Variable

A variable is a concept (construct) that has been so specifically defined that precise observations and therefore measurement can be accomplished.

Identifying the variables to be studied in a given project involves capturing only a portion of what the concept could convey. The researcher decides how to define the variable. The definition must be explicit and must convey the manner in which the variable will be measured. Clear identification of the variables under study gives clear direction to the research project. Although consumers may not be in agreement with the way in which a particular variable has been defined, if the definition is clear they can at least understand the results of the research. Figure 3.13 presents an example of the concept (construct) chair as a variable.

The concept *pain* is relevant to nursing practice. Figure 3.14 depicts how that concept might be described, viewed as a construct, and defined as a variable.

114

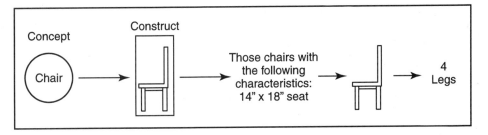

FIGURE 3.13 Concept-construct-variable

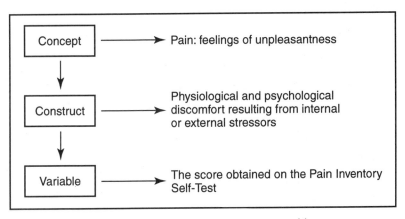

FIGURE 3.14 Concept-construct-variable

 PRACTICE

Concept-Construct-Variable

Select one of the following concepts, generate a definition, and then specify the construct and variable for that concept:

- Happiness
- Depression
- Restlessness
- Poverty
- Fatigue
- Energy
- Denial
- Well-being
- Joy

The process of identifying a *measurable concept* or variable ultimately leads to testing in the real world. The researcher must collect information using the definition provided under

115

the variable. By collecting observations, a researcher can determine the accuracy of the concepts and their relationship to each other as propositions. Collecting information or data to support a theory is dependent on the use of scientific reasoning.

CRITICAL APPRAISAL

Concept-Construct-Variable

- Are concepts defined in terms of their relationship to other concepts?

- Are the variables clearly defined?

- Are the constructs directly or indirectly observable?

- Are the variables defined in a specific manner?

- Are the variables measurable?

- Is the stated measurement of the variables logical?

Scientific Reasoning

The use of the research process is often likened to a particular manner of **reasoning**. There are two recognized categories of thinking or reasoning: an intuitive form of thinking, and a more structured, formalized approach. **Intuitive thinking,** unhampered by structure or specified expectations, can produce creative answers to questions. Past experience, in the form of emotions, actions, and thoughts, can be used in the resolution of a problem situation.

Although the intuitive manner of reasoning is helpful to the research process, particularly at the initial idea stage, the lack of information grounded in real-world experience hampers the formation of a sound study. Real-world experience in this context refers to information that has been gathered through a qualitative or quantitative research process or through expert clinical opinion. Students of the research process, regardless of their preferred method of reasoning, must adopt

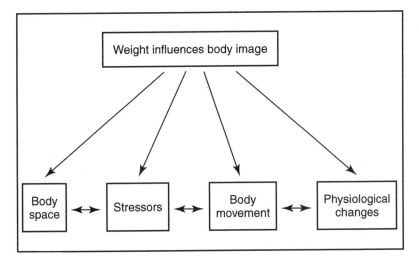

FIGURE 3.15 Working with a general belief: deductive reasoning

a **structured manner of reasoning** and apply it to their questions of interest.

Deductive

When a particular conceptual model or theory is selected to examine a problem, the model or theory provides direction in terms of expected observations. The model or theory provides a general belief about how or why a particular event occurs, and, based on those beliefs, details related to the event can be observed (see Figure 3.15). This type of reasoning is termed **deductive**.

WORKING DEFINITION

Deductive Reasoning

Deductive reasoning is a method of thinking that begins with a general statement of belief and moves to obtain specific observations. Reasoning moves from the general to the specific.

117

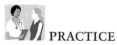 PRACTICE

Deductive Reasoning

Select one of the following general statements (propositions) and formulate four possible specific observations:

- Anxiety produces fear.
- Social support influences achievement.
- Touch influences development.
- Temperature influences healing.

Inductive

There are events of interest for which no theory can adequately explain their existence. In this case, observations related to the event can be collected and an explanation or theory can evolve from these observations (see Figure 3.16). This

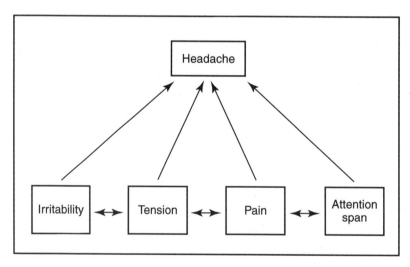

FIGURE 3.16 Working from observations to a theory: inductive reasoning

manner of reasoning is termed **inductive**, as opposed to deductive, in which the investigator begins with a model or theory.

WORKING DEFINITION

Inductive Reasoning

Inductive reasoning involves the collection of observations related to a particular event. From these observations, a theory or general explanation regarding the event can evolve. Reasoning moves from the specific to the general.

PRACTICE

Inductive Reasoning

Think of an event that occurs in your everyday life experience. Identify specific data/observations associated with that event. Formulate a general statement (pattern/trend) that could explain the event.

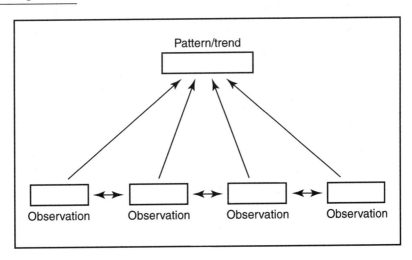

CRITICAL APPRAISAL

Scientific Reasoning

- Is the researcher using inductive or deductive reasoning?
- If an inductive approach is identified, is there an appropriate theory that could be used?
- If a deductive approach is identified, is it appropriate to the task at hand?

The Problem Statement

Returning to the idea of designing a house, it is understood that the architect may initiate the process by responding to an abstraction in the mind of the prospective buyer. The architect then outlines a design, constructs the roof and exterior walls, and continues to move in the direction of increasing detail. It is important to remember that the architect was probably aware from the beginning that the structure was going to be a two-story house as opposed to an apartment, or a brick house as opposed to a straw hut. There is, therefore, an awareness of some of the specifics from the beginning of the process.

Similarly, in identifying a problem for study, the researcher generally has at least one specific idea in mind, even though a plan of operation has not been developed. The formulation of the **problem statement** provides direction for the remainder of the process. When the formulation of the problem statement is effectively addressed, the remaining steps in the research process flow with relative ease. If the formulation of the problem statement is not adequately addressed, difficulties may follow, perhaps requiring a rethinking of the entire project. The steps related to formulating the problem statement are presented here to assist the consumer of research to understand the process involved. These steps are (1) specifying the topic of interest, (2) formulating the concept of interest, (3) designing a conceptual map, (4) identifying the research focus, (5) identifying the population, and (6) constructing the statement.

WORKING DEFINITION

The Problem Statement

The problem statement presents the topic under study, provides a rationale for the choice of topic, represents a synthesis of fact and theory, and directs the selection of the design.

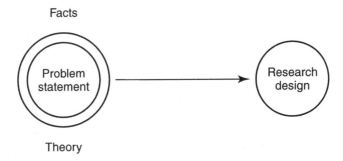

Specifying the Topic or Concept of Interest

The first step in the formulation of a problem statement is the specification of a **topic or concept of interest**. Some researchers may begin to formulate a problem statement from an identified topic. For example, an interest in the topic of alternative treatments for decubitus ulcers could be a starting point. Other individuals may begin to formulate a problem statement from an interest in a given concept. For example, an interest in the concept of stress could also be a starting point for the process (see Figure 3.17). Whether the researcher begins the formulation with a topic or with a concept of interest, it is important to identify the choice of starting point (topic or concept) and to specify both parts (topic and concept).

121

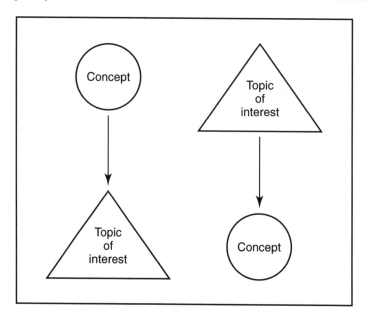

FIGURE 3.17   Topic or concept of interest

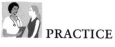 PRACTICE

Topic or Concept of Interest

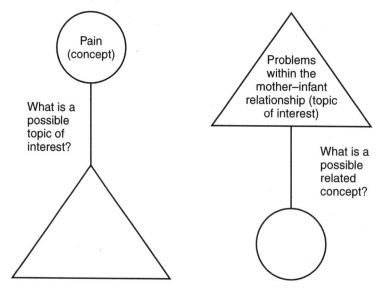

In order to understand fully either published or unpublished research, it is important to be able to identify the researcher's topic and concept of interest. If they are not clearly specified, the results of the study are diminished in power. For example, if the topic of interest in a given study is "the problems present in a mother-infant relationship," and an explanation is not presented as to whether the concept of interest is *stress* (the stressors involved), *care* (the care given at birth), or some other related concept, the results of the study cannot be easily applied. On the other hand, if the researcher chooses to study *pain* (concept) and does not identify the specific topic of interest, problems with measurement and analysis of the findings will ensue.

Topics and concepts of interest to researchers come from a variety of sources. A curious mind readily becomes involved in questioning information that comes from books, journals, friends, instructors, television, radio, conferences, and so on. The ability to identify readily both topics and concepts of interest sharpens both the researcher's and the consumer's research skills.

 PRACTICE

Topic or Concept of Interest

Specify a topic of interest and a concept of interest from one of the following:

- Nursing practice

- Friends

- Journals, books, magazines

- Television, radio, newspapers

- Theories

CRITICAL APPRAISAL

Topic or Concept of Interest

- Are the topic and concept of interest clearly identified?

- Is the relationship between concept and topic of interest readily apparent?

PRACTICE

Evaluating the Choice of Topic and Concept of Interest

Read the following excerpt:

> The concept of hope—that state of looking ahead to something pleasurable—is considered to be of great importance in relation to one's physical and mental well-being (Hutschnecker, 1981). Physiological changes may actually occur as a result of giving up hope or experiencing increased hope. The process of dealing with hope is therefore extremely important to nursing. How nurses define and utilize hope in their plan of care may have a powerful influence on a client's well-being.
>
> Unfortunately, hope, as a concept that influences nursing care, has not been defined, nor has a process of effectively utilizing hope within a plan of care been developed. Before recommending a definition or suggesting an appropriate utilization of the concept, it would seem important to examine nursing's present view of the concept. How do nurses relate to clients who look ahead to pleasurable events that may or may not exist? The following study was designed to examine these questions.

Answer the following questions:

- What is the concept of interest in this excerpt?

- What is the topic of interest in this excerpt?

124

- Is the concept clearly identified?
- Is the relationship between topic and concept apparent?

Concepts and Their Relationships

When formulating the problem statement, in addition to identifying a topic of interest and a related concept, researchers frequently need to understand the relationship of other concepts to their selection. For example, if researchers wish to study the perceived control of terminally ill patients, they might choose the concept of dying as a major idea. Other concepts, however, such as *learned helplessness* and *attribution*, might help the researcher develop a better framework for the study.

An effective approach to understanding the relationships among concepts is the use of a conceptual map. **Conceptual maps** help researchers to understand the breadth of the areas they are studying, as well as to place a specific problem within a larger framework of differing conceptual viewpoints. Conceptual maps can be highly complex or relatively simple. For the beginning researcher, four areas of concern are sufficient: (1) the original identified concept, (2) several concepts that are related to the original, (3) theories that relate to the concepts, and (4) the sources of information on all concepts and theories.

To draw a conceptual map, any graphic representation can be used—for example, straight lines, circles, and triangles. This visual presentation is often helpful in depicting the kinds of relationships that exist, as well as the relative importance of the various relationships. Figure 3.18, for example, visually depicts the central concept of dying, the related concepts (religion, death, aging, and helplessness), related theories (Christianity, stages of dying, learned helplessness, and developmental phases), and the sources of information (Bible; Kubler-Ross, 1969; Seligman, 1975; Burnside & Schmidt, 1994).

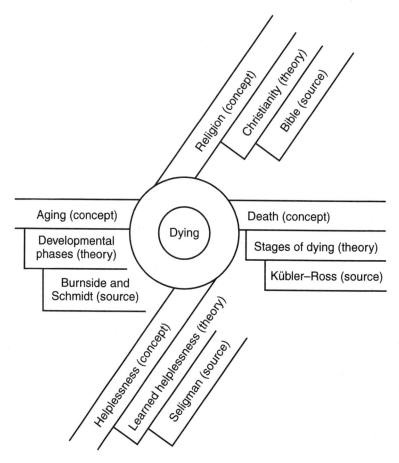

FIGURE 3.18 A conceptual map

 PRACTICE

Conceptual Map

Using a concept of interest, related concepts, theories, and sources, draw a conceptual map.

The Focus of the Study

As the processes of identifying a topic and concept of interest and examining conceptual relationships proceed, the focus of the study should become apparent. Some studies are designed to examine what exists; others are designed to assess the influence of a given activity. For example, if a researcher is interested in the problems encountered in a mother-infant relationship and has developed a framework around the concepts of *bonding, caring,* and *development,* the focus of the study might be on what exists. What are the problems encountered in a mother–infant relationship? How do they relate to bonding, caring, or development?

If, however, the researcher is interested in the problem of chronic back discomfort and has developed a framework around the concepts of *pain, rehabilitation,* and *learned helplessness,* the focus of the study may be on what activity will modify the discomfort. Will a particular intervention diminish the discomfort? How does the intervention relate to the selected concepts?

The topic or concept chosen does not direct the focus of the study. The researcher's goal or purpose will direct whether the focus is on what exists or on the influence of a given activity. Frequently, the problem statement will reflect the focus of the study. For example, the problem statement "What is the influence of biofeedback on chronic back pain" is obviously a study of a particular activity—biofeedback—on a physiological condition. Specifying the focus of a study is an important activity that occurs in the initial stages of the research process. Practice in formulating problem statements that reflect the focus is one way to learn this particular step.

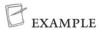 EXAMPLE

Study Focus

The researcher may choose to describe what exists or study the influence of a specified activity. Given the concept *pain* and the topic *postoperative discomfort,* the researcher needs to choose one of the following directions when designing a study:

- What are the characteristics of (1) postoperative discomfort? (2) nurses who care for patients experiencing discomfort? (3) two differing groups who experience postoperative discomfort?

- What will influence postoperative discomfort: therapeutic touch? client teaching? family support? range of motion?

The actual wording of a problem statement can reflect the investigator's ability to think clearly or, conversely, can represent a fuzzy approach to the topic under consideration. Time spent on the wording of the problem statement so that it is easily understood and the investigator's intent is readily apparent will be rewarded as the later stages of the investigation fall easily into place.

EXAMPLE

Study Focus

Phrases that help to describe what exists:

- What is/are . . . ?

- What are the differences between . . . and . . . among . . . ?

- Who is/are . . . ?

- Where is/are . . . ?

Phrases that help to describe the influence of an activity:

- What are the effects of . . . on . . . among . . . ?

- How does . . . affect . . . among . . . ?

PRACTICE

Study Focus

Write one problem statement or question for each of the phrases presented in the preceding example. Identify the topic and the focus when writing the problem statement.

128

CRITICAL APPRAISAL

Evaluating the Focus of the Study

- Is the focus of the study clear?
- Is the choice of focus logical?
- Is the choice of focus consistent throughout the research report?

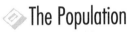

The Population

Although there are many factors related to the **population** under study, nurse researchers should be aware at the time of the formulation of the problem statement whom they will be studying. As the research process evolves, the investigator will continually specify desired characteristics of the selected population. At this point, however, a global idea of the group that will be examined is important.

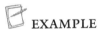

EXAMPLE

Problem Statements and Associated Populations

Problem statement: How does the loss of a loved one affect perceptions of control?

Population: Widows; widowers.

Problem statement: What are the effects of two differing treatments on decubitus care?

Population: Nursing home residents.

129

PRACTICE

Identifying the Population

Identify the population in each of the following examples:

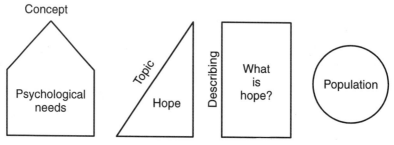

Problem statement: The perception of hope by a dying individual.

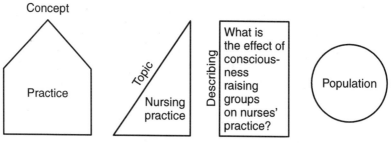

Problem statement: The effects of consciousness-raising groups on nurses' practice.

Critical Overview in Initiating a Study

Successful initiation of a study requires the selection of a topic that the investigator has the expertise to investigate, will sustain the researcher's interest, and is feasible to conduct. Once a topic is identified, the purpose needs to be clearly stated. As the consumer reads a research report, it is not difficult to spot areas that received insufficient attention. The purpose may not be clear or the kind of study attempted may not fit well with the information desired.

A well-planned project that will be successful will have identified a problem for study that involves detailing of conceptual models, theories, and methods of reasoning. In addition, a clearly written problem statement and the population to be tested are key elements in execution of a well-done study. A research report that makes these elements clear to the consumer helps to ensure that the project is not only doable and articulate, but of importance to nursing and most likely will help build a strong knowledge base in the discipline.

CRITICAL OVERVIEW
INITIATING A STUDY

Excerpt A

Two experienced clinical nurse researchers in a large metropolitan hospital design a study to determine the effectiveness of a psychosocial nursing intervention aimed at diminishing post-myocardial infarct anxiety. The intervention requires several interviews by clinic nurses over a period of six months postinfarct. The investigators have applied for and received funding to cover most of the expenses of the project.

The two investigators were asked by the hospital to design and carry out the project because there was considerable interest among the various health care professionals in developing an outpatient clinic to assist in the rehabilitation of cardiac patients. If the intervention is successful, funds could be forthcoming for the development of the clinic.

131

Activity 1

Critique the proposed project described in Excerpt A by making a judgment regarding the following:

- Is the project feasible as described?
- Is there reason to believe that the investigators will sustain interest in the topic?
- Is the project of importance to nursing?
- What is the purpose of the project?

Excerpt B

Within society, there are various systems that facilitate the achievement of common goals. These social systems reflect a set of values from which regulations regarding human behavior result. One such social system is the family unit (King, 1989). Each family unit has a set of values and a related system of regulations regarding family members' behavior. The family system provides an environment in which its members will reside for varying periods of time.

Various theorists and clinicians over the years have suggested means by which the family unit can provide an environment that is either more or less facilitative of individual growth. Some of these means have to do with roles played by individual family members; others are related to the dynamics or relationships that exist. *Bonding* is a concept that refers to a kind of relationship that exists between various family members. The term is used to represent the degree of connection that exists between people. How siblings connect or bond initially has obvious implications for their later relationships and possibly their individual development. This study was designed to examine the process of bonding. Will a child's bond or connection to a sibling be closer if the child was present at the sibling's birth than if he or she did not witness the event?

Activity 2

- Evaluate Except B by identifying the model, major concepts, theory (or theories), method of reasoning, problem statement, focus of study, and population.
- After identifying the factors in the excerpt, rank each on a scale of 1 to 5 (1 = poor; 5 = very good; N/A = not applicable) as to their clarity, importance to nursing, comprehensiveness, and logical presentation.

References

Abdellah, F. G. & Levine, E. (1986). *Better patient care through nursing research* (3rd Edition). New York: Macmillan.

Burnside, I. & Schmidt, M. G. (1994). *Working with older adults: Group process.* New York: McGraw-Hill.

Chinn, P. L. & Jacobs, M. K. (1998). *Theory and nursing: Integrated knowledge development* (4th Edition). St. Louis: Mosby Year Book.

Fawcett, J. (2000). *Analysis and evaluation of contemporary nursing knowledge: Nursing models & theories* (3rd Edition). Philadelphia: F. A. Davis.

Fitzpatrick, J. J. & Whall, A. (1996). *Conceptual models of nursing: Analysis and application* (3rd Edition). Englewood Cliffs, NJ: Prentice-Hall.

Hutschnecker, A. (1981). Hope. In *The dynamics of self-fulfillment.* New York: Putnam.

Johnson, D. E. (1980). The behavioral system model for nursing. In J. P. Riehl & C. Roy (Editors). *Conceptual models for nursing practice* (2nd Edition). New York: Appleton-Century-Crofts.

King, I. M. (1989). *A theory for nursing: Systems, concepts, process.* New York: Wiley.

Krieger, D. (1979). *Therapeutic touch: How to use your hands to help and heal.* Englewood Cliffs, NJ: Prentice-Hall.

Kübler-Ross, E. (1969). *On Death and Dying.* New York: Macmillan.

LoBiondo-Wood, G. & Haber, J. (1997). *Nursing research: Methods, critical appraisal and utilization* (3rd Edition). Boston: Mosby.

McMillan, J. H. & Schumacher, S. (1984). *Research in education: A conceptual approach*. Boston: Little, Brown.

Marriner-Tomey, A. & Alligood, M. R. (Editors). (1997). *Nursing theorists and their work*. St. Louis: C. V. Mosby.

Maslow, A. (1970). *Motivation and personality* (2nd Edition). New York: Harper & Row.

Meleis, A. I. (1991). *Theoretical nursing: Development and progress* (2nd Edition). Philadelphia: J. B. Lippincott.

Morse, J. M. (1992). If you believe in theories . . . (editorial). *Qualitative Health Research*, 2(3):259–261.

Neuman, B. (1994). *The Neuman systems model* (3rd Edition). Old Tappan, NJ: Pearson.

The Nursing Theories Conference Group. (1996). *Nursing theories: The base for professional nursing practice* (3rd Edition). Englewood Cliffs, NJ: Prentice-Hall.

Orem, D. E. (1985). *Nursing: Concepts of practice* (3rd Edition). New York: McGraw-Hill.

Oyster, C., Hanten, W. & Llorens, L. (1987). *Introduction to research: A guide for the health science professional*. Philadelphia: Lippincott.

Parsons, T. (1951). *The social system*. New York: Free Press.

Peplau, H. (1952). *Interpersonal relations in nursing*. New York: Putnam.

Polit, D. F. & Hungler, B. P. (1995). *Nursing research: Principles and methods* (5th Edition). Philadelphia: J. B. Lippincott.

Rogers, M. E. (1970). *An introduction to the theoretical basis of nursing*. Philadelphia: F. A. Davis.

Rogers, M. E. (1980). Nursing: A science of unitary man. In J. P. Riehl & C. Roy (Editors), *Conceptual models for nursing practice*. New York: Appleton-Century-Crofts.

Rogers, M. E. (1990). Nursing: Science of unitary, irreducible, human beings: Update 1990. In E. A. M. Barrett (Editor). *Visions of Rogers' science-based nursing*. New York: National League for Nursing.

134

Roy, C. (1989). The Roy adaptation model. In J. Riehl-Sisca (Editor), *Conceptual models for nursing practice* (pp. 105–114). Norwalk, CT: Appleton & Lange.

Roy, C. & Andrews, H. A. (1998). *The Roy adaptation model: The definitive statement* (2nd Edition). Englewood Cliffs, NJ: Prentice-Hall.

Seligman, M. (1975). *Helplessness*. San Francisco: W. H. Freeman.

Wilson, H. S. (1987). *Introducing research in nursing*. Menlo Park, CA: Addison-Wesley.

4

Review of the Literature

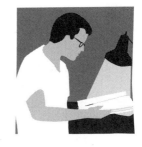

Goals

- *Describe the purpose of the review of literature.*
- *Identify the steps of the review process.*
- *Provide a method for retrieving important information from specific articles.*
- *Describe the process of writing a literature review.*
- *Provide a framework for evaluating the literature review process.*

Introduction

In order to understand fully a given area of interest, nurses need to read relevant clinical opinion and prior research on the topic. Clinical opinion refers to articles or books written by experts in a given field. These experts discuss a particular area within the context of their experience. Although references to research reports may be made in these articles and books, the major focus of the work is to elaborate on the individual's perspective as an expert in the field.

Research refers to those reports that describe the collection and analysis of data related to a given research question. Generally, research reports are found in professional journals or in unpublished theses. Research reports may focus on a specific topic, on the testing of an instrument, or on an overview of research in a given area.

Nurses who wish to improve their practice and those who want to be involved in conducting research need a sound knowledge base relative to their area of interest. Although nursing experience is an invaluable component of a sound knowledge base, a thorough examination of publications on a topic is essential to developing an understanding of a given area.

Overlooking the literature can lead to ineffective practice patterns and the development of research projects that will not serve to improve health care. For example, nurses who have not read the latest research on pain management will not understand that most patients do not need to suffer pain postoperatively. Designing a study to examine nurses' knowledge regarding pain management may be of little value, given the extent of prior research on this topic.

In addition to the problems that can occur when an investigator does not review the literature, there are certain advantages to reading about the topic of interest. Investigators may discover a variety of methodological approaches to the topic that can help assist them in designing a project. Alternative questionnaires, data collection procedures, or approaches to analysis may be found through examining the literature.

The assumptions or model used to describe the topic of interest must be considered when reviewing prior work. A model (conceptual framework, theory, assumption) reflects our view of the world and therefore influences the approach to practice and directs the research that is conducted. For example, if a group of investigators want to examine the effects of touch on the client within a Freudian framework, research based on a behavioral framework is unlikely to provide useful information. Freudian assumptions might lead the investigators to examine touch in terms of unconscious ideation, whereas a behaviorist approach would be more involved with responses to a given stimulus.

Information from the literature that can provide a foundation for research or enhance practice is analyzed in terms of the model used, the relevance of the particular opinion or data, the recency of the opinion or data, and the logic or methods used to arrive at conclusions. Although a comprehensive examination of the literature within a given area is essential to the review of literature, the analysis or the process of making sense out of the information retrieved is of equal importance if we are to further the development of nursing knowledge.

Steps in a Review of the Literature

The Initial Search

There are two phases to a review of the literature. In the first phase, the investigator quickly peruses pertinent publications and develops a somewhat superficial but sufficient knowledge base to make a decision about continuing in a particular area. For example, if an investigator wants to examine the effects of contraceptive education on teenage mothers, she could discover in an initial search of the literature that a comprehensive study has been conducted. The questions in the investigator's mind may have been answered satisfactorily and she will not pursue her idea, or she may question her original assumptions based on new information and proceed in a different direction. On the other hand, she may discover that little information is available and that she needs to proceed with her investigation.

In perusing the literature at any stage in the research process, journal articles are preferred over books because they are generally published more quickly than books and therefore represent more recent information. In addition, journal articles often reflect systematic investigations of areas of interest. Reports of research are preferred over expert opinion articles in that research reports suggest that a systematic investigation has been conducted. For example, titles of research reports might be "Differences in Attitudes toward Pregnancy between Mothers in Two Third World Countries," "The Psychosocial Needs of AIDS Patients, a Descriptive Study," or "The Development of a Tutor Evaluation Form, a Methodological Study." In each of these examples there is the suggestion that a systematic approach to examining the area under question has been taken. Reading beyond the title clearly identifies the systematic process and methods.

Examples of expert opinion articles would be "How to Deal with Families in the Critical Care Unit, One Nurse's Experience," "Suctioning Made Easy, What the Student Needs to Know," or "The Dying Experience, a Personal Diary." In each of these examples there is the suggestion that individuals who have had an experience (or years of experience) that could be important to others have written about that experience and published their perceptions.

WORKING DEFINITION

Initial Search of the Literature

The initial search of the literature is a cursory examination of available publications related to the major variables under study. This review is related to the area of interest and is conducted to assist the investigator in making decisions about proceeding with a given research idea.

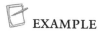

EXAMPLE

Initial Search of the Literature

Two graduate nursing students decide to examine the concept of self-actualization as it relates to self-disclosure among the well-aged. In an initial review of the literature related to the concept of self-actualization and the characteristics of the well-aged, they discover that the existing questionnaires, designed to measure both concepts, are not appropriate for this age group. They decide to rethink the direction of their project.

PRACTICE

Initial Search of the Literature

Identify one area of interest to nursing and gather five related publications. Make a decision based on the information gathered as to whether the area of interest should be pursued.

The Secondary Search

The second step in reviewing the literature involves an in-depth, critically evaluated search of the publications related to the area of interest. The guidelines for conducting an in-depth search include the following: (1) Identify all *relevant* publications related to the area of interest (publications may include articles taken from a number of fields that are related to nursing, e.g., sociology, psychology, anthropology, epidemiology, etc.); (2) review *primary sources* wherever possible; and (3) *critically evaluate* the information gathered.

WORKING DEFINITION

Secondary Search of the Literature

The secondary search of the literature involves an in-depth, critically evaluated search of all publications relevant to the topic of interest.

In conducting an in-depth search of the literature, the investigator needs to identify all relevant publications in the area of interest. Relevance refers to "how closely" the information relates to the topic of interest. Obviously, if an investigator reports on the psychological stages of development in childhood, that information will not be useful to the investigator who wants to examine depression in the older adult. On the other hand, information that focuses specifically on each of

141

the variables of interest is probably not available. For example, the nurse investigator who wishes to study the value of autonomy to nursing home residents in relation to their health status would try to find (1) research that has examined the same questions (e.g., "An Investigation of the Concept of Personal Control within the Nursing Home"), (2) research that has examined related questions (e.g., "Autonomy as a Factor in Institutional Life"), (3) information related to the concepts of autonomy and health status (e.g., "Autonomy as a Psychological Variable," "What Does Health Status Mean for the Elderly?"), and (4) information related to the characteristics of nursing home residents (e.g., "Demographic Characteristics of Nursing Home Residents").

The investigator starts with the most recent publications in order to find the most up-to-date information. *Recent*, in general terms, usually means within the last five years. For major works that are basic to the field, however, such as Sigmund Freud's (1910) writings on the unconscious or John Bowlby's writings on the concept of attachment, the date of publication would not be of concern (Alsop-Shields & Mohay, 2001).

Another consideration when searching the literature is the issue of primary versus secondary sources. A primary source refers to the publication in its original form. A secondary source occurs when an author writes about another author's work. An example of a primary source would be the books written by Abraham Maslow on the hierarchy of needs. Maslow originated the concept and published several works. An example of a secondary source would be a nursing text written by an author other than Maslow who described Maslow's hierarchy of needs. Primary sources are generally preferred because a distortion of ideas can occur in a secondary source (Polit & Hungler, 1999).

The investigator critically evaluates the information gathered by examining each component of the publication. Analysis of a clinical opinion article requires the reader to evaluate the logic used to validate the author's conclusion. When analyzing a research report, the reader must examine each component of the research process and make judgments about the appropriateness of the methods used in relation to the conclusions drawn.

Although knowledge of each component of the research process is essential for the reader to comprehend clearly the results of a research report, the naive reader can retrieve some useful information by applying principles of logic and knowledge gained from experience.

An example of using logic to evaluate a research article would be the concern expressed by orthopedic nurses who read the results of a study that claimed that sterile technique used in the process of changing dressings did not diminish the number of infections among patients. In fact, the investigator reported that the use of clean rather than sterile technique resulted in fewer infections. It did not make sense to these nurses—unless there were factors in the study that were not reported—that replacing sterile technique with clean technique would keep the number of wound infections stable or would decrease them. Even without being able to understand the kind of statistical analysis that was used in the particular study, these nurses were able to critically appraise the results.

When the consumer of research reads the literature review section of the research report, there are a number of concerns to be addressed. It is not sufficient merely to state the results of studies that agree with the basic premises of the investigator. If research is available that contradicts these premises, that information too must be included. It is also not sufficient to present the findings of prior research without describing some of the major components of the investigations, such as sample size, research design, and method of data collection.

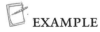 EXAMPLE

Secondary Search of the Literature

Following an initial search of the literature, two psychiatric nurses decide to evaluate the effectiveness of a behavior modification program on bulimic behavior (an eating disorder) among senior high school students. They identify 10 relevant research reports (e.g., "The Interaction between Exercise and Eating Disorders among 30 College Students"); 15 expert opinion articles (e.g., "Bulimia: A Feminist Concern"); and four books (e.g., *The Aftermath of an Eating Disorder*). All information gathered is subjected to an evaluation using clearly identified criteria.

PRACTICE

Secondary Search of the Literature

Select an area of interest and collect five research reports, five expert opinion articles, and two books related to the topic. Evaluate these works on the basis of common sense, experience, and logic.

CRITICAL APPRAISAL

The Literature Review

- Has an in-depth review been conducted (how many publications)?

- Has an evaluation of the prior research been presented along with the results?

- Are the criteria for evaluating each publication clearly identified?

- How recent are the identified publications?

- Have primary sources been used?

Identifying Publications

The two major methods for identifying publications are performing a computer search and examining books and periodicals one at a time (see Figure 4.1). Although a computer search

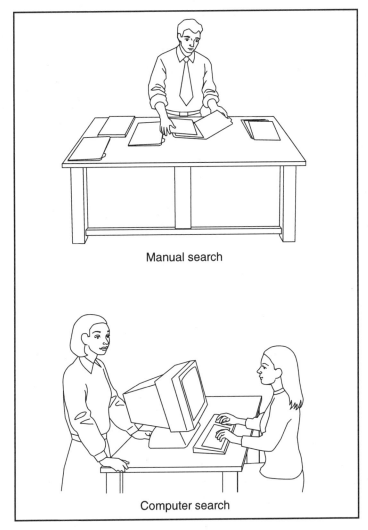

Manual search

Computer search

FIGURE 4.1 Two ways to identify publications

is a rapid method for discovering relevant information, the manual examination of books and periodicals is probably more thorough. A combination of the two methods can be fast and at the same time comprehensive.

A Computer Search

There are a number of computer-based searches of the litera-ture that are appropriate to health care research. MEDLARS

145

(Medical Literature Analysis and Retrieval System) provides access to innumerable journals located in the National Library of Medicine in Bethesda, Maryland. The computer search provides the investigator with a list of references, and sometimes additional information in the form of abstracts that relate to the topic under study. There are various databases located within MEDLARS that can assist the investigator in retrieving desired information. MEDLINE (MEDLARS Online) provides references to the biomedical journal literature and is probably the best known of these databases. *International Nursing Index* and *Index Medicus* are included in MEDLINE. CINAHL (*Cumulative Index to Nursing and Allied Health Literature*) is another database that is frequently used by nurses. CINAHL focuses more on nursing references than MEDLINE, but citations are available only since 1983, whereas citations within MEDLINE are available going back to 1966 (National Library of Medicine, 1985).

When conducting a *computerized* literature search, the investigator or clinician can work with a librarian or directly access a database. In either case, certain kinds of information are necessary to conduct a successful computerized literature search. Necessary information includes a clear and specific description of the topic, the names of authors who have written on that topic, and alternative terms that may be used to describe various concepts of interest.

Although computer searches of the literature are quick and relatively easy to perform, not all journals are available on databases and important information may be missed. A combination of a manual search and a computerized search will probably provide the most comprehensive coverage of a given topic.

Specifying an area of interest when conducting a computer search results in a list of articles and reports that will probably be more useful than if a broad concept is entered. For example, there are thousands of databased articles on the topic of pain. If the investigator is interested in acute rather than chronic pain and enters both "acute" and "pain," the number of articles gained from the search will be substantially diminished, thus saving considerable time and effort. Although computer searches can be accomplished by entering minimal information, the most effective searches include specific information regarding the topic, authors who have written on the topic, and terms that are acceptable to the specific database in use.

WORKING DEFINITION

A Computerized Search of the Literature

A computerized search of the literature involves the use of a computer to examine journals related to a specific topic in order to better understand an area of interest.

EXAMPLE

A Computerized Search of the Literature

Two nurse researchers design a study to examine nurses' use of visual analogue scales to assess acute and chronic cancer pain. They decide to conduct a computer search using MEDLARS and request access to the MEDLINE database (which contains biomedical journal articles). They provide the librarian conducting the search with the following information:

Topic: The management of acute and chronic cancer pain

Journal(s): Journal of Pain and Symptom Management

     Pain

     Pain Management Nursing

Author(s): Brockopp, Ferrell, Miaskowski

From this information, a skilled librarian can help the investigator develop other words, phrases, authors, and publications that will assist with the search.

PRACTICE

A Computerized Search of the Literature

Choose a topic of interest and identify the information necessary to conduct a computer search: *Title of Search* (using terms necessary for the appropriate database), *Suggested Journals*, and *Suggested Authors*.

A Manual Search

A manual search for information related to a given topic of interest requires the investigator to have an intimate knowledge of the workings of the library. Libraries have mechanisms (card catalogs, computers) for finding any publication in the library. Publications can be located by either author or subject.

In addition to the general holdings within the library, there are various mechanisms for finding specific categories of information. A variety of indexes such as *The Cumulative Index to Nursing Literature* and the *Index Medicus* list authors and subjects that may be useful to the nurse researcher. Abstracts—that is, brief descriptions of articles giving the author, title, and main ideas—are also available. Psychological abstracts and sociological abstracts are two examples that may be helpful.

As articles are located, the investigator can examine the references used and identify additional publications that may be relevant. The manual search, although time-consuming, can yield much that is pertinent to the area of investigation. Scanning individual articles for leads within the text as well as the reference list can produce information that may not be located in a computer search.

WORKING DEFINITION

A Manual Search of the Literature

A manual search of the literature requires the investigator to examine each of the mechanisms in the library—card catalog, indexes, and abstracts—for references relevant to the topic of interest.

 EXAMPLE

A Manual Search of the Literature

A nurse researcher and an epidemiologist decide to investigate the small proportion of clients who suffer negative side effects from DPT (diphtheria, pertussis, tetanus) immunization. The investigators begin with the card catalog, looking under the headings *DPT* and *immunization*. They move from there to all indexes related to health care. Because they find little related to their topic, they also check the psychological and sociological abstracts.

 PRACTICE

A Manual Search of the Literature

Choose a topic of interest and identify three relevant publications from the card catalog, three from an index, and three from a collection of abstracts.

Keeping a Record

As the investigator collects articles that are relevant to the topic for study, it is necessary to establish a systematic method for recording pertinent information. Although there are undoubtedly many methods for recording the data obtained, a frequent suggestion is that each article be entered separately on a card. Such information as author's name, date of publication, title of article, name of the journal or book, and library call number is often included. If a large card (4 × 6 or 5 × 7 inches) is used, a summary of the article and an evaluation of the content is possible (see Figure 4.2). The cards can be kept

Author's name: Black, J. Jones, R.	Title: Palliative Care: Reality or Delusion
Publication date: January 2001	
Journal: Health Science & Nursing	
Book: _____	Call number: _____
DESCRIPTION:	EVALUATION: (1) clear- (5) confused
Problem statement or topic: What proportion of dying patients receive palliative rather than curative care?	(3) Definition of dying unclear, population also unclear.
Conceptual framework:	No framework specified.
Hypotheses: (if applicable)	(4) A major portion (50%) of dying patients receive curative rather than palliative care.
Method of research: (if applicable)	(2) 300 patients from 5 large urban hospitals given less than 6 months to live examined in relation to medical and nursing care—convenience sample.
Instruments used: (if applicable)	(3) Questionaire devised for this study to evaluate care given is of questionable reliability, validity.
Data analysis: (if applicable)	(1) Dichotomous scores on questionnaires (palliation versus cure) tallied.
Findings or summary:	(1) 30% of patients received palliative care versus curative care.

FIGURE 4.2 Keeping a record

in alphabetical order by author or title for ease of use. For those individuals who have access to a computer, the same material can be entered into a computer.

Using the format depicted in Figure 4.2, an expert opinion article as well as a research report can be described and evaluated.

150

PRACTICE

Keeping a Record

Select an article related to a topic of interest, and, using the format depicted in Figure 4.2, briefly describe and evaluate its content. The following clues may be of some assistance.

Clues to Keeping a Record

- Organize entries alphabetically.

- Identify the author, title of article, journal or book title, call number, and date of publication.

- Identify the following components of the article: problem statement or topic, conceptual framework, hypotheses, methods, instruments, data analyses, and findings or summary.

Writing the Review of the Literature

The review of the literature sets the stage for the remainder of the article. It should be comprehensive and yet succinct and must reflect all sides of an issue. It must show how the evidence cited supports the conclusions reached. Expert opinion needs to be separated from research findings, and studies need to be clearly described.

For example, if nurse investigators want to examine the effect of patient teaching on patients labeled hypertensive, they need to address various viewpoints found in the literature. Descriptions of clinical opinion and research that both support the investigators' notions and contradict them must be included. If some evidence is supported by a thorough investigation on 100 subjects and other claims are supported by a less than systematic approach, the differences in methods used must be identified.

When writing the review of literature for a research report, decisions must be made regarding the studies that will be described. If considerable research exists on a given topic, only those studies that are most relevant to the investigation are included. If little research is available in an area, studies that have been conducted are reported in some detail.

Those studies that support the notions underlying the investigation should be described so that readers understand how confident they can be in the conclusions drawn. For example, Morris (2001) studied the relationship between spirituality and coronary heart disease. Morris refers to a study by Ornish and colleagues (1990) in his literature review as support for his research. It would be important for anyone interested in studying this area to become familiar with the Ornish study. This practice is particularly true when the area under investigation does not have a strong foundation in research.

Well-written reviews of literature include evaluative statements regarding the studies described. Comments about sample size, instruments used, research design, and other components of the research process can help the reader to better understand the value of the results of the investigations.

The written review of literature provides the reader with a context for the description of the study that follows. That context influences the nature of the study. This portion of the research report is therefore a basic and extremely important component of the research process.

WORKING DEFINITION

Review of the Literature

A review of the literature is a comprehensive description as well as an evaluation of the evidence related to a given topic.

EXAMPLE

Review of the Literature

Conflicting or confusing results often emerge from a literature review of a specific area of concern. For example, Todd, Samaroo, and Hoffman (1993) found that Hispanics were twice as likely as non-Hispanic whites to receive no pain medication in the emergency department. A follow-up study (Todd, Deaton, Adamo & Poe, 2000) showed no difference between Hispanics and non-Hispanic whites related to estimates of pain severity by the patients themselves and by physicians. From an examination of these two studies it is unclear as to whether there was bias on the part of physicians in the first study or Hispanics did not rate their pain as high as their white counterparts and, for that reason, did not receive similar doses of pain medication.

This example of a portion of a literature review related to bias and the management of pain shows how confusing or conflicting results can be discussed. The investigators from both studies were trying to determine whether racial bias influences patient care. Although the first study points in the direction of racial bias, the second study raises questions regarding that assumption. It is important to include both perspectives in the review of the literature.

 PRACTICE

Review of the Literature

Select a topic area and write a brief review of the literature using two studies that offer conflicting results.

 CRITICAL APPRAISAL

A Well-Written Review of the Literature

- Is the literature review comprehensive?

- Are all sides of the issue presented?

- Has the methodology of the studies been presented in the description?

153

- Has the evidence presented been evaluated in relation to design and method?

Critical Overview of the Review of the Literature

A group of nursing students are asked to evaluate the literature on a topic of clinical interest. They have not as yet learned all of the steps involved in the research process; therefore, they must examine the literature from a logical perspective. They choose the topic of bonding and select three articles to examine. They design the following chart to assist them in examining the literature.

CRITICAL OVERVIEW
THE REVIEW OF THE LITERATURE

Article 1: "Bonding Following a Normal Pregnancy in Mothers over Age 40," Brown, J. & Smith, A. (2001). Maternal Health Journal, 3(2):116–120.

1. Conceptual model—Maslow
2. Definition of concept—Bonding: The process of establishing a loving relationship between mother and newborn.
3. Focus of article (question addressed—To what degree do women over age 40 bond with their newborns?
4. Population studied—Fifty women over age 40 who gave birth in a large urban general hospital.
5. Means of measurement—A 10-item paper-and-pencil questionnaire measuring a mother-infant relationship.

6. Conclusion—The 50 women were divided as to educational level, income level, and number of children. Women with high educational and income levels with fewer than two children had a higher bonding score than women with low educational and income levels.

Article 2: "Encouraging Bonding in the Neonatal Unit," Jones, A. (2002). Neonatal Nursing, 4(8):98–201.

1. Conceptual model—Maslow
2. Definition of concept—The development of a close, loving relationship between mother and child during the first two weeks of life.
3. Focus of article (question addressed)—The experience of a neonatal nurse and her attempts to facilitate bonding between mothers and their preterm infants.
4. Population addressed—Mothers and their preterm infants in a large urban maternity hospital over a 10-year period.
5. Means of measurement—Personal observation.
6. Conclusion—The nurse is instrumental in providing reassurance as well as information to mothers of preterm infants and thereby facilitating the bonding process.

Article 3: "Bonding: Is It an Issue for the Working Mother?" Wells, S. (2002). Mother Child Health, 5(7):57–62.

1. Conceptual model—Maslow
2. Definition of concept—The development of a loving relationship between mother and child during the first month of life.
3. Focus of article (question addressed)—Do women who plan to return to work within two months after the birth of a child bond as successfully as those women who do not plan to return to work for six months?

4. Population addressed—A total of 120 women, 65 planning to return to work two months after childbirth, 55 planning to return after six months. Age range, 26–37.

5. Means of measurement—Each woman was interviewed using a predetermined format. Scores based on interviews.

6. Conclusion—There was no significant difference between the two groups of women.

Comparison of Three Articles on Bonding

1. Conceptual model—Each of the articles made reference to Maslow and used his assumptions on the hierarchy of need to frame the issue of bonding between mother and child.

2. Definition of concept—Definitions of bonding varied in terms of the length of time the process was expected to take.

3. Focus of article (question addressed)—Each article examined bonding from a different perspective: after age 40; how to facilitate the process in a neonatal unit; and how bonding can be affected when a woman plans to return to work.

4. Populations addressed—Three different populations were involved: women over 40, working women, and mothers of preterm infants.

5. Means of measurement—Three different measurement strategies were used: one paper-and-pencil test, one structured interview, and one personal observation.

6. Conclusion—
   • Perhaps lower levels of stress, as represented by higher income, higher educational level, and fewer other children, enhance the possibility for bonding.

- A nurse may be able to facilitate the process by providing information and reassurance.

- Planning to return to work after two months versus six months in and of itself does not seem to have an effect on the process. There are probably many variables involved in this complex concept.

Activity

Choose a topic of interest. Select four articles on one of the major concepts within the topic and complete a chart similar to the one depicted in the critical overview.

References

Alsop-Shields, L. & Mohay, H. (2001). John Bowlby and James Robertson: Theorists, scientists and crusaders for improvements in the care of children in hospital. *Journal of Advanced Nursing, 35*(1):50–58.

Freud, S. (1910). *The origin and development of psychoanalysis.* Toronto: Encyclopedia Britannica, Inc.

Morris, E. L. (2001). The relationship of spirituality to coronary heart disease. *Alternative Therapies, 7*(5):96–98.

National Library of Medicine. (1985). *The basics of searching MEDLINE: A guide for the health professional.* Bethesda, MD: Author.

Ornish, D., Brown, S., & Scherwitz, L. W. (1990). Can lifestyle changes reverse coronary heart disease? *Lancet, 336*(8708):129–133.

Polit, D. & Hungler, B. (1999). *Nursing Research Principles and Methods.* New York: Lippincott.

Todd, K. H., Deaton, C., Adamo, A., & Poe, L. (2001). Ethnicity and analgesic practice. *Annals of Emergency Medicine, 35*:11–16.

Todd, K. H., Samaroo, N., & Hoffman, J. R. (1993). Ethnicity as a risk factor for inadequate emergency department analgesia. *Journal of the American Medical Association, 269*:1537–1539.

5

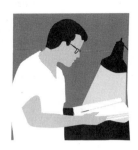

Protecting Research Participants

Goals

- *Describe the process of protecting research participants.*
- *Examine potential risks for research participants.*
- *Describe guidelines developed to protect research participants.*
- *Identify the role of research committees in safeguarding the rights of the research participant.*

Introduction

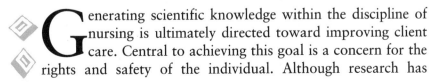

Generating scientific knowledge within the discipline of nursing is ultimately directed toward improving client care. Central to achieving this goal is a concern for the rights and safety of the individual. Although research has undoubtedly produced significant health care benefits, potential and actual risks exist for those who volunteer as research participants. It is important for nurses to be able to distinguish between research designed to protect the individuals' rights and research that may violate the rights of research participants.

This chapter examines those areas of a research project that are relevant to the protection of research participants. These areas include guidelines that have been developed to assist in the protection of participants, an examination of informed consent, the individual's right to anonymity, the issue of confidentiality, withdrawal from a study, dealing with deception, debriefing procedures, the role of research review committees, and the process of submitting a proposal to a review committee. An examination of each of these areas is crucial to ensuring that the individual is protected from harm while participating in a research project. Whether directly or indirectly involved in research, the nurse has a professional responsibility to protect the rights of all research participants and to speak out when violations become apparent.

Guidelines for Conducting Research

Research is concerned with answering questions. In a discipline like nursing, where people and their health experience are the primary focus, the interest in research lies in generating information that can ultimately be applied to the clinical situation. In the struggle to conduct a research study, the researcher may be tempted to contemplate shortcuts that would speed up the research project. Pressures to finish the project quickly can arise from both external and internal sources. Funding deadlines, academic deadlines (if the study is in fulfillment of degree requirements), and tardiness on the part of co-researchers are but a few of the external pressures. Internal sources of pressure include personal expectations for completion, as well as the researcher's past experience in conducting research.

Shortcuts in the research process can sometimes unintentionally affect the wellbeing of the individuals who participate in the research project. Because nursing deals almost exclusively with human participants in conducting research, there is an ongoing concern that individuals be protected from any harmful effects that might result from their participation. Adequate protection of research participants may require a delay in the proposed schedule or a change in the completed research design. In either case, such changes are necessary if the safety of the human participants is involved.

Guidelines for conducting research have been developed after careful consideration of past innocuous, as well as blatant, abuses of research participants. In an effort to "advance science," countless incidents of individual abuse have been recorded. Administering hallucinogenic drugs to unknowing individuals to determine human response, withholding treatment of syphilis to learn more about the untreated disease, administering live cancer cells to elderly infirm patients, engaging alcoholics in a study that claimed to use behavioral modification to rehabilitate subjects so that they could "drink socially," injecting individuals with radioactive material in the 1950s and 1960s, and the horrifying Nazi atrocities, many performed under the guise of "medical experimentation," are but a few of the more highly publicized violations that have occurred in recent times. Apart from these, however, many more subtle and less well known abuses have been identified.

Professional Guidelines

Although the advancement of nursing knowledge is crucial to the development of the profession, it should never be held in higher regard than the rights of the individual. Many disciplines have attempted to develop guidelines to ensure the protection of research participants when members of the profession are conducting research. The basic documents that have been used to develop guidelines within the nursing profession are based on two historical papers: the Nuremberg Code of 1947 and the Helsinki Declaration of 1964 (revised in 1975).

The Nuremberg Code (Articles) was developed in response to the Nazi war crimes in order to outline a basic set of standards for judging the physicians and scientists who had conducted biomedical experiments on concentration camp prisoners. These standards were then applied to the cases brought to trial regarding the sadistic experiments conducted by Nazi physicians and scientists under the guise of medical research and scientific advancement. This document identifies the inalienable rights of human research participants.

The Helsinki Declaration was drafted in an effort to establish clinical research guidelines for physicians. The crux of this document centered on the need for individuals to be informed when their participation in a particular research project might be harmful to them or at least of little direct benefit.

These two documents have served as the prototype for the development of codes for the conduct of research in several disciplines, including nursing. The codes, which consist of "rules" that are intended to guide the researcher in carrying out research, are helpful to those who are responsible for reviewing the research work of others. The American Nurses Association (1985) has produced a publication titled *Human Rights Guidelines for Nurses in Clinical and Other Research*. This document focuses on the human rights of health care recipients, the rights of persons who are involved in research within the health care arena, and the responsibility of the nurse in providing care where research investigations impinge on health care. Adhering to these guidelines minimizes the likelihood that the rights of research participants might be violated. Figure 5.1 summarizes key points addressed in the document.

Federal Guidelines

The federal government has also established guidelines and policies related to how certain research protocols must be conducted, as well as regulations to be followed in using research participants (DHEW, 1978; DHHS, 1981). Abusive research methods in past studies have led to federal government participation in many research projects conducted in the United States. Federal participation can range from involvement in the design of the research study to approval or denial of funding.

Conducting a research investigation can be a costly undertaking. Many researchers seek federal funding for assistance in scientific endeavors. In addition, many agencies (academic institutions, extended care facilities, hospitals, etc.) receive fed-

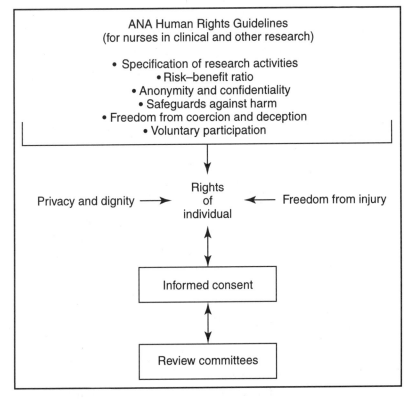

FIGURE 5.1 ANA human rights guidelines. (*Source:*
"Human Rights Guidelines for Nurses in Clinical and Other Research" by
American Nurses Association. Copyright © 1985 by American Nurses
Association. Reprinted by permission.)

eral funds in one form or another. Any researcher who is seeking direct federal research funding or who is associated with
an agency receiving federal monies must comply with federal
research guidelines, in addition to guidelines established within
the profession. The monitoring of the project to ensure compliance with federal guidelines is usually done by an **institutional review board (IRB)**.

An IRB is composed of representatives from the professional
groups providing health care at a facility. The committee meets
to provide a review of all proposed research investigations.
The primary concern of the board is to make a determination

163

regarding the adequacy of human participant protection and to ensure that informed consent will be obtained, that adequate follow-up of research participants will be conducted, and that sufficient documentation of the process will be produced.

 WORKING DEFINITION

Institutional Review Board (IRB)

The IRB is a committee established by each agency (institution) for the express purpose of evaluating all research conducted in that facility. The IRB is concerned with the protection of human rights and evaluates research proposals in accordance with federal guidelines.

Research Participants at Risk

A basic responsibility of the individual researcher, as well as review committees and those assisting in carrying out the project, is to protect all research participants from harm while they are participating in an investigation or as a result of the study. The researcher makes every effort to protect research participants by carefully identifying all possible risks for harm as well as any benefits that may be incurred by individuals during the course of the study. This is often referred to as the **risk–benefit ratio** and should include a determination of all the obvious and not-so-obvious risks and benefits.

Risks and benefits from participating in a research project may involve physical, emotional, spiritual, economic, social, or legal aspects (Figure 5.2). Benefits may include monetary gain, access to a treatment not otherwise available, increased knowledge about their situation or condition, or something as simple as increased attention or meals. Risks may include untoward side effects from a treatment, time required to participate, financial cost (e.g., babysitters, transportation, meals), or distress from dealing with potentially sensitive or personal issues. Research review committees are particularly concerned that

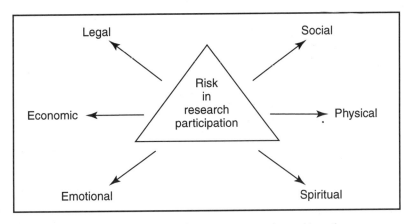

FIGURE 5.2 Research participants: Risks and benefits

the risks of research be minimized whenever possible. When the risks far outweigh the benefits and the study has limited merit, the researcher should reconsider the project. This may mean totally redesigning the project, making significant alterations, or dropping the project altogether.

 WORKING DEFINITION

Research Participants at Risk

Research participants at risk are individuals who may be harmed physically, emotionally, spiritually, economically, socially, or legally through participation in a research study.

Although protection of all research participants is of concern, some individuals are inherently at higher risk by virtue of circumstances, their particular health problems, or their developmental level. Whether the nurse is involved in research as the principal investigator, involved as an assistant in carrying out the research design, or not directly involved but caring for a research participant, careful attention should be paid to the protection of the rights of the individual.

165

PRACTICE

Research Participants at Risk

For each of the following areas of risk, identify one example of how a participant in a research project could be harmed:

- Physical
- Economic
- Emotional
- Social
- Spiritual
- Legal

Individuals who are limited in their capacity to enter freely into a study with full understanding of the possible consequences are at higher risk, and the nurse needs to be particularly vigilant about protecting their rights. Prisoners, children, the elderly, those with emotional or cognitive deficits, students, and hospitalized patients are examples of particularly vulnerable individuals in a research situation (Figure 5.3). These individuals may be coerced into participating in a study or may agree to participate because they lack the ability to make a clear and free decision.

PRACTICE

Vulnerable Populations

Identify three groups of individuals who would be at increased physical, emotional, spiritual, economic, social, or legal risk. Describe possible reasons why they might choose to participate in a research study.

EXAMPLE

Vulnerable group: Members of the armed forces.

Reasons for participation: Fear of reprisal from those in authority, desire for preferential treatment or favors, need for compensation (if offered).

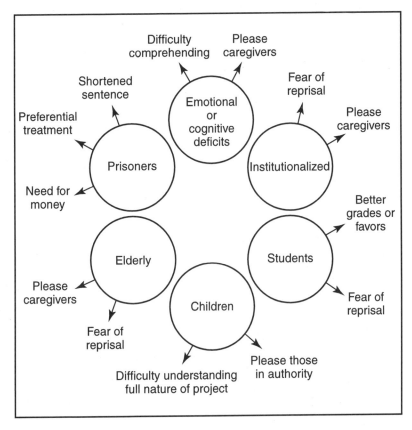

FIGURE 5.3 Vulnerable populations: Why they participate

Although it is sometimes necessary and desirable to study vulnerable populations, the responsible researcher uses participants who are not at increased risk of harm whenever possible. Responsible researchers do not choose a vulnerable population to study simply because its members are easily manipulated or readily available. When studying vulnerable populations, the researcher may have to devise additional safeguards to ensure adequate protection for the individuals. For example, a faculty member could protect a group of students under study by engaging a research associate who was neither an instructor of those students nor in any other manner influential with them to give information about the study to the students and enlist their consent to participate. Similarly, if a researcher wanted to study women in active labor, participants should be solicited

167

prior to labor, when their ability to weigh risks versus benefits is not impaired by undue pressure and stress. In any event, the research safeguards should be fully addressed and discussed in the development of the project, and the IRB should approve the final research plan.

CRITICAL APPRAISAL

Research Participants at Risk

- Has the researcher identified the necessity for using a population that is at increased risk (or vulnerability) for harm or injury?

- Could the researcher have used a less vulnerable population and still have gained the same knowledge?

- Does the researcher clearly describe the type of risk or harm to which the participant is particularly vulnerable?

- Have emotional, physical, spiritual, economic, social, and legal risks been assessed?

Informed Consent

One of the fundamental responsibilities that the investigator has to human research participants is to ensure that each individual understands the nature of the research project and the implications of participation and that the individual is able to decide freely whether to participate in the project, without fear of reprisal. The idea that individuals have the right to decide their destiny and control their own activities is referred to as the principle of **self-determination.** Self-determination is central to the process of **informed consent,** which seeks to clarify the individuals' understanding of the project and to obtain their freely given consent to participate (Commission for the

Protection of Human Subjects for Biomedical and Behavioral Research, 1978).

Informed consent is the researcher's conscious and deliberate attempt to clearly and fully provide the potential participant with information about the study. After participants have been given the necessary information about the project, they can decide whether to become involved in the research. Together the researcher and the participant can reach an agreement about the rights and responsibilities of each during the investigation.

 WORKING DEFINITION

Informed Consent

Informed consent is the process of providing an individual with sufficient understandable information regarding his or her participation in a research project. It includes providing potential participants with information about their rights and responsibilities within the project and documenting the nature of the agreement.

Informed consent may be obtained by allowing individuals to read materials and make a decision on the basis of their understanding of what they have read or by discussing the proposed research project with the researcher or research assistant. The advantages of discussion are obvious. Personal contact allows the material to be presented at a level and rate best suited to the individual's needs and situation. A discussion also permits immediate feedback in response to the concerns of the individual regarding the study. Nurses can possess considerable power over populations that may be vulnerable because of their health care needs. Nurses have a responsibility, therefore, to ensure that potential research participants are given the information in a manner facilitating maximum understanding.

In addition to presenting information in a written or verbal form, taping devices may be used. An audio or video tape recording may be used to present the information about the study to the individual. Regardless of the method used, the agreement reached between researcher and participant must be documented. The method to be used should be selected after careful consideration of the potential research participants' cognitive abilities and developmental level, the best way to present the information, and the size of the sample required.

The information that should be conveyed to potential research participants when seeking informed consent includes the following:

- A clear description of the purpose of the document, discussion, or tape (i.e., seeking informed consent)
- The title of the research project
- The researcher's title and position
- The purpose of the project
- What population is under study and why it was selected
- What will be happening to the participant during the research project
- A description of any changes in usual health care procedures or daily activities that may occur as a result of participation in the project
- Possible risks of participating in the study
- What financial compensation (if any) participants can expect and when they would receive it
- What benefits (other than financial) are available to participants (counseling, treatments, etc.)
- How the data will be handled to ensure individual anonymity and confidentiality
- The voluntary nature of participation; for example, individuals may withdraw at any time without reprisal
- The name of the contact person, in case participants should need to talk to someone regarding their participation

- A clearly delineated area for the signatures of both researcher and research participant

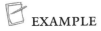

EXAMPLE

Consent Form

Study to Determine Fathers' Experience of Pregnancy

This is to verify that I have been informed about a study concerning how <u>first-time fathers experience the pregnancies of their spouses. Pat Arbot, Ph.D., R.N., nurse researcher at the parent-child nursing clinic,</u> explained that my participation is <u>voluntary</u> and that I may <u>withdraw</u> at any time without jeopardy to myself or family.

Dr. Arbot has discussed with me the nature of the study, informing me that there are <u>no known risks</u> in participating. There are <u>no known benefits</u> either, and it is unlikely that I will experience any direct benefit. However, the information the study produces may be of assistance in helping other fathers cope with the pregnancies of their spouses.

I will receive <u>no financial compensation</u> for my participation; however, discussions with the researcher may help me to better understand my feelings about the experience of pregnancy.

My <u>participation will mean</u> that I will need to meet with Dr. Arbot for two 30-minute interviews, and complete three paper-and-pencil tests. My <u>name will not appear</u> on materials—only a code number will identify me as a participant in the study. All information I share with Dr. Arbot will be kept <u>confidential</u>.

- TITLE

- PURPOSE
- STUDY POPULATION
- RESEARCHER's QUALIFICATIONS
- VOLUNTARY NATURE AND WITHDRAWAL RIGHTS

- RISKS
- BENEFITS

- COMPENSATION

- WHAT WILL HAPPEN IN THE STUDY

- ANONYMITY

- CONFIDENTIALITY

I have been given a copy of the summary of this agreement for my review. If I have any further questions, <u>I may contact Dr. Arbot at 555-0000, ext. 123</u>.

• CONTACT PERSON

I will receive information about the results of my participation in the study either by phone or by mail at the conclusion of the project.

• DEBRIEFING

_____

PARTICIPANT'S SIGNATURE   DATE

• DATED SIGNATURE OF
  RESEARCH PARTICIPANT
  AND RESEARCHER

_____

RESEARCHER'S SIGNATURE   DATE

Individuals involved in a research project should receive a copy of a document that has been signed by both parties and signifies that informed consent has been obtained. Additional information describing key points relating to the research (a checklist or summary) can be given to participants so that they may review the information at will.

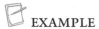

EXAMPLE

Checklist

Study to Determine Fathers' Experience of Pregnancy

❑ Study of first-time fathers' experiences of their spouse's pregnancy.

❑ Pat Arbot, Ph.D., R.N., is the nurse researcher.

❑ Voluntary participation.

❑ Participants may withdraw at any time without jeopardy.

❑ No known risks in participating.

❑ No direct benefits to the participant, but may help nurses to better assist other fathers to cope with their spouses' pregnancies.

❏ Participation involves two 30-minute interviews with Dr. Arbot and the completion of three paper-and-pencil tests.

❏ The name of the research participant will not appear on any materials (anonymity); a code number will be used to identify a participant's materials.

❏ All information shared with Dr. Arbot will be kept confidential.

❏ No financial compensation will be given; however, participants may better understand their feelings about their spouse's pregnancy as a result of their participation.

❏ If there are further questions, Dr. Arbot may be reached at 555-0000 ext. 123.

❏ Results of the study will be given to research participants either by phone or by mail.

❏ Signature indicating agreement.

 EXAMPLE

Summary Sheet

Study to Determine Fathers' Experience of Pregnancy

• A study of first-time fathers' experiences of their spouse's pregnancy.

• Participation involves two 30-minute interviews with the researcher and the completion of three paper-and-pencil tests.

• Participation is voluntary and without known risks or benefits to participants, although other fathers may be helped to cope better with their spouses' pregnancies. Individuals may withdraw at any time without fear of reprisal or jeopardy.

• No financial compensation will be given; however, participants may better understand their feelings about their spouse's pregnancy as a result of their participation.

- Results of the study will be fully discussed with each participant after completion of the study. This will be done either by phone or by mail.

- The researcher, Pat Arbot, Ph.D., R.N., is a nurse researcher at the parent-child nursing clinic and may be reached at 555-0000 ext. 123 if there are any further questions. Dr. Arbot will keep all information confidential, and every research participant will remain anonymous, identified only by a code number.

Some potential research participants may be unwilling or unable to sign a form documenting that they are giving informed consent for their participation in the project. Some individuals, for example the elderly, may be wary of signing forms, and others, such as small children and individuals who have certain physical handicaps, may be unable to sign. The researcher needs to decide regarding informed consent whether or not the individual has given permission to be involved and what is the best way for permission to be documented. For example, in cases where individuals cannot write, a tape-recorded consent may be obtained. In the case of a child, the parent or legal guardian can sign a document.

Legally, children (all minors under 18 years of age) are not considered competent to provide informed consent (Langer, 1985; Siantz, 1988). However, when children are involved in research the researcher should obtain both informed consent of the parent/legal guardian and assent of the child, when possible. "Assent" means a child's affirmative agreement to participate in the research protocol. Failure of the child to object cannot be construed as assent.

 PRACTICE

Obtaining Informed Consent

Survey back issues of *Nursing Research* and identify two studies that utilize research participants unable to give written informed consent. Describe how the researcher obtained informed consent and the extent to which the participants participated in the decision.

CRITICAL APPRAISAL

Informed Consent

- Does the researcher indicate whether informed consent was obtained?

- Does the researcher outline how informed consent was obtained?

- Is the method used to obtain informed consent appropriate for the developmental and situational needs of the participant?

Confidentiality and Anonymity

Individuals who agree to participate in research have a right to expect that the information collected from or about them will remain private. It is the researcher's responsibility to devise a method for ensuring that **confidentiality** is maintained.

WORKING DEFINITION

Confidentiality

Confidentiality refers to the researcher's responsibility to protect all data gathered within the scope of the project from being divulged to others.

Mechanisms used to protect the data that are collected in a research study include using a locked file, limiting access to the data to those individuals who are intimately involved in the research, and destroying the list of participant names at the conclusion of the project.

Responsibility in maintaining confidentiality is very important. Researchers must understand and provide confidentiality, especially when the topic under study is sensitive, deals with a vulnerable population, involves participants that others are likely to be interested in, or involves an area of investigation where traditional efforts to maintain confidentiality have been inadequate. To help provide additional protection, a *certificate of confidentiality* has been develop by the Department of Health and Human Services (DHHS) (Dunn & Chadwick, 1999). The certificate is issued to researchers to protect against compelled identification of scientific research participants. The certificate, however, does not provide exemption from certain mandatory reporting laws, such as instances of child abuse.

Anonymity is another essential concept related to protection of participants in research. Participants have the right to remain anonymous throughout the research project. Information related to participants or to the fact that certain individuals have participated in a study should not be available to anyone beyond the immediate research team. At the conclusion of the study, any means for identifying particular research participants should be destroyed.

 WORKING DEFINITION

Anonymity

Anonymity refers to the act of keeping individuals nameless in relation to their participation in a research project.

Mechanisms used to ensure participant anonymity include keeping the master list of participant names and matching code numbers in separate locations, under lock and key, after providing each participant with a number or code name; destroying the list of actual names; and using code names when discussing data. Figure 5.4 provides an example of how both anonymity and confidentiality could be maintained.

Research designed so that data are collected at one point in time presents few problems in terms of anonymity. When data are collected at one sitting, the use of names is unnecessary. By contrast, research that is designed to compare individual per-

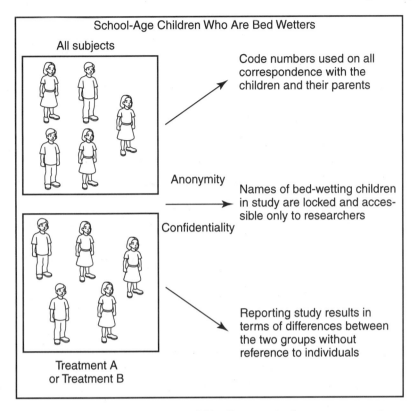

FIGURE 5.4   An investigation of the effectiveness of a new treatment for bedwetting

formance over time presents a challenge in relation to ensuring participant anonymity. For example, a nurse researcher may want to study a new teaching method designed to facilitate the practice of breast self-examination. The researcher may need to make a list of participants so that they may be contacted at a later date to ascertain the success of the teaching method. Having a list of names in this instance would be necessary for follow-up but poses increased potential for the violation of the individual's right to anonymity.

One method that has been suggested as a means of protecting anonymity and confidentiality is to have the participants generate their own identification code (Damrosch, 1986). The researcher never records the participant's name; rather, the

177

participant's code is obtained. This method allows the researcher to connect sets of data with any given participant who has responded, while allowing only the individual participant to know the name represented by the code number.

EXAMPLE

Subject-Generated Identification Codes

A nurse researcher is conducting a study to determine nursing students' attitudes toward abortion before and after clinical experience on the abortion unit. The nurse researcher wants to maintain anonymity for the students but needs to conduct a pretest and posttest. To analyze the data, the two test scores must be related to each participant.

To protect participant anonymity, the nurse researcher asks each student to generate her or his own user-specific code number at the time of the pretest. Based on the researcher's instructions regarding the code format, one participant generated the following code number:

Participant's middle initial	R
Mother's middle initial	M
Gender (M= male; F = female)	F
Month of birth	May
Number of older sisters	3
Number of younger brothers	0

In this example, the subject-generated identification number is *RMFMAY30*. At the time of the posttest, the participant would be asked to recall the same data. Thus the researcher could link this participant's two test scores for analysis without ever having recorded the participant's name.

Each participant in a research study should be told verbally or in writing of the right to anonymity and confidentiality and informed on how the investigator will ensure that both are maintained. Anonymity and confidentiality are important not only during the process of investigation but also when results are presented and perhaps published.

EXAMPLE

Protecting Anonymity and Confidentiality

The researcher might say the following: "This study will take every precaution to protect your right to privacy. Your name will not be used directly on any materials. Only a code number will identify you as a participant. A list that matches code numbers and names will be kept in a separate, locked location, accessible only to the researcher. Your name will not be used in the reporting and publishing of the results of the study. The report will discuss only the findings as they relate to all participants or in a general way. All information you share with the researcher will remain confidential."

EXAMPLE

Protecting Anonymity and Confidentiality

The researcher might write the following in the consent form: "All information collected that pertains to my participation in the research project will be identified by my code number, not by my name, and the researcher will keep my name separate from the responses I give. The list that matches my name with my assigned code number will be kept separately, under lock and key. When reporting the results of this study my privacy will be further protected by the reporting of aggregate (group) data only."

In the presentation of findings, the researcher must remember to camouflage the individual participant's identity. Certain descriptors applied to participants in a study could suggest the identity of particular individuals. For example, nurse researchers might study a group of fathers who are expecting

179

the birth of their first child. If in reporting the results of the study, they described the occupations of each of the participants and one of them was identified as a new state senator, anonymity would have been breached.

 PRACTICE

Protecting Anonymity

Select one of the following groups of participants that might be used in conducting a research study. Write a statement that could be used to describe that particular group in presenting the results of the research.

- 22-year-old persons with AIDS

- Single parents in a support group

- Adolescents who frequent video arcades

- Women over 65 with a rare blood disorder

- Hmong immigrants in a southwestern rural community

Example

Study population: Farmers who have experienced bankruptcy.

Description of participants: Participants were a group of farmers from a Midwestern state who had experienced bankruptcy between two and six months ago.

 CRITICAL APPRAISAL

Anonymity and Confidentiality

- Has the researcher informed participants of their right to anonymity and confidentiality?

- Have steps been taken to protect the individual's privacy, anonymity, and confidentiality?

- Have data been reported so that the participants' anonymity is protected?

- Have data results been discussed only as they relate to the study's purpose?

Participant Withdrawal

All consent forms need to assure potential participants of their right to **withdraw** from a research study at any time. It must be stressed that leaving the study or choosing not to participate at all will in no way jeopardize clients or influence the care they would normally expect to receive. Some participants, because they did not fully understand what participation would mean or because their personal situation has changed (e.g., lack of a babysitter, lack of transportation, death or injury of a loved one, added job stressors, or a change in their own health status), may elect to leave the study.

It is not unusual in any research study for one or more participants to withdraw before the completion of the project. Depending on the complexity of the participant's involvement (amount of time and energy spent in relation to intrinsic or extrinsic rewards), many or few individuals may withdraw before the end of the study. In order to obtain meaningful results from the research project, it is important that the investigator keep a careful record of each individual who has agreed to participate and has then withdrawn.

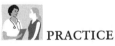 PRACTICE

Participant Withdrawal

Of the following research investigations, identify those that are likely to have high participant withdrawal:

- Feelings about impending abortion in adolescent females

- Success in quitting smoking after attending a 15-week counseling program

- Dietary calcium intake in young, middle-aged, and elderly females

- Parental concerns prior to the circumcision of their infant sons

- Surgical patients' reporting of pain and rate of wound healing in single- versus multiple-occupancy hospital rooms

CRITICAL APPRAISAL

Participant Withdrawal

- Has the investigator informed potential participants of their right to leave the study at any time?

- Has the investigator informed participants that withdrawal from the study will not affect them negatively?

 Deception

Deception refers to the practice of withholding accurate information about the study or giving potential participants inaccurate information regarding their participation in the project. The danger inherent in deceiving potential participants is that harm may result from their involvement in the study that they were unable to evaluate prior to their participation. Hence deceived participants are unable to make an informed decision regarding their involvement.

WORKING DEFINITION

Deception

Deception involves a failure to adequately inform potential research participants about the full nature of the research, thereby preventing them from making an informed decision on their participation.

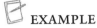 EXAMPLE

Deception

A nurse researcher is investigating the relationship of therapeutic touch (Krieger, 1981) to discomfort from breast engorgement in postpartum women. The researcher will randomly assign participants to one of two treatment groups: one to receive therapeutic touch and one to receive no touch. Because knowing what treatment they were receiving might influence the participants' responses, the researcher does not provide full information about this aspect of the study. The researcher would share details when the study has been completed or when the individual requests information.

It is occasionally necessary when conducting research to consider how the results might be affected if the participants were informed of all aspects of the study. For example, a researcher examining the effectiveness of a new pain medication would be concerned with the validity of the research if the participants knew about the expected results of using the drug. In this study, the researcher might wish to withhold that information. The concern in a situation like this is the violation of the participant's right to information.

If full disclosure of the nature of the study cannot be given in the process of obtaining informed consent, then participants are informed that they are not being told all pertinent aspects regarding the nature of the study. Incomplete disclosure, however, is justified only when there are no other research alternatives to obtain the information sought and when there are minimal risks to participants. In any case, the IRB would be involved in evaluating these studies in detail, and careful attention would be given to the benefits versus the risks of participation. Regardless of whether full disclosure or incomplete disclosure of the details of a study is possible, every effort needs to be made to answer direct questions posed by potential participants.

CRITICAL APPRAISAL

Deception

- Does the researcher use every possible means of protecting the participant from deception?

- Does the research project seem straightforward; that is, is there no hidden agenda in the study's purpose?

- If full disclosure is not possible, is the participant so informed?

Debriefing

If the participant has not been given full disclosure of the nature of the research, then the researcher needs to inform the individual that details will be given following completion of the study. Similarly, all participants, even those who were given full disclosure, need to have an opportunity to review the findings of the research project. The process of instructing the research participant about key aspects of the study that had previously been withheld or informing research participants about the findings of the study is referred to as **debriefing**.

WORKING DEFINITION

Debriefing

Debriefing refers to the process of providing participants with information about the study that had previously been withheld to protect the validity of the research. Debriefing also refers to sharing the results of the study with all participants prior to publication or public presentation.

Plans for debriefing are best made as the study is designed. At that time, plans can be made for providing participants with information that was previously withheld as well as the results of the study. This information may be communicated to participants through a written summary or letter, a phone conversation, or a personal meeting.

CRITICAL APPRAISAL

Debriefing

If full disclosure is not given prior to the study, does the researcher describe plans for doing so?

Role of the Research Committee and IRB

In an effort to protect human research participants and ensure that professional and federal research guidelines are met, many agencies have an established mechanism for reviewing each individual research proposal. Although the process of review differs among various agencies, the following steps describe one possible approach.

A nursing departmental review may be the first step in the process. The ANA research guidelines are often used by a departmental committee to evaluate submissions as to their appropriateness in answering the question posed, as well as how well the rights of research participants are protected. This committee may then either forward the proposal to the agency's **institutional review board (IRB)** for final approval or return the proposal to the investigator with suggestions for change.

The IRB is generally composed of individuals from several different disciplines. Ethicists, nurses, physicians, social workers, and pharmacists are but a few of the possible professions that might be represented. A lay person is also sought in an

185

effort to represent fairly the interests of clients in that facility. This committee usually meets at regularly scheduled intervals to evaluate submissions, and the researcher may expect the review process to take one to two months.

The IRB has the primary responsibility for ensuring that federal research guidelines are followed in any research project implemented within the institution. Committee members evaluate the merit of each proposal, as well as the extent to which human research participants are protected from harm through the use of informed consent procedures. Studies that involve a high risk to participants, incomplete disclosure, or questionable benefits to participants are less likely to be approved.

Committees that review proposals for research projects frequently ask that the investigator attend either some or, in some cases, all of the meetings dedicated to review and discussion of that particular proposal. Although the experience of participating in a review of one's own proposal can be anxiety producing, it can also be rewarding. If viewed in the spirit of constructive criticism, suggestions from a diverse group can be invaluable in strengthening the research proposal and ensuring that the rights of participants are fully protected. Researchers, scientists, and scholars who are not directly involved in a given project can frequently offer insight into potential problems that the researcher may not be able to see. Incorporating suggestions made by these committees can help save valuable time, while also providing maximum protection to research participants involved in the project.

It is important for nurses to sit on IRB committees to assist members from other disciplines in understanding nursing research and to experience the process of reviewing proposals. Understanding the research process as a reviewer can improve the evaluative skills of the consumer as well as those individuals who assist in the planning of research projects. Because nursing has a relatively brief history in relation to the systematic pursuit of nursing knowledge, many IRB committees may not include nurses on their membership lists.

PRACTICE

The Research Review Committee

Call a health care agency or educational institution and ask to attend a research review committee meeting or an IRB meeting.

 CRITICAL APPRAISAL

The Research Review Committee

- Have appropriate agencies been consulted for review of the research proposal, and have measures been taken to protect research participants?

- Does the researcher identify how informed consent procedures were carried out?

Critical Overview of Research Participant Selection and Protection

Whether the nurse is conducting a research study as the investigator, assisting the researcher in the collection of data, or providing care to an individual who is involved in a research project, protecting individual human rights is a crucial role. Potential and actual abuses are a constant threat to a patient who is at increased vulnerability because of a health alteration. The nurse, in the role of patient advocate, must seek to protect the patient from harm while simultaneously encouraging the discovery of knowledge crucial to the development of the discipline of nursing.

Professional nurses who assume an entry-level position in nursing will typically find themselves involved in carrying out research activities designed by another investigator or caring directly for a patient who is a participant in another researcher's study. In the role of research consumer, the nurse must make an effort to ascertain the nature of the study and whether the study has been reviewed by the appropriate review committees. When possible human rights violations are

187

noted in the course of an investigation, the nurse needs to report the concern to both the researcher and the review committees. Similarly, the nurse should not assume that the rights of research participants have been adequately addressed in a research study unless the exact nature is specified. It is incorrect to assume that the rights of the individual and the process of informed consent have been dealt with adequately unless the procedures for doing so are clearly articulated.

CRITICAL OVERVIEW
PARTICIPANT SELECTION AND
PROTECTION

Excerpt A

A baccalaureate nursing student has been caring for a patient on a medical-surgical floor who is a participant in a medical research project. The patient has been experiencing considerable intractable back pain since a job-related injury occurred several years earlier. One morning, while the student is providing regular nursing care, the patient complains about being a participant in the research project.

Because the nurse is unsure about the project, she speaks to the head nurse to ascertain the exact nature of the study. The head nurse tells her that the patient is part of a double-blind study where some of the participants are receiving a placebo medication and some a new analgesic medication. All patients were to receive a summary sheet of the study, as well as a copy of the informed consent document. The length of the study was to be three weeks.

Upon speaking to the patient again, the nurse inquires about what materials the patient received relating to the project. The participant states that he

188

can't remember receiving any summary sheet and says he doesn't know why he "had to be in this doctor's research." He denies knowing anything about the nature of the project, and can't locate a copy of the informed consent document.

Activity 1

Decide what the nursing student should do to help in protecting the individual's right to self-determination. Provide a rationale for your decision.

Activity 2

Describe what debriefing in this study should include.

Excerpt B

A nurse researcher is interested in examining the relationship between auditory stimulation and weight gain in premature infants. The nurse has noted that weight gain seems to be more rapid in cases where the primary nurse plays a recorded audiotape made by the parents on a daily basis.

The nurse obtains two groups of premature infants that are matched for age, weight, and health status. One group hears a recorded audiotape message made by their parents twice a day. The other group of infants receives the usual nursing care, but no recorded audiotape message. Both groups of infants are weighed on a daily basis.

Activity 1

Write a consent form for the investigation described above.

Activity 2

Develop a summary sheet describing the key aspects of the study to give to the parents of the participants.

References

American Nurses Association. (1985). *Human rights guidelines for nurses in clinical and other research*. Kansas City, MO: American Nurses Association.

Commission for the Protection of Human Subjects for Biomedical and Behavioral Research. (1978). *The Belmont report: Ethical principles and guidelines for the protection of human subjects of research*. Washington, DC: Department of Health, Education, and Welfare, Publication No. (05)78-0012.

Committee on Scientific and Professional Ethics and Conduct of the American Psychological Association. (1977). Ethical standards of psychologists, *APA Monitor, 8*: 22.

Damrosch, S. P. (1986). Ensuring anonymity by use of subject-generated identification codes. *Research in Nursing and Health, 9*(1) (March): 61–63.

Department of Health, Education, and Welfare (DHEW). (1978). Code of federal regulations and certain other related laws and regulations on use of human subjects, *Federal Register, 43*(November 3): 515.

Department of Health and Human Services (DHHS). (1981). Final regulations amending basic HHS policy for the protection of human research subjects. *Federal Register, 46*(January 26): 8366.

Dunn, C. M. & Chadwick, G. (1999). *Protecting study volunteers in research*. Boston: CenterWatch.

Krieger, D. (1981). *Foundations for holistic health in nursing practice: The renaissance nurse*. Philadelphia: J. B. Lippincott.

Langer, D. H. (1985). Children's legal rights as research subjects. *Journal of the American Academy of Child Psychiatry, 24*, 653–662.

Siantz, M. L. DeL. (1988). Defining informed consent. *American Journal of Maternal Child Nursing, 13*(2), 94.

Note

In June 1988, the American Nurses Association (ANA) House of Delegates passed a resolution concerning the responsible use of animals in nursing research. Proposed by the ANA Cabinet on Nursing Research, the resolution provides broad guidelines for researchers who use an animal model. Additionally, the American Psychological Committee on Precautions and Standards in Animal Experimentation has developed *Rules Regarding Animals* (1977). These adopted guidelines can be used as an adjunct to guide the nurse researcher when animals are used in research.

Unit 3

Answering the Research Question: Quantitative Designs

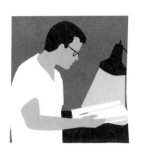

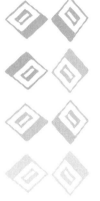

6

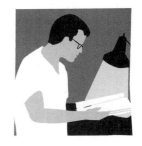

Measurement

Goals

- *Analyze the levels of measurement.*
- *Describe the key concepts related to measurement.*
- *Describe knowledge necessary to evaluate adequately the use of instruments.*

Introduction

The goal of research is to provide accurate answers to questions of interest. Questions of interest within nursing are developed from nursing concepts, namely, those thoughts, notions, or ideas that relate to nursing or nursing practice. Nursing concepts are then translated into observable facts or events. Translating a nursing concept into an observable fact or event permits the investigator to measure the event(s) of interest. The key word in relation to measurement is *accuracy*. The selection of a method of sampling influences the degree to which findings can be generalized; the measurement process influences the degree of accuracy of the results.

Concerns related to measurement include the following:

1. What level of measurement is used (**nominal, ordinal, interval, ratio**)?

2. What strategy is used to measure the variables under study (paper-and-pencil questionnaire, interview, etc.)?

3. To what degree can a measurement strategy provide accurate information (**reliability, validity, normative data**)?

4. What factors related to data collection enhance or diminish the accuracy of the results?

5. Given the measurement strategies used in a particular study, what methods of data analysis are most likely to provide accurate information?

This chapter deals with each of these concerns and discusses the importance of appraising the literature from a measurement perspective.

Measuring Variables

The number of variables appropriate for examination by nurses is almost limitless. Any of the physiological and psychosocial concepts that are a part of nursing practice are open to systematic examination. Specific variables that may be identified in nursing research can include age, sex, measures of pain, blood pressure readings, a psychological attribute such as perception of control, and others too numerous to mention (see Figure 6.1). Although a major focus of nursing research at present is the development of a scientific body of knowledge as the underpinnings for practice, in nursing as a whole there is tremendous diversity among the variables appropriate for study.

Regardless of the variables under study, in order to make sense out of the data collected, each variable must be measured in such a way that its magnitude or quantity can be clearly identified. A variety of measurement methods are available for use in nursing research. The specific strategies chosen depend

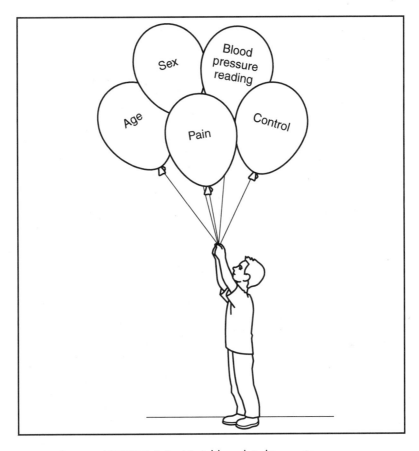

FIGURE 6.1 Variables related to nursing

on the particular research question, the sample under study, the availability of instruments, and the general feasibility of the project. One measurement strategy is not necessarily better than another. Four scales or levels of measurement have been identified: nominal, ordinal, interval, or ratio. Each level of measurement is classified in relation to certain characteristics. When investigators' data fall within the first level of measurement, the range of choice relative to statistical analysis is limited. Data that fall within the fourth level of measurement can be analyzed using a broad array of statistical techniques.

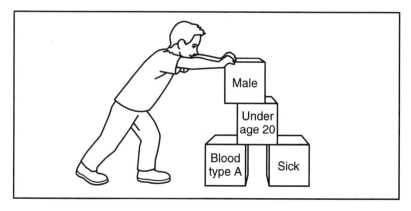

FIGURE 6.2 The nominal level of measurement: Discrete categories

The Nominal Level of Measurement

The first or **nominal** level of measurement is characterized by variables that are discrete and noncontinuous. These variables are categorical and include such examples as sex (male, female), marital status (married, unmarried), blood types (0, A, B, AB), and health state (sick, well). Examples are shown in Figure 6.2.

Expressions commonly used to denote this level of measurement include *nominal scale*, *categorical data*, *nominal data*, and *nominal measurement*. In each instance the expression describes categories that are discrete, named, and therefore mutually exclusive.

 WORKING DEFINITION

The Nominal Level of Measurement

The nominal level of measurement is the most primitive method of classifying information. Nominal replies that categories of people, events, and other phenomena are named, are exhaustive in nature, and are mutually exclusive. These categories are discrete and noncontinuous.

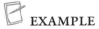

EXAMPLE

The Nominal Level of Measurement

A nurse researcher investigated the effects of an educational package dealing with diabetes on the teenage diabetic's compliance with dietary restrictions. The following data were collected three months after the educational presentation:

Exposure to educational package: 65

Compliance. Males, $N = 38$
                       Good, $N = 15$
                       Poor, $N = 23$

            Females, $N = 27$
                       Good, $N = 18$
                       Poor, $N = 9$

To analyze the data, the researcher used a method of statistical analysis appropriate to the nominal level of measurement (chi-square).

In this example compliance is measured in a discrete fashion; that is, the participants were either compliers or noncompliers. A focus of the research was on sexual differences, males versus females. The nominal level of measurement implies that there are named categories–for example, male, female; that the categories are mutually exclusive—for example, male–female, compliers–noncompliers; and that the categories are not ordered in any fashion. There are not, for example, degrees of maleness or femaleness, nor are there degrees of compliance, as defined in this study.

The choice of the appropriate statistical method with which to analyze data is a crucial factor in the eventual worth of the research project. When a nominal level of measurement has been used, the choice of statistical methods that will provide meaningful results is limited.

PRACTICE

Identifying Nominal Variables

From the following research questions, identify those variables that are most likely to be measured using a nominal scale:

• What is the relationship between gender and the incidence of diabetes?

• *Variables:* Gender, incidence of diabetes

• How does paying a shift differential affect absenteeism among nurses on a critical care unit?

• *Variables:* Shift differential, absenteeism

• How do age and sex affect compliance in a cardiac rehabilitation program?

• *Variables:* Age, sex, compliance

 CRITICAL APPRAISAL

The Nominal Level of Measurement

If a nominal level of measurement is used, does it seem appropriate given the topic under study?

The Ordinal Level of Measurement

The second or **ordinal** level of measurement is characterized by variables that are assessed incrementally. For example, pain can be measured as slight, moderate, or intense. Exercise can be measured in terms of frequency—that is, often, sometimes, or never. In each case, there are increments or intervals in the scale, but these intervals cannot be considered equal (see Figure 6.3).

As with the nominal variable, it is not some innate value of the specific variable that causes it to be ordinal, but the manner in which it is measured. Pain or exercise could be meas-

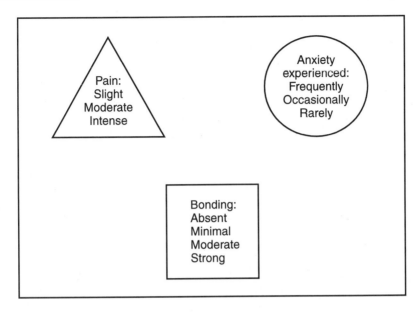

FIGURE 6.3 The ordinal level of measurement: Continuous variables, increments not of equal value; variables can be rank-ordered from highest to lowest

ured using a scale that denotes equal intervals. Exercise could be assessed in terms of the number of miles run or the amount of weight lifted.

Expressions commonly used to denote this kind of measurement include *ordinal scale, ordinal variables, ordinal data,* and *ordinal measurement.* Unlike the nominal level of measurement, the ordinal level of measurement suggests an ordering of variables. Within the ordinal level of measurement, an event is assigned to a category based on the amount of a particular attribute. This level of measurement can be described as the ranking of events in terms of the relative amounts of a specified characteristic. Pain can be ordered or ranked in terms of the intensity of the experience—namely, intense, moderate, or mild—thus reflecting an ordinal approach. Sex is usually perceived as male or female without an ordering of sexual characteristics, thus reflecting the nominal level of measurement.

WORKING DEFINITION

The Ordinal Level of Measurement

The ordinal level of measurement is second in terms of its refinement as a means of classifying information. *Ordinal* implies that the values of variables can be rank-ordered from highest to lowest.

EXAMPLE

The Ordinal Level of Measurement

A team of nurse researchers designed a research project to compare the degree of social support (SS) perceived by 100 teenage girls diagnosed as bulimics with a group of nonbulimic girls of the same age, educational level, family size, and placement within the family. Each participant responded to a paper-and-pencil test. The following data were collected:

	Considerable SS	Moderate SS	Little SS
Bulimics	13	30	57
Nonbulimics	35	55	10

To analyze the data, the researcher used a method of statistical analysis appropriate to the ordinal level of measurement (chi-square).

In this example, the variable of social support is rank-ordered. Some participants felt that they had considerable social support; others had moderate social support; and still others had little social support. Even though social support is measured in an incremental fashion (considerable, moderate, little), a consistent number cannot be associated with the distance between considerable, moderate, and little. The data collected, therefore, are ordinal and are somewhat limited in relation to the statistical techniques available for data analysis.

PRACTICE

Identifying Ordinal Variables

How could the following variables be measured at the ordinal level?

Example: Pain—using a scale that measures pain as absent, moderate, strong, or intense.

Variables: Depression, skin turgor, helplessness, grief, stress, confusion, nausea.

CRITICAL APPRAISAL

The Ordinal Level of Measurement

If an ordinal level of measurement is used, does it seem appropriate given the topic under study?

The Interval Level of Measurement

The third or **interval** level of measurement is characterized by a scale that is quantitative in nature. Increments on the scale can be measured, and they are equidistant. An individual's temperature is measured in terms of numbers of degrees. Between a temperature of 97 and 100 degrees Fahrenheit, there are three equal increments of one degree each (Figure 6.4).

An interval scale, though quantitative in nature, does not have an absolute or actual zero. Temperature is a good example of an interval scale in that zero changes depending on the scale used—Fahrenheit or Celsius. Expressions commonly used

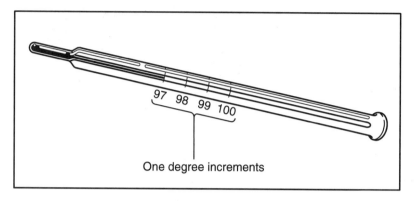

FIGURE 6.4 The interval level of measurement: Continuous variables, increments of equal value

to denote this kind of measurement include *interval scale,
interval variables, interval data,* and *interval measurement.*

 WORKING DEFINITION

The Interval Level of Measurement

Interval measurement refers to the third level of measurement
in relation to the complexity of statistical techniques that can be
used to analyze data. Variables within this level of measurement
are assessed incrementally, and the increments are equal. Many
statistical techniques can be used to analyze interval variables.

 EXAMPLE

The Interval Level of Measurement

A nurse researcher investigated the psychological status of 60
abused women before and after an intervention designed to
enhance their feelings of independence. A psychological test
was given before and after the intervention, and test scores

were then compared using a paired *t*-test. Examples of the data collected are given below:

Abused woman	Before	After	Difference
1	36	42	6
2	25	40	15
3	39	45	6
4	40	40	0
5	41	44	3
6	35	40	5

The scores on the psychological test represent interval data. To analyze this data the researcher could choose any one of many statistical methods appropriate for use with interval data.

 PRACTICE

Identifying Interval Variables

Identify those variables that are most likely to be measured using a nominal scale, an ordinal scale, or an interval scale:

- How does assertiveness training affect the lifestyle patterns of abused women?

  Variables: Assertiveness training, lifestyle patterns

- What effect does health education have on compliance with a low-fat diet on men diagnosed with hypertension?

  Variables: Health education, compliance

- How does extended visitation on the neonatal unit affect the bonding process between father and infant?

  Variables: Extended visitation, bonding process

CRITICAL APPRAISAL

The Interval Level of Measurement

If an interval level of measurement is used, does it seem appropriate given the topic under study?

The Ratio Level of Measurement

The fourth or **ratio** level of measurement is characterized by variables that are assessed incrementally with equal distances between the increments and a scale that has an absolute zero. Obvious ratio scales include time, length, and weight (Figure 6.5).

Even though the variables of time, length, and weight are obvious examples of ratio scales, they can also be measured using a nominal or ordinal scale. For example, the nurse researcher who chooses to measure the time it takes nursing students to perform a given task could divide time into two categories: less than five minutes and more than five minutes. These two categories could then be represented by Time 1 and Time 2, nominal variables necessitating statistical analysis appropriate to that method of measurement.

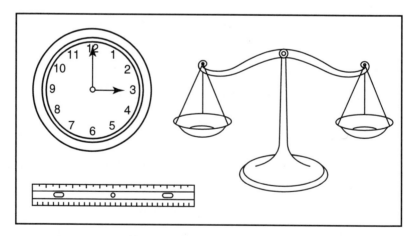

FIGURE 6.5 The ratio level of measurement: Continuous variables, increments of equal value, absolute zero exists

WORKING DEFINITION

The Ratio Level of Measurement

The ratio level of measurement is the fourth and least primitive method of classifying information. *Ratio* implies that the variables reflect the characteristics of ordinal and interval measurement and can also be compared by ratios; that is, the number representing a given variable can be compared by describing it as two or three times another number or as one-third, one-quarter, and so on. The ratio level of measurement, unlike the other three levels, has an absolute zero.

EXAMPLE

The Ratio Level of Measurement

A team of nurse investigators designed a research project to determine the effect of a support group on the weight loss of 35 morbidly obese women motivated to comply with a specific diet. Both the experimental and control groups were weighed one week before the initiation of the support group, and participants in both groups agreed to try the specified diet. The following data were collected and data analysis completed using statistical procedures appropriate to the ratio level of measurement.

	Experimental group	Control group
Sample size	35	35
Mean weight loss	26 lbs.	19 lbs.
Standard deviation	2 lbs.	4.5 lbs.

The advantage of interval and ratio levels of measurement compared with nominal and ordinal levels of measurement is

205

that more complex statistical techniques can be used to analyze the data collected. The result of having an increased number of options for the analysis of data is that the description of what has actually happened in the study is more precise.

PRACTICE

Identifying Ratio Variables

Formulate four research questions and incorporate the four levels of measurement in the methods of measurement proposed.

>   *Example:* What is the relationship of teenage anorexia to weight, sex, emotional status, and family structure?
>
>   *Variables and proposed measurement level:*
>
>   Weight—ratio
>
>   Sex—nominal
>
>   Emotional status—interval
>
>   Family structure—ordinal

CRITICAL APPRAISAL

The Ratio Level of Measurement

If a ratio level of measurement is used, does it seem appropriate given the topic under study?

Methods of Measurement

The Instrument

The term **instrument** is used in research to describe a particular method of collecting data. Instruments used in research include paper-and-pencil tests, structured interviews, puzzles, mechanical equipment, direct observations, and the like. Instruments may provide a total score or may consist of a series of items that must be analyzed independently. The instrument is the device that is used to measure the concept of interest. The construction of an instrument is a complex and time-consuming undertaking. The development of an effective instrument requires an in-depth knowledge of the content area under study and considerable skill in the area of measurement theory. Beginning researchers are advised to use instruments that have already been developed and have had their effectiveness established wherever possible. Consumers of research are advised to carefully appraise the instruments used when reviewing a research report.

Whether the instrument is a paper-and-pencil test, a piece of equipment, or a direct observation, there are characteristics of the instrument that are important in terms of the accuracy and meaning of the results. The two major characteristics that are essential in relation to the meaning and accuracy produced by a given instrument are **validity** and **reliability**. When appraising the literature or designing a study, it is important to evaluate the validity and reliability of the methods of measurement used in the research.

 WORKING DEFINITION

An Instrument

An instrument is a device used to measure the concept of interest in a research project. An instrument may be a paper-and-pencil test, a structured interview, or a piece of equipment.

When measuring attributes of interest, a norm-referenced or a criterion-referenced approach may be used. The norm-referenced approach is one in which a participant's performance can be evaluated against the performance of others in similar circumstances. For example, many of the achievement tests taken by high school students have been taken by thousands of students, and statistical information has been gathered that describes the distribution of scores among that group of individuals. Any individual taking the test can then be measured against similar individuals.

The criterion-referenced-approach involves the identification of certain attributes of interest—for example, a set of standards for a nursing intervention—and then the construction of an instrument to measure how well participants meet the standards. In this instance, comparing participants' performance without standards would be irrelevant (Cozby, 2000).

EXAMPLE

An Instrument

A team of nurse investigators plan to examine the association between attitudes toward health and the performance of routine breast self-examination. The investigators choose a paper-and-pencil test (the instrument) that requires individuals to answer "agree" or "disagree" to 25 items designed to measure attitudes toward health. A total score on attitudes toward health is calculated. Participants are also asked to identify whether they perform routine breast self-examination.

PRACTICE

Identifying instruments

Identify five instruments used in various nursing studies, and describe the differences in their approach to measurement by answering the following questions:

1. Does the investigator want to compare the results with a set standard?

2. Does the investigator want to compare the results of one group with another group?

3. Does the investigator design the instrument specifically for a particular study?

4. Is the instrument one that has been used many times in a variety of studies?

5. Does the instrument provide a total score, or is it a series of items that must be analyzed independently?

Errors of Measurement

Whenever a variable is measured, there is the potential for errors to occur. Some of the factors that can influence the outcome can be controlled, others cannot. The score obtained from using a particular instrument in a particular setting consists of two parts—the true score and the error. A concerted effort should be made to limit the error portion of the score.

The following list consists of potential sources of error when measures of specific attributes are taken.

1. *Instrument clarity:* Frequently, participants will respond to an instrument inappropriately—for example, placing a check-mark in a box when "yes" or "no" was required. If the instructions for taking the instrument are not clear, participants cannot respond appropriately and the information received is not accurate. Similarly, if the items themselves are not readily understood, responses may not reflect the participants' perceptions and the resultant information is of limited value.

2. *Variations in administration:* If some participants are allowed to respond to an instrument at their leisure while others are given time constraints, the information received is not comparable. If some participants are assisted in responding to an instrument while others are not, again, the information received may be different.

3. *Situational variations:* If an instrument is administered under differing environmental conditions—unpleasant versus pleasant surroundings, or threatening versus non-threatening conditions—responses may vary according to the situation.

4. *Response set biases:* Frequently, participants will give an answer that is socially desirable. For example, questions about an individual's sexual practices, views on religion, or politics may produce responses that are untrue but are chosen because they are considered acceptable by the

majority of individuals in society. Another problem is the tendency of some individuals to consistently respond in an extreme fashion. On a scale of I to 5, some people will consistently respond at one end of the scale, regardless of the topic.

5. *Transitory personal factors:* Participants' mood, state of mind, and level of stress at the time of responding to the instrument may affect either their answers or their desire to participate in the project.

6. *Response sampling:* The content of the instrument—that is, the sampling of items—may affect the participant's score. Depending on the items selected, a nurse might perform well on a pain knowledge questionnaire or poorly on the same questionnaire.

7. *Instrument format:* The order of items on a questionnaire and the kind of questions asked (open-ended or closed) can affect the responses given.

Validity

The concept of **validity** in relation to research is a judgment regarding the degree to which the components of research reflect the theory, concept, or variable under study (Streiner & Norman, 1996). The validity of the instrument used (how well it measures what it is supposed to measure) and the validity of the research design as a whole are important criteria in evaluating the worth of the results of the research conducted.

Instruments may not be designed in such a way that the concept under study is reflected in the items. For example, a group of nurse researchers may want to design an instrument that measures stress. In examining the literature related to stress, it may become apparent that the items are really assessing anxiety rather than stress. In this instance the instrument would not be valid. It does not measure what the investigators want it to measure.

In relation to the overall research design, the term validity can refer to the likelihood that the experimental manipulation was indeed responsible for the differences observed. This kind of validity is termed *internal validity.* Another kind of validity used in relation to the research design is termed *external validity* and refers to the extent to which the results of a study can be generalized to the larger population (Polit & Hungler, 1999).

The Validity of an Instrument

Four types of validity are used to judge the accuracy of an instrument: (1) content validity, (2) predictive validity, (3) concurrent validity, and (4) construct validity. Using these categories, it is important for the consumer of research and the investigator designing a study to evaluate the instruments used.

Content validity is a judgment regarding how well the instrument represents the characteristics to be assessed. Instruments with a high degree of content validity are as representative as possible of all the items that could be included to measure the concept under study. For example, to design a questionnaire on individuals' attitudes toward eating but forget to ask anything about the importance of food in their lives would be an oversight. The content validity of the instrument would be in question.

Judgments about content validity are subjective. Objective methods for measuring the areas of concern that must be reflected on an instrument are not available. Judgments are generally based on prior research in the field and on the opinions of experts.

Predictive validity is a judgment as to the degree to which an instrument can accurately forecast the future. For example, certain achievement tests can predict the academic futures of students. Some personality tests can predict behavior patterns. The assessment of predictive validity is an objective task and can be accomplished through comparing one instrument with another of known predictive validity, or through examining the outcome in terms of available data. For example, a lifestyle questionnaire aimed at identifying women who are likely to develop osteoporosis could be evaluated in terms of its predictive validity by following identified individuals to see whether they indeed develop the disease.

Concurrent validity is a judgment as to the degree to which an instrument can accurately identify a difference in the present. Such questions as "Can the instrument accurately determine the difference between the learning disabled child and the normal child?" or "Can the piece of equipment identify those individuals who are hypertensive?" reflect the degree of concurrent validity of a particular instrument. Concurrent validity suggests that the instrument in question can indicate a specific behavior or characteristic in the present. Judgments can be made through assessing the literature and using multiple criteria to examine results.

Construct validity refers to the extent to which a participant actually possesses the characteristic under study. For example, nurse investigators may choose to examine the concept of pain among children diagnosed with leukemia, and they may want to design an instrument to measure pain in this setting. They will want to know if their instrument is actually measuring pain (construct validity) or if it is in fact assessing something else (e.g., anxiety). In order to determine whether their instrument is measuring pain, these investigators can use multiple measures to assess the same construct, namely, a questionnaire, a structured interview, and direct observation. In judging construct validity, theoretical considerations come into play. The investigator needs to be able to make predictions about the construct in terms of other related constructs. For example, the degree of pain expressed may be a function of the kind of social support perceived.

The validity of an instrument (how well it measures what it is supposed to measure) is essential to the success of any research endeavor. If the investigator designs a study to examine parenting skills but uses an instrument that is actually measuring general coping skills, the results of the study are of little value. Similarly, if an investigator decides to examine the relationship between effective nursing care and a particular kind of nursing education, and yet the instrument used actually measures attitudes toward nursing as a profession, the results can be either misleading or meaningless.

 WORKING DEFINITION

The Validity of an instrument

Validity describes the usefulness of an instrument given the context in which it is applied. It reflects how well an instrument has measured what it was supposed to measure given a particular set of circumstances. The following kinds of validity are frequently assessed in trying to make a judgment about a given instrument.

Content: All important areas of concern are reflected.

Predictive: Events are accurately predicted.

Concurrent: Accurate differences are shown in the present.

Construct: The attribute of interest is actually being measured.

The characteristic of validity is one that frequently takes years to ascertain. As instruments are used and tested repeatedly, information about exactly what they are measuring can be gathered and assessed. Unfortunately, nursing does not have a long history of instrument development, and therefore it is frequently difficult to find an instrument measuring a nursing concept of interest that has adequate data on its validity.

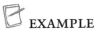 EXAMPLE

Assessing the Validity of an Instrument

A team of nurse investigators design a lifestyle questionnaire to identify those women who are at risk of developing osteoporosis. In order to validate the instrument, they take the following steps:

1. Obtain from the literature, as well as from experts in osteoporosis, those lifestyle factors that are believed to predispose an individual to osteoporosis (content validity).

2. Incorporate all lifestyle factors believed to predispose individuals to osteoporosis within the instrument (content validity).

3. Involve experts in the field of osteoporosis in the formulation of the instrument (content validity).

4. Give the instrument to a randomly selected sample of individuals and follow them to see if those identified as at risk do, in fact, develop osteoporosis (predictive validity).

213

5. Give the instrument to a randomly selected group of individuals along with another accepted measure to see if this instrument identifies the same individuals as being at risk (concurrent validity).

6. Give the instrument to a group of women who have osteoporosis and a group of women who do not have osteoporosis (construct validity).

Designing an instrument that is capable of accurately measuring a specific concept takes a considerable amount of effort and time. When an instrument does not accurately measure what it is supposed to measure, the results of a study can be misleading or meaningless. An important process in appraising the literature or in designing a study is the assessment of the instruments used in relation to their validity.

 PRACTICE

Assessing the Validity of an instrument

Select three published nursing studies and identify the information given in relation to the validity of the instruments used. List possible concerns about the instruments used based on the information provided.

 CRITICAL APPRAISAL

Assessing the Validity of an Instrument

• Is sufficient information available in regard to the instrument's validity; that is, does it seem to measure what it purports to measure?

• Does the instrument cover all of the important factors related to the topic?

• Is there evidence that using this instrument to collect data can help the investigator to predict an occurrence in the future?

- Is there evidence that the instrument can identify the desired characteristic(s) in the present?

- Does the instrument measure the construct that it claims to measure?

Reliability

The **reliability** of an instrument reflects its stability and consistency within a given context. For example, a scale developed to measure attitudes toward pain among the elderly might not be reliable if used with young adults. Because the consistency and stability of responses to questions asked is such an important concept, instruments must be evaluated for their reliability.

Three characteristics of reliability are commonly evaluated: (1) stability, (2) internal consistency, and (3) equivalence (Figure 6.6). *Stability* refers to the degree to which research participants' responses change overtime. Ideally, we would like participants to respond to an instrument measuring their self-esteem in a similar fashion on any number of occasions unless intervening events occur to change their perceptions.

Stability is measured by giving the same individuals an instrument on two occasions within a relatively short period of time (two to three weeks apart is often suggested) and then examining their responses for similarities. This method for determining reliability is termed test–retest. A correlation coefficient is calculated to determine how closely participants' responses on the second occasion matched their responses on the first occasion. Reliability coefficients range from −1 to +1.00. A coefficient of .60 shows a moderately strong relationship, .20 a weak relationship, and 0 no relationship. We rarely find perfect relationships (1.00).

If a group of adolescents respond to a questionnaire that asks them to examine their level of confidence on two occasions and the resulting correlation coefficient is .15, we know that the construct of level of confidence is not stable over time as measured by that instrument. Problems with the notion of test-retest as a measure of reliability include the fact that some may respond to the instrument the second time on the basis of

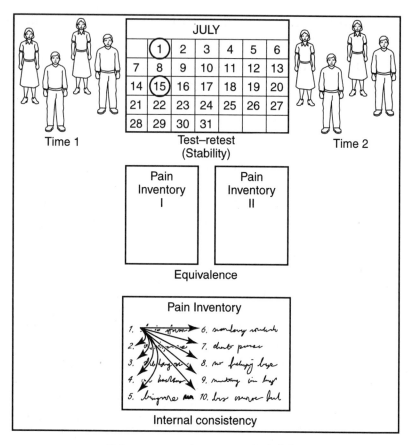

FIGURE 6.6 Three types of reliability

their memory of their first exposure to the instrument; participants may change as a result of responding to the instrument the first time; and, knowing that they have already responded to the instrument, participants may not answer questions carefully. In addition, an assessment of test–retest reliability is not useful for constructs that we know change over time, such as pain, anxiety, and anger.

Internal consistency is a measure of reliability that is frequently used with scales designed to assess psychosocial characteristics. An instrument is describe as internally consistent to the extent that all of its subparts measure the same characteristic. This method of reliability assessment deals with error made in relation to the sampling of items. If an instrument is designed to assess self-esteem and a few of the items actually measure depression, individuals are likely to answer those questions differently. The instrument as a whole will not be internally consistent.

Instruments can be assessed for internal consistency using a split-half technique (i.e., answers to one half of the items are compared with answers to the other half of the items) or by calculating an alpha coefficient or using the Kuder-Richardson formula. In the case of the alpha coefficient and the Kuder-Richardson formula, a coefficient that ranges from 0 to 1.00 generally results.

The notion of *equivalence* is often a concern when different observers are using the same instrument to collect data at the same time. For example, three observers may be using a checklist to identify the mood states of preschool children. Each observer needs to understand what constitutes the characteristics listed—happy, sad, angry, and so forth. In this instance, interrater reliability is calculated on information gathered by the various observers. When appropriate, a coefficient can be calculated or other statistical and nonstatistical procedures can be used.

An important practical note regarding the assessment of reliability is that the testing of an instrument is done before the study is initiated and on individuals not participating in the study. If a few individuals participated in a test–retest of an instrument and were then included in the study they would have responded to the instrument on three occasions, and other participants would have only one chance to respond.

 WORKING DEFINITION

Reliability

Reliability is a characteristic of an instrument that reflects the degree to which the instrument provokes consistent responses.

There are three characteristics of reliability that are commonly evaluated:

Test–retest: Degree of consistency when individuals respond on two separate occasions

Equivalence: Degree of consistency in providing measurements of same attributes

Internal consistency: Degree of consistency among responses to items

EXAMPLE

Establishing Reliability

A team of nurse investigators designs an instrument to identify the population at risk for developing eating disorders. They review the literature and work closely with experts in the field while formulating the items. Their questionnaire contains 10 items, and participants are asked to respond using a 5-point scale.

Sample Item:

(Scale: frequently = 5, often = 4, sometimes = 3, rarely = 2, never = 1)

I am critical of my appearance   <u>5</u>   <u>4</u>   <u>3</u>   <u>2</u>   <u>1</u>

The research team takes the following steps to establish the reliability of the instrument:

- Ten volunteers from a support group for bulimics respond to the items at the same time and place and then repeat the experience two weeks later. A correlation coefficient is calculated, and the test–retest reliability is considered adequate.

- Ten volunteers from a different support group for bulimics respond to the items at the same time and place. An alpha coefficient is calculated, and the internal consistency of the instrument is considered adequate.

PRACTICE

Reliability

- Identify a nursing concept of interest and develop three related items. Administer the three items to a small group of people on two separate occasions and examine the results for consistency (visually examine the responses).

- Find two studies published in nursing journals that give an acceptable description of the reliability of the instrument used.

CRITICAL APPRAISAL

Reliability

Is sufficient information available in regard to the instrument's reliability; that is, is there consistency over time, is there consistency relative to a parallel form of the instrument, and is there internal consistency?

Critical Overview of Measurement

The manner in which variables are measured can make the difference between useful and meaningless results. When instruments used are of questionable validity and reliability, the data collected cannot be considered accurate. In addition to the concepts of validity and reliability, a knowledge of the various levels of measurement is important because appropriate statistical analysis is dependent on such an understanding.

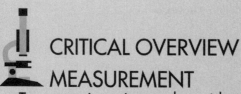

CRITICAL OVERVIEW
MEASUREMENT

Two nurse investigators have identified the following research question: What are the predisposing characteristics of osteoporosis for women 19 years of age? They identify three factors as important to their study: diet, exercise, and family incidence.

Activity 1

Given the variables of diet, exercise, and family incidence, identify which levels of measurement are possible.

Activity 2

Formulate four items related to each of the following: diet, exercise, and family incidence. Divide the items in half (two on each topic on separate sheets of paper) and give the two forms of the questionnaire to two different groups of students. Scan the responses within each category to see if they are similar.

References

Cozby, P. C. (2000). *Methods in Behavioral Research* (7th Edition). Toronto: Mayfield Publishing Co.

Polit, D. F. & Hungler, B. P. (1999). *Essentials of nursing research* (6th Edition). Philadelphia, J. B. Lippincott.

Streiner, D. & Norman, G. (1996). *PDQ Epidemiology* (2nd Edition). St. Louis: Mosby.

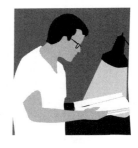

7

Quantitative Designs in Research

Goals

- *Describe basic research designs used in quantitative research.*
- *Analyze the key elements of experimental and nonexperimental research designs.*
- *Provide a rationale for selecting a particular design.*

Introduction

Once nurse investigators have identified their area of research interest, they need to decide how they will proceed to answer their research questions. Some will decide to conduct a qualitative study, others will use quantitative methods. The topic under investigation, the amount of information available on the topic, and the individual's philosophy may guide the choice of methodology. Some nurse researchers believe that certain areas of investigation, particularly those having to do with human qualities, can be studied only in a qualitative fashion. Others believe that new areas of investigation need to be examined in a qualitative manner before conducting a quantitative investigation. Still others support the use of both methods when conducting research in order to produce results that can best enhance our knowledge of a given area.

This chapter deals with research designs that reflect a quantitative approach to examining phenomena. The quantitative approach is characterized by beliefs that objective data can be gained in the psychosocial as well as the physical world, that the same research procedures can be used to study both inanimate and animate objects (human beings), and that a structured research design is able to produce objective results. These beliefs stem from positivistic or mechanistic notions of the universe and are questioned by many nurses who challenge the idea that structure produces objective results and that the same research procedures can be used successfully for people, animals, and other objects of study.

Clearly, quantitative approaches to research have produced valuable information in many psychosocial as well as physical fields of study. Although there are problems inherent in the quantitative approach and in the specific research designs, our knowledge has increased and can continue to do so through application of a quantitative methodology.

In this chapter, experimental and nonexperimental designs are described. The key elements of each design are identified, and an analysis of the strengths and weaknesses of the designs is proposed.

Experimental Designs

The Experiment
The **experiment** is a design that is commonly used in the natural or basic sciences. This design permits the researcher to

establish cause-effect relationships and therefore accurately predict and explain phenomena. In conducting an experiment, the investigator attempts to ensure that the results of the study can be accurately attributed to the manipulation of the variables under examination. In order to ensure that the results of the study can be attributed to the intervention, a comparison between a **treatment group** and a **control group** is required. Experiments are easier to conduct in the natural or basic sciences than in the social sciences because the objects or units involved can be more readily controlled and manipulated.

Designing an experiment in which people are a focus of the research question is more difficult than designing an experiment in which chemicals, elements, or even animals are under examination. The number of variables that need to be controlled in order to conduct an experiment in which people are the focus of the investigation is frequently so great that this particular design cannot be used. Additional requirements of the experiment can also limit its usefulness in the areas of interest to nurse investigators.

Characteristics of the Experiment   In order to conduct an experiment, a comparison of two or more *groups* is required. The groups under study must be the same so that the results of the project can be attributed to the *manipulation* of the variable and not to differences between the groups. For example, if nurse researchers want to study the effect of postpartum home visits on the anxiety levels of new mothers and they design a project in which one group of new mothers experiences the visits and the other group does not, the groups need to be the same in every possible way prior to the intervention. If some of the women in one group have had training in caring for babies and in the other group no one has been trained, the differences in the groups could affect the results of the study. These differences may be resolved through *randomly* assigning participants to the experimental and control groups (see Figure 7.1).

The experiment involves the manipulation of the independent variable. The investigator decides how the study groups will experience the intervention. For example, a group of nurse researchers could design three educational packages for post-myocardial infarct patients in an attempt to diminish the

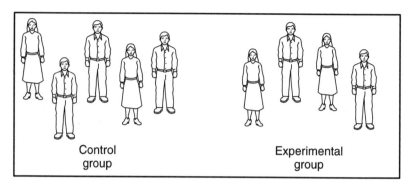

FIGURE 7.1 Forming equivalent groups

occurrence of depression in this population. One group of patients might experience Package A: a one-afternoon session with a group leader and the distribution of two pages of helpful information. Another group might experience Package B: a four-week, one-hour-per-week seminar providing information and opportunities for discussion of ten key points. A third group might experience Package C: a weekend retreat with a psychiatric nurse specialist examining problems that have occurred as a result of the infarct. (Technically an experiment has a control group that does not experience the intervention; however, in nursing it is often more appropriate to describe the control group as receiving traditional or routine care as the alternative to the intervention.)

The educational package is the *independent variable*, and it is manipulated by the researchers. Depression is the *dependent* variable. The researchers decide to assign the participants randomly to Groups 1, 2, and 3 and identify which group will experience which of the three packages (see Figure 7.2). The educational package is the independent variable manipulated by the researchers to examine its effect on occurrence of depression among post-myocardial infarct patients. The effect of the educational package is measured, and, using appropriate statistical procedures (inferential statistics), the data are analyzed to determine the probability that the intervention has had an effect.

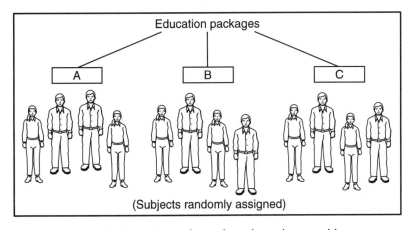

FIGURE 7.2 Manipulating the independent variable

Controlling **extraneous variables** is an important character-istic of most research endeavors. In the experiment, a con-certed effort is made to ensure that one or more extraneous variables are not directly responsible for the results of the study. For example, nurse researchers might decide to investi-gate the effect of a comprehensive educational seminar on pain management on nurses' responses to patients in pain. There is evidence to suggest that nurses' knowledge of opioids can affect their care of patients (Ferrell & McCaffery, 1997). Vary-ing differences in opioid knowledge could, therefore, influence study results. The variable "opioid knowledge" would be con-sidered an extraneous variable. This variable could influence nurses' responses to patients in pain, thereby contaminating the results of the study.

One possibility for negotiating the influence of extraneous variables is collecting data on the variable of concern and excluding individuals based on that variable. In relation to the pain study above, an opioid knowledge questionnaire could be given to all participants. Data could be analyzed to see if, in fact, knowledge did influence the results of the study. Another option would be to limit participants in the study to those nurses who have a predetermined level of knowledge.

225

WORKING DEFINITION

The Experiment

An experiment is a research design that is characterized by a comparison among groups that are as equal as possible, the manipulation of an independent variable, the use of inferential statistics, and stringent control of extraneous variables.

Although the experiment provides the investigator with the best mechanism for determining cause and effect, the complexity of the human experience often makes conducting an experiment difficult, if not impossible. In order to exert the kind of control that characterizes the true experiment, human subjects may need to be placed in an artificial setting. There are two problems with this approach: (1) the setting itself may influence individuals to respond in an abnormal fashion, and (2) placing individuals in an artificial setting may be neither practical nor possible. For example, individuals placed in a room containing video equipment may respond to the equipment in a self-conscious manner unlike their usual way of being, thereby affecting study results. Frequently it is not possible to randomly assign patients to hospital rooms in order to conduct a study on some aspect of patient care. Another example would be if moving patients out of their in-hospital setting to a different environment increased their anxiety. In this case, the setting might affect the outcome of the study.

In a study in which nurses wish to examine the functional level of schizophrenic patients after a series of behavior modification classes, they may be able to control the environment during the classes but probably cannot control patients' experiences between classes. The between-classes experiences could affect the outcome. The project may be conducted and may be designed in such a way that the basic requirements of an experiment appear to be met. Given the complex nature of human participants, however, the requirements probably will not be met as stringently as they should be to meet the criteria for an experiment.

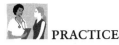 PRACTICE

The Experiment

Identify from the nursing literature one study that could be termed an experiment. Describe the characteristics that make this study an experiment.

The consumer of research, as well as individuals who assist in the development of a research project, can evaluate those studies that are described as experiments in relation to their adherence to the basic requirements of that particular research design. How stringently these requirements have been met can also be assessed and related to the value of the results obtained.

 CRITICAL APPRAISAL

The Experiment

When reviewing an experiment ask the following questions:

- Is there a comparison between or among groups?

- Is there equivalence between or among groups?

- Is there manipulation of the independent variable?

- Are extraneous variables controlled to the greatest extent possible?

An Example of an Experimental Design: Pretest–Posttest Control Group Design This research design can be described by the four major steps used in carrying out the project. The first step is to assign research participants randomly to the experimental or control group in order to establish as well as possible the equivalence of groups (see Figure 7.3).

The second step is to pretest all participants regarding the dependent variable. If anxiety is the variable of interest, all

227

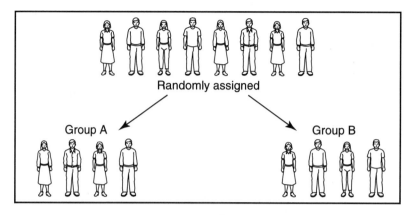

FIGURE 7.3 Random assignment

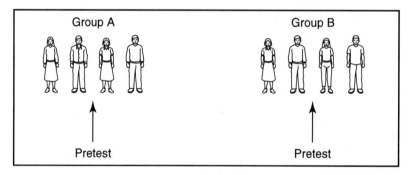

FIGURE 7.4 Pretesting

participants would respond to an instrument measuring anxiety (see Figure 7.4).

The third step is to expose the experimental group to the intervention (see Figure 7.5).

The fourth step is to posttest all participants on the dependent variable. The data collected are then statistically analyzed to determine whether the intervention produced a difference in the outcomes of the groups (see Figure 7.6).

A **pretest–posttest** comparison group design differs only in that some level of the intervention is given to each group. For example, three forms of relaxation therapy may be given, one to each group, and the effects of these therapies on anxiety compared. Another option is to provide different forms of the

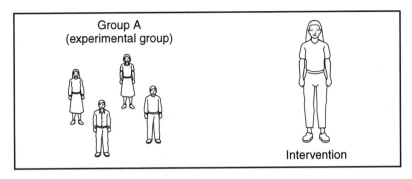

FIGURE 7.5 Intervention

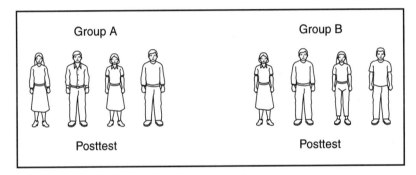

FIGURE 7.6 Posttesting

intervention to each group and include a control group as well. This research design would be termed a pretest–posttest control/comparison group design.

Another variation in the experiment occurs when participants are not pretested. Because the purpose of randomization is to equalize the groups under investigation, a pretest may not be necessary if the groups are sufficiently large (>15). This design would then be termed a posttest-only control group design.

The Quasi-experimental Design

Within nursing research, the randomization of participants to experimental and control groups is frequently not possible. There is a design, however, termed **quasi-experimental**, that permits a reasonable degree of control but does not adhere to the requirements of the experiments. Researchers who design quasi-experiments can feel more confident regarding the validity of their results than investigators who use preexperimental (descriptive) methods. They cannot, however, infer causality.

WORKING DEFINITION

The Quasi-experimental Design

Quasi-experimental designs require the manipulation of the independent variable but may lack randomization to the control group or may not have a control group.

Much of nursing research involves preexisting groups of patients whose members cannot be assigned to experimental and control groups. In order to conduct research with these individuals, the use of nonequivalent groups must be accepted. In some instances, a control group will not be used.

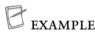

EXAMPLE

The Quasi-experimental Design

A group of nurse researchers decides to investigate the effects of a six-month nursing intervention that includes home visits on the quality of life of heart failure patients who present regularly to the emergency department for care. They measure quality of life at weekly intervals for two months before instituting the new regimen and measure quality of life in the same manner following the intervention. Differences in quality of life before and after the regimen are analyzed.

PRACTICE

The Quasi-experimental Design

A group of nurse researchers designs a study to examine the effects of an educational intervention aimed at assisting high school students to stop smoking. The researchers divide senior high school students into two groups, the control group and the experimental group (classes A, B, and C are in one group; classes D, E, and F are in the second group). The experimental group experiences the intervention; the control group does not. Smoking rates for both groups are measured before and after the intervention.

What makes this study quasi-experimental rather than experimental?

As with any research design, when evaluating a quasi-experimental design it is important to identify those factors that were not controlled and that could have influenced the outcome of the study. All research designs are flawed to some degree. The challenge for both the consumer and the individual assisting with the design of a project is to identify those factors outside of the study that could have been partially or completely responsible for the outcome.

CRITICAL APPRAISAL

Quasi-experimental Designs

When reviewing a quasi-experiment ask the following questions:

- Is there manipulation of the independent variable?

- If a control group is lacking, how might that omission have affected the results?

- If participants were not randomly assigned to an experimental group and a control group, how might the omission of that process have affected the results?

Nonexperimental Designs

Nonexperimental research is generally present-oriented; that is, it describes what exists at a given point in time. Data obtained are analyzed, and the results may lead to the formation of **hypotheses** that can then be tested experimentally. Variables are not deliberately manipulated, nor is the setting controlled. Within a quantitative framework, the observations are represented by numbers that can be statistically analyzed. Data are generally collected through the use of a questionnaire, interview, observation, literature review, or critical incident technique.

Nonexperimental research can provide a rich source of data that can be used to generate questions best answered by experimental designs. Areas of research interest that have not been examined in any depth may be best understood by conducting a descriptive study.

There are different kinds of nonexperimental, or what is frequently termed descriptive, research. Some investigators want to simply explore what exists (often termed *exploratory research*) and may ask questions like "What is the quality of life of individuals who have experienced their first surgery for colorectal cancer?" Other investigators may want to explain (often termed *explanatory research*) a particular phenomenon and ask "What is the difference in confidence level regarding nursing skills between nurse practitioners and clinical specialists?" Correlational designs are a third kind of nonexperimental design that is frequently used by nurses. Questions asked using this kind of design pose relationships; for example, investigators may ask, "What is the relationship between the extent of individuals' spiritual life and their overall well-being during the last six months of life?"

 WORKING DEFINITION

Nonexperimental

Nonexperimental research is generally present-oriented. It attempts to describe what exists. Variables are not deliberately manipulated, nor is the setting controlled. The analysis of data often leads to the formation of hypotheses that can then be tested experimentally.

A consideration when conducting or evaluating descriptive research is that the results cannot be generalized to the larger population.

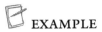

EXAMPLE

Nonexperimental

A group of nurse researchers decided to investigate the possibility that obese college women were suffering from depression. They enlisted the support of a campus weight reduction clinic and were able to administer a scale designed to measure depression to 45 female college students. They discovered that 87% of their participants were depressed.

The problems in using the findings in this example are obvious. Although the results may lend some credence to the investigator's belief that obesity and depression are related, many questions need to be raised. For example, what other factors at this particular college might be inducing depression among its students? Would nonobese female college students show an equally high rate of depression? Might the interventions used in this particular clinic influence depression?

PRACTICE

Nonexperimental

Two nurse researchers are interested in identifying the level of social support perceived by single pregnant adolescents in their last trimester. They want to identify the adolescents' perception of both the magnitude and the kind of support available.

What factors suggest that this study is descriptive in nature?

An important consideration when evaluating a descriptive study is to be certain that causation is not implied. The findings of these studies may be invaluable in building a base of knowledge; however, they do not possess the design characteristics necessary to attribute causation to a particular phenomenon.

CRITICAL APPRAISAL

Nonexperimental

When reviewing a nonexperimental study, ask the following questions:

- Are the findings inappropriately generalized to the larger population?

- Do the study findings provide information that can be useful in further examination of the particular area of interest?

- Are controls applied to the study to the greatest extent possible?

Key Concepts in Quantitative Designs

Three key concepts are related to the development of a quantitative research design. Depending on the design selected, the researcher needs to answer the following questions:

- What do you think will happen?
- What are you studying?
- How will you get your research participants?

The **hypothesis** answers the question, "What do you think will happen?" Hypotheses are formulated in experimental research. In some nonexperimental correlational studies, hypotheses may also be developed. For example, the researcher may believe that a strong correlation will be found between pain and anxiety among patients undergoing their first surgical procedure.

The question "What are you studying?" is answered by a careful and thorough description of the concepts under examination. These concepts are termed variables in research, and there are different kinds of variables, depending on the design of the study. Finally, the question of how participants will be identified is answered through an understanding of **sampling** methodology. To conduct an experiment the researcher must follow stringent rules for selecting a sample. The rules are less stringent for the investigator conducting nonexperimental research, although great care must still be taken in identifying participants for study.

Key Research Concepts

Hypothesis Formation

In many research designs, the investigators predict a particular outcome. They make an educated guess, or formulate a hypothesis, regarding the results of the study. The hypothesis succinctly suggests a relationship between or among variables and provides a focus for the research process. Hypotheses may be directional or nondirectional. A **directional hypothesis** predicts an outcome in a specific direction—for example, that participants in the experimental group will have less pain than participants in the control group. A **nondirectional hypothesis** simply states that there will be a difference between the two groups.

Other examples of hypotheses formulated by nurses as they designed research projects include the following:

- Children ages 5–12 who are provided with prior information about their tonsillectomy will experience less postoperative anxiety than children of the same age who do not receive information.

- Women ages 25–40 who are prone to experiencing migraine headaches report fewer headaches if they follow a regular regimen of relaxation therapy than women of the same age who have not followed the relaxation regimen.

- There will be a difference in the number of individuals diagnosed with depression between adult male aphasics who relate to others through a communication board (CB) and adult male aphasics who do not use a CB.

PRACTICE

Hypothesis Formation

Identify a research problem relevant to nursing practice and formulate one or more research hypotheses. For example, consider a problem that is often encountered with adolescent diabetics—their reluctance to adhere to dietary restrictions. Perhaps a group experience in which group members discussed their concerns about diet would help. Participants could be divided so that some experienced a group session and others did not. On the basis of this approach, a research hypothesis could be formulated.

CRITICAL APPRAISAL

Hypothesis Formation

- Does the research problem and design require the formation of a hypothesis or hypotheses?

- Are hypotheses clearly and succinctly stated?

Identifying Variables

When a concept has been defined and its method of measurement has been identified, it is referred to as a **variable**. For example, academic success—the ability to achieve in a university setting as measured by the student's grade point average—is a variable in a study investigating two different educational approaches to nursing.

Variables are differentiated on the basis of the part they play in a particular study. Independent variables are antecedents to other variables. An **independent variable** is perceived as contributing to or preceding a particular outcome. This outcome, or **dependent variable**, is the focus of the study and must be measured or assessed in some way.

When studying a relationship, the dependent variable is the consequence of a preceding (independent) variable. The dependent variable is thought to vary in relationship to the independent variable. The investigator identifies the focus of the study and, therefore, the dependent and independent variables. For example, a particular kind of nursing care for a decubitus ulcer is seen as preceding a change in the state of the ulcer. The nursing care in this example is the independent variable that affects the state of the ulcer, or dependent variable. Socioeconomic status may be an antecedent (independent variable) to certain attitudes toward health promotion (dependent variable). In an experimental or quasi-experimental design the independent variable is the variable that is manipulated in order to observe its effects on the dependent variable.

As an example, consider the hypothesis that states, "The social support available to new mothers is related to the length of their hospital stay." Social support in this case could be considered an independent variable. It is the social support that is being used (manipulated) to discover its effect on the length of hospital stay. The length of the new mothers' hospital stay is considered the dependent variable or focus of this study.

In this study, an intervention is designed to provide social support to one group of mothers immediately after birth. Another group of mothers does not experience the intervention, and all mothers are assessed as to their length of stay in the hospital. The social support intervention is used (manipulated) by the investigators to determine its effect on the length of stay in hospital. This manipulation of a variable (social support) in order to determine its effect on another variable (length of stay in hospital) identifies social support as the independent variable.

It is important to understand that there is nothing about a variable that causes it to be inherently independent or dependent. The use of the variable is the important factor. For example, another group of nurse investigators formulate the following hypothesis: "Conveying information about the normal grieving process to bereaved individuals enables them to increase their social support" (Figure 7.7). In this study, an intervention is designed to convey information about the normal grieving process to one group of bereaved individuals. Another group of bereaved individuals does not experience the

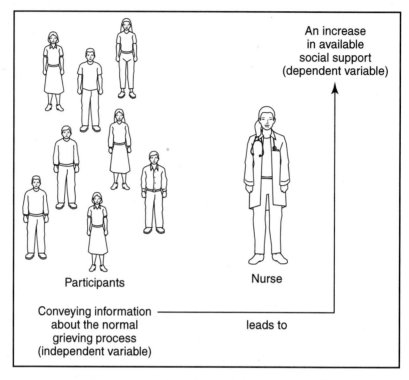

FIGURE 7.7   Independent and dependent variables

intervention. The effects on social support are measured for all bereaved individuals in the study. In this instance, the intervention designed to provide the participants with information on grieving is the independent variable. Social support in this study is the dependent variable.

WORKING DEFINITION

Independent and Dependent Variables

The independent variable (often referred to in an experimental or quasi-experimental study as the experimental or treatment variable) is an antecedent to other variables. In an experiment

238

or quasi-experiment, it is the variable that is manipulated, and its effect on the dependent variable is observed.

The dependent variable represents the area of interest under investigation. It reflects the effect of or the response to the independent variable.

 EXAMPLE

Independent and Dependent Variables

A group of nurse investigators formulate the following hypothesis: "Female clients diagnosed with schizophrenia who attend a support group on a weekly basis will adhere to their medication regimen better than female schizophrenics who do not attend a support group."

Independent variable: The variable that is manipulated in this study is the support group. It is the effect of this variable on the clients' adherence to their medication regimens that is under consideration.

Dependent variable: The variable being examined in the study is the adherence to medication regimens.

 PRACTICE

Independent and Dependent Variables

From the following research questions, identify the independent and dependent variables:

- Is there a relationship between family discord and adolescent suicide attempts?

- Is the degree of personal control experienced by elderly nursing home residents related to their overall satisfaction with the facility?

- What is the relationship between length of stay in an institution for the mentally ill and ability to function independently in the community?

CRITICAL APPRAISAL

Independent and Dependent Variables

- Is the independent variable adequately specified?

- Is the dependent variable adequately specified?

Defining Terms

Variables under study must be described clearly so that consumers of research understand the process used to arrive at conclusions. The dependent variable—the variable of interest—is defined so that readers know how data was collected. Two kinds of definitions are generally required: (1) a dictionary or conceptual definition and (2) an **operational definition**. A conceptual definition conveys the investigator's perspective on a given concept but is not sufficient because it does not specify how the variable is to be measured—that is, the specific steps the researcher must take in order to gather the required information. For example, in the hypothesis "An educational program on hypertension will increase patient compliance with medication schedules," **compliance** is a variable that must be defined. The dictionary or conceptual definition of *compliance* is "a tendency to give in readily to others" (*Webster's New World Dictionary*, 1984). This definition does not assist the consumer to understand how compliance is measured in the study. The operational definition of *compliance*, "as measured by the percentage of prescribed medication taken over a one-month period," describes the specific meaning of compliance within the project. The operational definition of a variable defines it narrowly, resulting in increased objectivity in observation and precision in measurement.

WORKING DEFINITION

Operational Definition

An operational definition assigns meaning to a variable and describes the activities required to measure it.

In those studies in which paper-and-pencil tests are used, operational definitions frequently include the name of the specific test chosen to measure the variable in question. For example, an operational definition of *anxiety* might be "as measured by the XYZ Anxiety Inventory."

EXAMPLE

Operational Definition

A group of nurse researchers decide to examine the effect of patient-controlled analgesia on cancer patients' physical activity level. They operationally define *activity level* as the score on the Brown Physical Activity Inventory.

PRACTICE

Operational Definition

In each of the following examples, formulate an operational definition and a dictionary or conceptual definition for the italicized variables.

- What is the effect of relaxation therapy on *pain* experienced following abdominal surgery?

- What is the effect of preabortion counseling on the *incidence of postabortion emotional trauma*?

- What is the relationship between *state anxiety* and *quality of life* among women diagnosed with breast cancer?

241

CRITICAL APPRAISAL

Operational Definition

Does the operational definition specify the method for measuring the variable?

There are other variables in addition to the independent and dependent variables that can have an undesirable effect on a particular study. These variables are termed extraneous (Figure 7.8). **Extraneous variables** are relevant to the area under study but are not the focus of the study. They cannot be ignored because they can influence the outcome of the investigation. In the study in which an intervention was designed to provide social support for mothers immediately after birth and then to measure its effect on length of hospital stay, marital status might be an extraneous variable. Whether or not a woman was married might affect the length of hospital stay, quite apart from the social support that was provided following birth. Marital status in this case is a confounding variable in that it could confound (confuse) the results.

The most common extraneous variables are those that relate to the characteristics of the participants in the study. Polit and

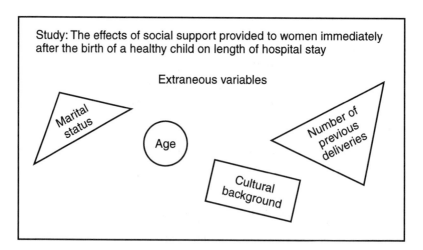

FIGURE 7.8 Extraneous variables

Hungler (1999) have identified six methods for controlling extraneous variables related to subject characteristics: (1) ensuring that subjects are homogeneous in relation to variables considered extraneous (e.g., studying only married or unmarried mothers in the study previously described); (2) including the extraneous variables as independent variables (e.g., studying the effect of marriage on length of hospital stay); (3) matching subjects in relation to extraneous variables (e.g., the same number of married and unmarried mothers in experimental and control groups); (4) using statistical procedures to control undesirable variables; (5) randomly assigning subjects to experimental and control groups; and (6) using a repeated measures design.

Neither the statistical procedures used to control extraneous variables nor the repeated measures design is described here. Interested readers can consult advanced texts on statistics and design. The important point for the beginning researcher to understand is that efforts can be made to control extraneous variables.

 WORKING DEFINITION

Extraneous Variable

Extraneous variables are those variables that can influence the relationship between the independent and dependent variables. They must be controlled through statistical analysis or research design.

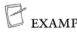 EXAMPLE

Extraneous Variable

Two community health nurses formulate the following hypothesis in preparation for designing a study: "Prenatal nutrition classes have a positive effect on the dietary habits of mothers after delivery."

Extraneous variable: A possible extraneous variable in this study is the kind of delivery experienced by each of these subjects. The mother who has experienced an emergency cesarean section may not be as likely to spend as much time and energy on dietary concerns as the mother who has a normal vaginal delivery and feels well immediately following the birth.

 PRACTICE

Extraneous Variable

A group of nurse researchers is interested in examining the problem of obesity among female preadolescents. They believe that repeated unsuccessful attempts to lose weight lead to a decline in self-esteem. They identify their population of interest as young women ages 8 through 11 who are 20 pounds or more overweight and who have made three or more structured attempts to lose weight (e.g., following a planned diet, attending a weight loss group). They plan to measure self-esteem through a paper-and-pencil self-report questionnaire.

Identify factors (extraneous variables) in addition to the attempts to lose weight that could influence the scores on the self-esteem questionnaire.

 CRITICAL APPRAISAL

Extraneous Variable

Are the extraneous variables identified or taken into account in the design of the study?

 ## Sample Selection: Choosing Participants

Probability Sampling

When planning a study, researchers designate a population—that is, a group of persons or objects that meet specific criteria.

The population of interest may be anorectic females of a given age, newborn males, elderly residents of nursing homes, or—in the case of objects—particular devices for measuring physiological processes. The participants who are chosen from a particular population for a research project are called a **sample**. The usual purpose in selecting a sample is to gather and analyze data from a small group so that findings can then be generalized to the larger population. If generalizations are to be made, the sample must represent the larger population as closely as possible. The selection strategy most useful in assuring that the sample is representative of the larger population is the process of random selection.

The process of random selection is based on probability theory—that is, the possibility that events occur by chance. The probability of selection is the same for each individual in a randomly selected sample. Random sampling is in fact often termed probability sampling. The advantages of using probability sampling are: (1) statistical techniques can be applied that will show to what degree the sample actually represents the population, (2) an unconscious bias toward selecting a particular segment of the population can be avoided, and (3) an appropriate sample size can be statistically derived (Munro, 2001).

 WORKING DEFINITION

Population

The population is the entire group of persons or objects that is of interest to the investigator. The population is often designated by specific criteria such as age, sex, and illness state.

 WORKING DEFINITION

Sample

The sample is a subset of the population selected by the investigator to participate in a research project.

245

WORKING DEFINITION

Random Sampling

Random sampling is a selection process that ensures each participant the same probability of being selected. Random sampling is the best method for ensuring that a sample is representative of the larger population.

To randomly select a sample, investigators take the following steps:

1. They define the population.
2. They calculate the sample size.
3. They assign a number to each participant (unit) in the population (or use numbers that are already assigned, e.g., social security numbers).
4. They use a table of random numbers (see Table 7.1) to select the desired number of participants. Alternatively, numbers can be pulled from a hat, or cards containing the numbers can be shuffled thoroughly and then the desired number of participants drawn. When a name or number is drawn it is coded and replaced to ensure that each participant has an equal chance of being chosen on each selection. Random assignment tables can also be generated by computer.

To use a table of random numbers, the following procedure is suggested (see also Figure 7.9):

1. Arbitrarily select a column from the table.

◈ TABLE 7.1 A Table of Random Numbers

13	45	78	75	32	09	21	10	27
26	24	99	06	55	20	01	89	72
75	17	83	62	12	56	39	48	36

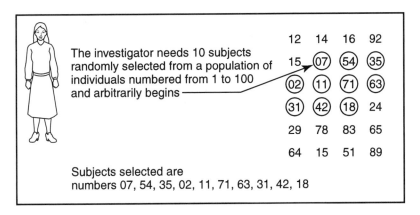

FIGURE 7.9 Random sampling

2. With eyes closed, select a number in that column.

3. Beginning with the number selected, continue in a systematic fashion (choose a direction—horizontal, diagonal, etc.) to select the desired number of participants.

4. If a number occurs within a column that is not represented in the population, exclude that number and move to the next.

The procedure described here is termed **simple random sampling**. Depending on the particular area of investigation, there are two additional methods of random sampling that can be used: stratified random sampling and cluster sampling.

Stratified random sampling describes a method in which the investigator defines the population to be studied and then identifies areas of interest (strata) that run across the population. For example, if the area of study is cancer, areas of interest may include several diagnoses of cancer—leukemia, Hodgkins, lymphoma, and so on. The investigator randomly samples a number of participants from each diagnosis (stratum). The number of participants in each stratum should reflect the distribution of that particular diagnosis in the population under study (the percentage of leukemia patients among all cancer patients, etc.).

In some instances in which the distribution of cases within the population under study provides too few cases to draw meaningful conclusions, a disproportionate number of cases may be selected. For example, in the study of cancer using

247

diagnostic labels, if only two cases of lymphoma represented the proportion of that diagnosis within the population, as opposed to 50 in other diagnostic categories, additional cases of lymphoma would need to be added. A process of weighting is used to identify the exact number of cases to be added.

Cluster sampling is often used when natural groupings occur within the population under study. If investigators wish to study all cancer patients across the country, they may identify groups (clusters) of cancer hospitals in various regions of the country. A sample of cancer hospitals could then be drawn, from which a sample of patients could ultimately be selected.

 EXAMPLE

Random Sampling

A group of nurse investigators design a study to examine the effect of an educational package on the prevention of AIDS on grade 9 students in their community. Each grade 9 student in the eight local schools is given a number from 1 through 317. Using a table of random numbers, a sample of 72 students is selected.

There are two occasions when the concept of probability is used in relation to participant selection. The sample that is selected from the larger population can be randomly selected to represent that population. In addition, the participants, once selected, can be "randomized" to either the control or the experimental group.

 PRACTICE

Random Sampling

Identify an area of interest within nursing practice and the population to be studied. Outline a method for selecting a random sample from that population.

CRITICAL APPRAISAL

Random Sampling

- If random sampling was used, has the process been described?

- Are there any factors related to the process that may have caused the sample to be biased (nonrepresentative of the larger group)?

Nonprobability Sampling

In nursing research, it is frequently impossible to make a random selection of a sample from a given population. For example, it is unlikely that nurse investigators who wish to study the effects of primary nursing care versus team nursing care on adult inpatients can randomly select a sample of inpatients to experience the intervention. There are too many factors that influence patient placement on specific units, and therefore the researchers would probably compare units that are similar in nature (surgical, medical, etc.). The participants studied probably would not represent all inpatients in the hospital.

Accidental (convenience), **quota**, and **purposive** sampling are methods used by investigators when random sampling is not possible. An accidental or convenience sample is obtained by selecting those participants that are readily available. Asking individuals at a shopping mall to respond to a health care questionnaire would be an example of selecting an accidental or convenience sample.

Quota sampling refers to a selection process in which the investigator imposes a set of criteria on the selection procedure. For example, nurse investigators studying the psychosocial needs of patients suffering from a particular chronic debilitating illness may be aware that the ratio of men to women suffering from the disease is 4:1. The investigators will then choose four men to every woman in selecting their sample.

Purposive sampling requires the investigators to make judgments regarding the selection of participants. If a given institution is known for its effectiveness in a particular area, practitioners in that institution may be selected for study.

249

Depending on the procedure used, **systematic sampling** can be classified as either probability or nonprobability sampling. Systematic sampling refers to a process in which the investigator chooses a number and selects a sample based on that number (every *n*th subject). For example, an investigator decides to study the relationship between scores on college entrance exams and the grade point average of graduating nurses from three university programs. Instead of using a table of random numbers, the investigator selects every tenth (or fifth, or eleventh, etc.) individual to be involved in the study.

Systematic sampling can be a problem if the lists used are not homogeneous in nature. If, for instance, all of the male students are grouped on the lists in such a way that they would be missed completely by choosing every tenth individual, then the sample selection is not truly representative of the larger population.

To use systematic sampling so that a random sample is drawn, you divide the size of the population by the size of the sample. This number is termed the *sampling interval*. You randomly select the first element (subject) using a random table of numbers, and then select other elements based on the sampling interval.

For example, if the population is 400 and the sample size is 80, the sampling interval is 5. Starting with a randomly selected number (e.g., 12), the next four subjects would be numbers 17, 22, 27, and 32.

 WORKING DEFINITION

Nonprobability Sampling

Nonprobability sampling is a selection process in which the probability that any one individual may be selected is not equal to the probability that another individual may be chosen. The probability of inclusion and the degree to which the sample represents the population are unknown.

A major problem with nonprobability sampling is that there is little confidence that the sample will truly represent the larger population. When a sample does not represent the larger population, *sampling bias* is said to have occurred. When sampling bias exists, generalizations from sample to population are questionable.

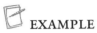

EXAMPLE

Nonprobability Sampling

In a neonatal intensive care unit, a group of nurse investigators design a study to examine the effect of open visitation for parents on the bonding between father and child. They select all those families who have a child on the unit within a specified period of time (one month).

CRITICAL APPRAISAL

Nonprobability Sampling

Are generalizations made that are not warranted given the sampling procedure used?

Validity in Relation to the Research Design

There are two kinds of validity related to research design: internal and external validity. **Internal validity** refers to whether the independent variable actually made a difference. Did the intervention or treatment lead to the results or were the results a response to extraneous variables?

Seven extraneous variables have been identified that can negatively affect the internal validity of the research design. According to Campbell and Stanley (1966), history, maturation, testing, instrumentation, statistical regression, differential selection bias, and experimental mortality can jeopardize the

251

internal validity of the research design. Using the example of a research project in which nurse investigators are examining the effect of an educational package on the willingness of teenage diabetics to comply with a healthy diet, the following factors could affect the internal validity of the study:

History: If a group of teenage diabetics describe their diet before the educational package and then again six weeks after the intervention, an occurrence within that period of time may have had more effect on their compliance than the educational package. For example, if examinations were given during that period, they might not have had the usual opportunities to get out to eat and therefore stray from their diets.

Maturation: If the teenagers are at different maturational levels, the realization that their future health may be dependent on their present activities may influence the more mature individuals to comply, even without the educational package.

Testing: The act of having to write down everything they eat before the educational package is presented may have an effect on the compliance of the teenagers, without their ever taking part in the educational offering.

Statistical regression: If a score were given to each participant based on the degree of compliance and a group was chosen because they rarely complied with their diets (and thus had extremely low scores), their scores on the second compliance test would tend to be higher. There is a tendency for scores at either extreme to move closer to the mean or average score. This phenomenon is termed *regression toward the mean.*

Selection bias: If the teenagers were not randomly assigned to their groups, a number of biases could be introduced into the study. A group of particularly passive individuals certainly could be more compliant because of their personalities rather than the intervention. Similarly, a group of teenagers whose major interest is losing weight might comply with the diet for that reason rather than as a response to the intervention.

Experimental mortality: If the teenagers are randomly selected and then assigned to a control and an experimental group, some of the participants may drop out of the study before it is completed. The loss of these participants can influence the accuracy of the results and bias the findings in a particular direction.

These extraneous variables can seriously affect the internal validity of a study. The definition and possible effects of each variable are presented in Table 7.2.

External validity refers to the extent to which the results of a study can be generalized to the larger population. Threats to external validity include both population and ecological factors. Results of a study can only be generalized to a population that possesses the same (or similar) characteristics as the sample studied. A specific intervention may be effective with one age and not another, one sex and not the other, and so on. Ecological factors that can jeopardize external validity refer to the conditions under which the research was conducted. For example, the fact that participants are involved in a study may in and of itself affect the outcome. In addition, the time of day or year, together with the particular setting in which the study was conducted, may affect the outcome.

Critical Overview of Quantitative Designs in Research

A group of nurse investigators are interested in designing a study to evaluate three different approaches to providing prenatal care through education to third world immigrants. One approach is a large group lecture using audiovisual aids; one approach uses a small group discussion format without visual aids; and the third is a small group format using visual aids.

◈ TABLE 7.2   Threats to Internal Validity

Factor	Definition	Possible effects
History	Events occurring from the beginning of data collection to its completion	Occurrences during the period of data collection can influence the results of the study.
Maturation	The developmental stage of participants	Differences in development among participants may influence the results of the study.
Testing	The effect of taking a pretest on the posttest	The actual process of responding to an instrument may influence the results of the test.
Statistical regression	The tendency of scores that represent either end of a continuum to move toward the mean on repeated tests	If participants are asked to respond to an instrument on more than one occasion, the scores at either end of the continuum are likely to regress toward the mean regardless of the influence of the intervention.
Selection	Nonrandom formation of groups	Without random assignment, a particular characteristic may be introduced to the sample that can influence the results of the study.
Experimental mortality	The loss of participants during a study	The loss of participants can influence the results of a study even though the sample was randomly selected—the responses of lost subjects could have influenced the results of the study in a different direction.

CRITICAL OVERVIEW
QUANTITATIVE DESIGNS IN
RESEARCH

Activity 1

- Formulate an appropriate hypothesis (or hypotheses) for this study.
- Operationally define prenatal care.
- Identify the dependent and independent variables.

Activity 2

- Briefly outline an appropriate design for the prenatal care study.
- Comment on each of the seven threats to internal validity.
- Comment on the two factors governing external validity in relation to the prenatal care study.

References

Campbell, D. & Stanley, J. (1966). *Experimental and quasi-experimental designs for research,* rev. ed. Chicago: Rand McNally.

Ferrell, B. & McCaffery, M. (1997). Nurses' knowledge about equianalgesic and opioid dosing. *Cancer Nursing, 20*(3):201–212.

Munro, B. (2001). *Statistical Methods for Health Care Research.* New York: Lippincott.

Polit, D. F. & Hungler, B. P. (1999). *Nursing research: Principles and methods* (6th Edition). Philadelphia: J. B. Lippincott.

Webster's New World Dictionary of the American Language. (1984). David B. Guralnik, editor in chief. New York: New World Dictionaries/Simon and Schuster.

Bibliography

Cozby, P. C. (2000). *Methods in Behavioral Research* (7th Edition). Toronto: Mayfield Publishing Co.

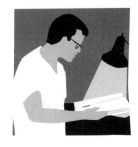

8

Epidemiologic Research

Goals

- *Describe the purpose of epidemiology.*
- *Describe major concepts of epidemiologic research.*
- *Analyze the key elements of epidemiologic research.*
- *Analyze differences in epidemiologic research as compared to other kinds of quantitative research approaches.*

Introduction

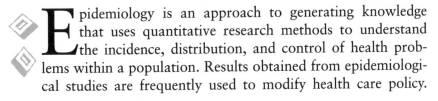

Epidemiology is an approach to generating knowledge that uses quantitative research methods to understand the incidence, distribution, and control of health problems within a population. Results obtained from epidemiological studies are frequently used to modify health care policy.

Classical epidemiology is concerned with observing and hypothesizing. Clinical epidemiology focuses on intervening and improving. Together these two components form an investigative branch of health care that seeks to examine and address major health care problems (Streiner & Norman, 1996).

Epidemiologic studies can be categorized as observational or experimental. *Observational studies* include cohort, case control, cross-sectional, and ecological designs. The two most common *experimental designs* are the randomized controlled trial and the cross-over design.

An example of a *cohort* study is when a group of individuals who smoke and a group of individuals who do not smoke are followed in order to assess a number of health outcomes. *Case control* approaches involve assessing participants who represent a given outcome, such as determining which individuals who have been diagnosed with AIDS had unprotected sex. *Cross-sectional* studies are designed to examine an outcome, such as hypertension and exposure to a predisposing factor at the same time. *Ecological designs* are used to identify different rates of an outcome by geographic area. For example, researchers might want to know how many cases of a particular disease (e.g., childhood leukemia) are present in a given county or state. In addition to these designs, epidemiologists also conduct *methodological* studies in order to produce psychometrically sound instruments to measure variables of interest.

Randomized controlled trials are used to test a particular intervention/treatment relative to a health care concern. These studies require strict adherence to the principles of experimental research. *Cross-over* designs are similar to randomized controlled trials except that both the control and experimental groups receive the treatment and the placebo. In the usual trial only the experimental group receives the treatment.

There are three major concepts related to epidemiology that are important to understand: population health, causation, and risk. Although the methods used in epidemiology are similar to methods used in any quantitative research project, epidemiology has its own focus and overall concerns.

258

Population Health

The health of populations is the focus of epidemiology. The population is the group of individuals for whom the results will be applicable. Populations are generally very large so epidemiologists study a subset or sample that represents the population. This subset or sample is often called a *cohort*. A cohort is a group of people who share a common attribute, for example, age.

WORKING DEFINITION

Cohort

The term *cohort*, as it relates to epidemiologic research, is a group of individuals who share a common attribute. For example, age, belonging to a specific group (e.g., an experimental group in a clinical trial), or sharing a specific diagnosis, can result in referring to that group as a cohort.

EXAMPLE

Cohort

A nurse researcher examines the effect of an educational program on the immunization behaviors of parents in a specific geographical region. A cohort of parents selected on the basis of their health beliefs experience the intervention. The common characteristic shared by these parents is that they believe in immunization, even though they may not follow through with immunizing their children.

PRACTICE

Cohort

From your reading of the literature, select five cohorts and the attribute that makes them an identifiable group.

259

Epidemiologists assess the health of populations, plan interventions to address health problems, and evaluate the interventions used. These studies have identified new syndromes and their causes (e.g., toxic shock syndrome), changes in known diseases (e.g., treatment-resistant tuberculosis), risks of health problems (e.g., environmental pollutants), and effects of treatments (e.g., lumpectomy vs. mastectomy among breast cancer patients). Epidemiology also identifies health service needs and trends. Overall, the purpose of epidemiology is to estimate the relationship between exposure and outcome and to try, where possible, to ascertain causation.

 WORKING DEFINITION

Population Health

The health of populations is the major focus of epidemiology. A population may be defined by age, gender, race, socioeconomic status, or other similar descriptors.

 EXAMPLE

Population Health

Given a concern that childhood diseases were on the increase in rural areas, a group of nurse epidemiologists examined the percentage of infants in Appalachia who receive appropriate immunizations.

This data could provide a foundation for interventions that might diminish the incidence of childhood diseases. For example, if a large number of children are not being immunized, educational programs might increase immunization activities.

 PRACTICE

Population Health

Identify an epidemiological study and the population it addresses. Describe the characteristics of that population.

Populations addressed in epidemiological studies may have age, a specific disease entity, and/or a particular lifestyle (e.g., eating habits) as a common factor. Outcomes of these studies are aimed at improving the health of the identified population.

CRITICAL APPRAISAL

Population Health

- Is the study focused on a particular health care issue within a specified population?

- Are the characteristics of the population clearly described?

- Are desired health care outcomes evident?

Causation

Within epidemiology, causes are frequently grouped under the following headings: lifestyle issues, environmental factors, genetic factors, and weaknesses within the health care system. Lifestyle issues such as smoking, overeating, or leading a stressful or sedentary life can lead to serious health problems. Similarly, pollutants and genetic predispositions can cause disease. The health care system, if it does not effectively address health care concerns, can also lead to increased disease.

WORKING DEFINITION

Causation

Causation within the epidemiological framework refers to the degree to which we can suggest that a particular cause or set of causes leads to a particular outcome.

It is important to note that most health problems, even diseases once thought to have one cause, are the result of multiple causes. It is also important to understand that no one criterion can provide a strong case for causation. We need to meet a number of criteria in order to validate causation. Even then, changes in notions regarding causality may occur.

 EXAMPLE

Causation

A nurse epidemiologist completes an intervention study investigating the effect of diet change on the incidence of second cardiac events among older adults in one Midwestern region. She is able to apply five of the nine causation criteria (see Table 8.1) to her findings and thus concludes that the change in diet contributed to a decrease in second cardiac events.

 PRACTICE

Causation

Find an epidemiological intervention study and identify how many criteria for causation are available.

 CRITICAL APPRAISAL

Causation

- If causation is implied in a report, have several criteria been met?

- Are multiple causes considered?

To determine whether there is a cause-and-effect relationship between an exposure and an outcome, a number of studies must be evaluated. For example, if you were interested in trying to determine if use of Hormone Replacement Therapy (HRT) causes breast cancer, research that has addressed this issue would be evaluated to determine whether the relative risk of developing cancer among women who use HRT is statistically significantly. If there is a significant association, the researcher considers the extent to which biases and confounding variables have been eliminated by the studies, as well as the reason for elevated risk.

If there is no association between an exposure and an outcome, there is little reason to evaluate causation. If there is an association, the researcher needs to ask: Is the magnitude of the relationship meaningful? If it is determined that a significant relative risk exists and that it is not likely the result of bias or confounding variables, further evaluation of the relationship should be done. The nine criteria proposed by Sir Austin Bradford-Hill (Hill, 1965) can be used to determine the existence of a cause-and-effect relationship. Table 8.1 describes Bradford-Hill criteria for determining the existence of a cause-and-effect relationship and explains each criterion.

The researcher can answer the question of whether use of HRT causes breast cancer in women by analyzing the data across various studies and using appropriate statistical outcomes to evaluate risk.

The question that needs to be asked is, "Is the evidence good enough to allow the drawing of causal inferences from the data?" At present, there is not enough evidence to say that use of HRT causes breast cancer. There is, however, some evidence that use beyond five years may be associated with the development of breast cancer. When reviewing evidence in an attempt to determine the strength of an association, it is important to consider the influence of biases or confounding factors. A meta-analysis of all studies pertaining to the area of interest helps to ascertain the strength of a given relationship. Using specified guidelines such as the Bradford-Hill Criteria (see page 264) reviewers can delineate information from a number of studies and come to a conclusion regarding the strength of the association.

TABLE 8.1   Bradford-Hill Criteria for
Determining Cause-Effect Relationships

Criterion	Example
Strength of the association	If the specific relationship between cause and effect is strong (e.g., height and weight) the overall relationship is likely to be strong. The larger the risk, the more likely it is not due to bias.
Consistency of the association	The relationship between the perceived cause and effect should be apparent across a number of studies. The same result has been repeatedly observed in different groups and studied in different ways by different investigators.
Study's specificity	In an ideal world, one cause would lead to one outcome. When this phenomenon occurs a powerful argument for causality can be made. Unfortunately, life is usually more complicated than a one-to-one relationship.
Temporal relationship	We tend to think that factor A must precede factor B if A has caused B. Sometimes we believe that a particular event/virus/bacteria causes a chronic condition when perhaps a genetic predisposition is the actual cause. Temporality, therefore, is an important issue in supporting causation. An exposure cannot cause a disease unless the exposure precedes the onset of the disease. Two issues here: 1) When was the exposure? and 2) When was the disease diagnosed?
Biologic gradient	The biologic gradient suggests that if more exposure to a causal factor leads to more severe disease, then causation is strengthened (i.e., does the risk of disease rise with increasing duration of exposure or dose?).
Biologic plausibility	If the finding makes sense from a biological perspective, causation is enhanced. The findings fit the known biology of the disease, providing a physiologic explanation.
Coherence	If findings do not conflict with present knowledge about the specific area, causation is strengthened. Do all the data reasonably fit together?
Evidence from experiments	If randomized controlled trials have provided similar findings, causation is strengthened.
Analogy	Analogies are weak criteria at best. If we find a cause of a disease that fits in a particular category of disease then we might assume that the same cause will be appropriate for other diseases in that category.

Meta-analysis

Meta-analyses are often conducted on topics that have been researched in some depth. A meta-analysis involves an examination of studies conducted in a particular area to try to better understand the overall outcomes of available research. Criteria are usually developed regarding the research methods used. For example, the author of a meta-analysis may only review randomized controlled trials. Judgments need to be made as to whether the criteria limit the information gained from prior research. It is particularly important when research influences treatment that all available research is reviewed before conclusions are drawn. The results of an individual study may suggest one variation on treatment while a review of all research may show that the particular variation is not efficacious. Thus, when all the appropriately selected studies are analyzed together, the larger analysis can be helpful in clinical decision making and can sometimes avoid the need for larger studies.

WORKING DEFINITION

Meta-analysis

Meta-analysis is a technique where the findings from several small clinical trials are analyzed together. Although the findings from each study alone may not be powerful enough to allow for decisions affecting clinical practice, when analyzed together, the findings may be much more powerful.

EXAMPLE

Meta-analysis

Eight clinical trials are located that have examined exposure to video games and Attention Deficit Hyperactivity Disorder (ADHD) in children. The findings from these studies are analyzed together and it is determined that there is no statistically significant increase in the RR.

265

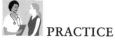

PRACTICE

Meta-analysis

Search the literature for a published meta-analysis report. Make a chart listing the studies that were examined in the meta-analysis. Detail the main finding from each study and the final conclusion drawn from the meta-analysis.

CRITICAL APPRAISAL

Meta-analysis

- Are the studies included in the meta-analysis clearly identified?

- Is there clear discussion on why studies were included in the analysis?

- Were the individual study findings similar to the findings from the meta-analysis?

- Does the weight of the evidence from the meta-analysis lead to the conclusion that there is a cause-and-effect association?

Risk

Epidemiology has contributed a great deal to the identification of risks to health. Investigators have found that exposure to some noxious agents lead to health problems. They have also shown that exposures often believed to cause problems are not responsible for suspected outcomes. For example, studies have shown that smoking, nitrates in food, a diet high in cholesterol, and exposure to a number of chemicals can lead to serious health problems. They have also discovered that previously considered noxious agents such as formaldehyde foam insulation, video display terminals, and silicone breast implants do not pose a serious risk.

Identification of risk factors can lead to effective identification and treatment of health problems. Probably the most important factor related to the identification of risk is that preventive measures can be suggested when risk is clear.

WORKING DEFINITION

Risk

Risk within the framework of epidemiology refers to the possibility of developing a health problem.

EXAMPLE

Risk

A group of nurse epidemiologists are interested in the effect of smoking on lung disease among young adults. They plan a five-year study to examine smoking habits within this population and diagnoses of lung disease. After five years, if the study is well designed, data from this research may support the notion that young adults who smoke are at risk for lung disease.

PRACTICE

Risk

Identify five health problems and the known risks associated with them.

CRITICAL APPRAISAL

Risk

What evidence supports the notion that a particular factor poses a risk?

267

Incidence and Prevalence

For purposes of epidemiological research, morbidity often refers to anything that can disable an individual or categorize a person as having a health problem. This expanded definition would include diseases, injuries of all types, accidents, and so on. *Incidence* is a means by which we measure morbidity. This measure tells us how many new cases of an illness or other event occurred within a given period of time. For example, since the first case of AIDS was diagnosed it has been extremely important to understand the incidence of this dis-ease in various parts of the world for specific time periods. This information enables us to better deal with the disease, develop prevention models, and prepare for the future.

Prevalence is another measure of morbidity. Whereas inci-dence reflects new cases in a population, prevalence reflects all morbidity in a given population. Point prevalence refers to all cases at a given point in time; period prevalence refers to cases within a particular period.

WORKING DEFINITION

Incidence

Incidence is a mathematical reflection of the number of cases of a health problem in a given population. The term inci-dence describes the number of new cases within a specific time period.

EXAMPLE

Incidence

A nurse investigator interested in the increase in diagnoses of tuberculosis compares the number of new cases in the present year with the incidence of tuberculosis or the number of new cases diagnosed over the past five years.

268

WORKING DEFINITION

Prevalence

Prevalence is a mathematical reflection of the number of cases of a health problem in a given population. The term prevalence describes all cases of a health problem in a population.

EXAMPLE

Prevalence

A nurse investigator interested in the increase in diagnoses of tuberculosis examines the number of all cases of tuberculosis in the population during the present year.

PRACTICE

Prevalence

Identify a health care problem and calculate or find the prevalence of the particular problem in your geographical area.

CRITICAL APPRAISAL

Prevalence

- Is prevalence correctly calculated?
- Is this concept appropriately used?

 Rates and Ratios

Rates and ratios are measures of frequency that are commonly used in epidemiology to characterize data collected. A *ratio* is the relationship in quantity, amount, or size between two or more things. A *rate* is a fixed ratio between two things. Attack rates are a specific kind of rate that reflects the number of individuals who develop a health care problem in relation to the number who were exposed. Adjusted rates reflect the number of cases of a health problem in a population, taking into account a descriptor of that population. For example, certain occurrences (death, certain diseases) may occur more frequently at one age than another. The population will therefore be described in terms of number of cases at a given age.

For example, we may want to know the number of teenage girls who smoke in relation to all of the girls in the high school (ratio—number of girls who smoke divided by the total number of girls in the high school). If we wanted to know how many teenage girls smoked in relation to all high school students, we would have a proportion (girls who smoke divided by all high school students). A rate is determined when we want to know how many teenage girls among the total number of girls in a high school smoked in a particular year.

Epidemiologists frequently describe their findings in terms of the following ratios: relative risk (RR), attributable risk (AR) and/or relative odds (RO). The *RR* refers to the likelihood that a target event (e.g., disease or death) will occur in individuals exposed and not exposed to the agent of interest (e.g., an environmental pollutant). The rate of disease in the exposed group is divided by the rate of disease in the unexposed group. If the relative risk is above 1.0, then there is a positive association between the exposure and the disease; if it is less than 1.0, then there is a negative association. The larger the risk, the more likely it is not due to bias. The *AR* describes the increase in the target event (e.g., death) attributed to the cause (environmental pollutant). The *RO* is used when case-control studies are conducted. In this instance, epidemiologists want to examine situations in which the likelihood of developing a particular disease is low or there is a long latency period before the disease is clinically apparent. A group of individuals who have the disease are matched with individuals who do not, and their exposure to risk factors is assessed. Risk factors are calculated for both groups and a ratio is determined. The RO is only an approximation of the RR.

WORKING DEFINITION

Rates and Ratios

Rates and ratios are numerical representations of data collected by epidemiologists. They describe population parameters of interest and assist with the determination of risk and causation.

EXAMPLE

Rates and Ratios

Nurse epidemiologists examine the effect of a statewide smoking cessation educational program on the number of new smokers ages 14 to 18. They calculate an attributable risk ratio that reflects the decrease (or increase) that can be attributed to the educational program.

PRACTICE

Rates and Ratios

From your reading of the literature, find a rate or ratio and discuss the meaning within the context of the study.

CRITICAL APPRAISAL

Rates and Ratios

- Have ratios and rates been calculated correctly?
- Do the calculations provide useful information?

Frequently Used Concepts in Epidemiology

The concepts described below may be a part of any quantitative research project. The underlying issues when conducting research remain the same—how do we describe events related to a population using a subset of that population in the most accurate manner?

Statistical Estimates: Confidence Intervals

Epidemiologists often use confidence intervals to describe their findings. A confidence interval identifies the population mean within certain limits. Those limits are traditionally set as 95% or 99%. For example, if a researcher wants to know the survival rates of individuals with end stage AIDS, they will calculate a confidence interval based on their data; the result could be a range of months or weeks. The numbers (e.g., five to eight months) reflect the mean survival time of the individuals assessed. That range of survival times at the 95% level of confidence suggests that the mean survival time will fall between five and eight months 95% of the time.

Bias

Researchers draw inferences about a population from studying a sample from that population. Even when every effort is made to see that the sample is similar to the population, differences will occur. The ways in which the sample differs from the larger population is referred to as bias. If investigators are not aware of the existence of bias they may draw inappropriate conclusions from their work. Conclusions may be accurate for the sample studied but will not be appropriate for the larger population. For example, if epidemiologists are studying survival rates among AIDS patients and include only men over age 40 who are homosexual, they could not apply their findings to the larger population of men and women of all ages who are heterosexual as well as homosexual.

Other means of introducing bias include using instruments that do not accurately measure the variable under study, losing a number of participants during the study, and using methods of data collection that require recall (memories can fade). The concept of bias is important in all research, and evaluations of any study need to include an examination of potential bias.

Confounding Variables

Confounding variables are those variables that can influence the outcome of a study in ways that are not intended by the investigator. Age, gender, and educational level are obvious variables that could sway results. In epidemiological research investigators need to pay close attention to issues of accurate diagnosis, factors that may be involved in both diagnosis and morbidity (e.g., smoking), treatment differences, and environmental factors.

WORKING DEFINITIONS

Confidence Intervals, Confounding Variables, and Bias

A confidence interval is a statistical method of describing data. Confounding variables are variables that can inappropriately influence the outcome. Bias implies that methods have been used that may inappropriately influence the outcome.

EXAMPLE

Confidence Intervals, Confounding Variables, and Bias

An investigator reviews a meta-analysis on the subject of survival with breast cancer and its relationship to prior hormone replacement. It is obvious from the meta-analysis that age was not adequately considered (confounding variable), and the process of collecting the data on who did or did not take hormones was questionable (bias). In some of the studies reviewed, confidence intervals were used to describe the mean survival rate.

PRACTICE

Confidence Intervals, Confounding Variables, and Bias

Design a study to examine a health concern. Identify potential confounding variables, possible bias, and how you would use a confidence interval.

 CRITICAL APPRAISAL

Confidence Intervals, Confounding Variables, and Bias

- Is the confidence interval interpreted as the frequency with which the population mean lies between the stated limits?

- Are all confounding variables taken into account?

- Is there any evidence of bias in relation to the methods used?

Critical Overview of Epidemiology

Epidemiologists use quantitative methods to better understand the health of populations. They are interested in the number of cases of a particular disease within selected parameters, such as age or gender, what treatments work for a given problem, what causes health problems, and how our health care system can respond in an effective manner.

274

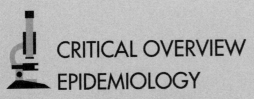

CRITICAL OVERVIEW
EPIDEMIOLOGY

Select an epidemiological study in an area that interests you.

- Describe the approach to the study: What is the investigator trying to accomplish?

- Is the study descriptive or experimental?

- What effect might the study have on the health care system?

References

Hill, A. B. (1965). The environment and disease: Association or causation? *Proc R Soc Med*, 58:295–300.

Streiner, D. L. & Norman, G. R. (1996). *PDQ Epidemiology*. St. Louis: Mosby.

9

Data Analysis

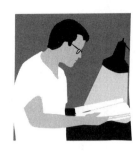

Goals

- *Describe the logic underlying the analysis of data.*
- *Analyze different methods of processing data in relation to research design.*
- *Describe basic statistical tests and their use.*

Introduction

The purpose of this chapter is to enable both the consumer of research and nurses who participate in a research project to understand the basic concepts involved in analyzing data. The intent is not to prepare individuals to conduct advanced statistical analyses but to help them understand the kinds of techniques used to reach particular goals. Simple formulas and calculations are described; complex statistical manipulations are not presented. The underlying logic of the most frequently used statistical techniques is explained.

Although the traditional undergraduate nursing research course has required students to understand the statistical procedures of chi-square, t-tests, correlation, and perhaps one-way analysis of variance, packaged statistical computer programs have enabled nurse researchers to use more advanced techniques. Consumers therefore are increasingly faced with deciphering advanced techniques in the articles they read. For this reason, descriptions of *factorial analysis of variance, analysis of covariance, multivariate analysis,* and *regression analysis* are also presented. Consumers can then understand the results section of a research publication and may also be able to contribute to discussions about the appropriate kinds of statistical analyses to use given specific conditions.

The purpose of analyzing the data collected in a study is to describe the data in meaningful terms. The alternative approach—that is, for the interested person to examine pages of scores of one variety or another—would be extremely time consuming, and would not provide a reasonable conclusion regarding the research. Depending on the kinds of variables identified (*nominal, ordinal, interval, ratio*) and the design of a particular study, a number of statistical techniques are available to analyze the data. These statistical techniques are designed to identify systematic variations between or among groups within the sample. The variations in data are the result of an intervention (treatment) or the effects of one set of measured variables on another variable (or variables).

For example, an intervention aimed at decreasing pain may be studied in a particular sample. After the statistical analysis of the data has been carried out, a significant decrease in pain may occur in the treatment group as compared to the control group. In this instance the variation in the outcome resulted from an intervention or treatment (see Figure 9.1).

In another study of the psychological needs of hospice patients, the variable, age, may have an effect on the particular needs that are identified as important. In this example an intervention is not used; however, for purposes of analysis, the sample is divided into groups based on age, and a statistical technique is

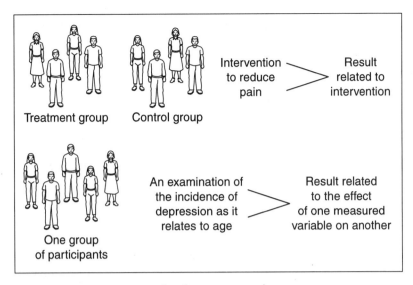

FIGURE 9.1 Identifying variations between groups

applied. In this instance it is the effect of the variable *age* that produces the variation in the results (see Figure 9.1).

There are two approaches to the statistical analysis of data: the *descriptive* approach and the *inferential* approach. The descriptive approach simply describes the data in a form that is readily understandable. Descriptive statistics convert a collection of data into a picture of the information that has some meaning for the consumer. The inferential approach allows the investigator to decide whether the outcome of the study is a result of factors planned within the design of the study or determined by chance. The inferential approach permits the investigator to infer that particular characteristics in a sample exist in the larger population.

These approaches are often used sequentially in that first, data are described (descriptive), and then additional statistical manipulations are performed to make inferences about the likelihood that the outcome was due to chance (inferential). When a descriptive approach is used, terms such as *mean, median, mode, variation*, and *standard deviation* are used to communicate the analysis of the data. When an inferential approach is used, *p* values (the probability that the outcome was due to chance) are used to communicate the significance or lack of significance of the results (Norman & Streiner, 1996).

Basic Concepts in Descriptive Statistics

Descriptive Measures

Pictorial Displays A researcher using the quantitative approach (i.e., using numbers to organize, analyze, and interpret data) must make sense out of a set of numbers and communicate them in some logical fashion to the consumer. The investigator who is examining the pain response of patients suffering from a particular form of cancer may have a set of scores from a pain scale. A pictorial display is a relatively simple technique for describing and communicating results. Frequently used pictorial displays include a pie graph, a bar graph, a histogram, and a frequency polygon. The pie graph is a circle that represents the entire sample. Divisions within the pie graph reflect specific areas of concern. The *bar graph*, *histogram*, and *frequency polygon* use the vertical scale to record the frequency of an event and the horizontal scale to reflect the categories of interest. A frequency polygon is depicted by marking the center of the top of each column and drawing connecting lines. In each case, the frequency of the occurrence of each category under study is plotted so that the reader can view the overall results in a meaningful fashion.

The pictorial displays in Figure 9.2 reflect data that might be collected from a study designed to measure the pain levels in a sample of 14 patients diagnosed with cancer.

Measures of Central Tendency Pictorial displays of data require the investigator to calculate percentages and to determine how many observations fit into various categories, but other descriptive methods of analyzing data require additional calculations. When describing quantitative data, measures of central tendency or "measures of the middle" are often used. The mean, median, and mode are measures of *central tendency*, and they provide information about central characteris-

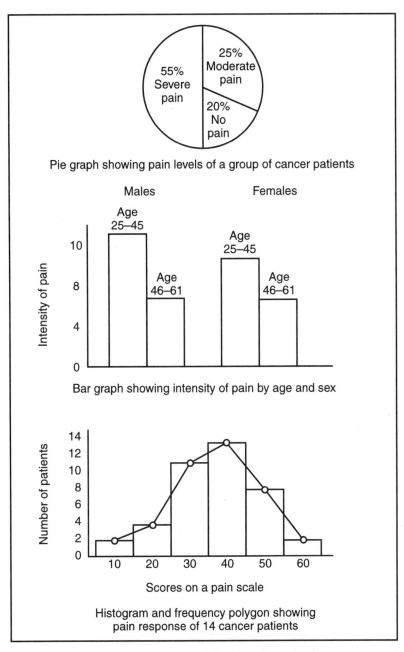

Pie graph showing pain levels of a group of cancer patients

Bar graph showing intensity of pain by age and sex

Histogram and frequency polygon showing
pain response of 14 cancer patients

FIGURE 9.2 Pictorial displays of pain levels

tics of the data. For example, to describe the scores of six patients on a pain scale that ranges from 0 to 25, the investigator can calculate the *mean* (add all the scores and divide by the number of patients), the *median* (identify the score that divides the set of scores in half), and the *mode* (identify the most frequently occurring score).

In a study to assess levels of pain, the following six scores on the pain scale are obtained: 12, 17, 14, 5, 12, 3. The mean is calculated by adding these scores and dividing by 6: that is, 63 divided by 6, or 10.5. The median is the score that lies between the two middle scores, that is, 12 (3–5–12–12–14–17), and is therefore the most typical score. When there is an even number of scores, the median lies between the two middle scores; when there is an odd number of scores, the median is the middle score. The mode is the most frequently occurring score, that is, 12 (3, 5, 12, 12, 14, 17) (Munro, 2000).

 WORKING DEFINITION

Measures of Central Tendency

Measures of central tendency—the mean, median, and mode—are calculated to identify the average, the most typical, and the most common values, respectively, among the data collected.

 EXAMPLE

Measures of Central Tendency

A group of nurse investigators design a study to assess the level of helplessness among children of alcoholics. To test their instrument they obtain helplessness scores on ten participants. Possible scores on the instrument range from 6 to 36. From the following scores they calculate the mean, median, and mode (hypothetical data):

Scores: 8   17   10   12   13   11   17   22   24   21

Mean: 8 + 17 + 10 + 12 + 13 + 11 + 17 + 22 + 24 + 21
divided by 10 = 15.5

Median: 24   22   21   17   17   13   12   11   10 8 = 15

Mode: 24   22   21   17   17   13   12   11   10 8 = 17

These measures of central tendency are more or less appropriate, depending on the kinds of variables examined in the study. The mode is the best measure of central tendency when nominal variables are used; the median is the best measure when ordinal variables are used; and the mean is the best measure when interval or ratio variables are used. Investigators who want to determine the self-care ability of the majority of women 24 hours postpartum would calculate the mode; if they want to identify the typical number of calories ingested per day by 13-year-old females, they would calculate the median. In order to conduct a statistical analysis to determine the difference between two groups of subjects who have been exposed to different nursing interventions, the mean would be calculated.

There are some obvious difficulties in relying on measures of central tendency to describe the findings of a study accurately. For example, although the mean in the study of the helplessness levels of the children of alcoholics provides an average level of 15.5, it does not show that one child scored as low as 8 and another scored as high as 24. An intervention designed to assist the child who scored 24 might not be effective with the child who scored 8. Similarly, the median and mode give limited information as to the actual makeup of the entire group.

 PRACTICE

Measures of Central Tendency

The following scores were obtained from eight patients on a dialysis unit who responded to a psychological test evaluating their ability to cope with their disability (hypothetical data). Calculate the mean, median, and mode.

Scores: 42 35 38 31 43 29 38 27

In communicating the results of a study when the findings are described using measures of central tendency, the consumer needs to evaluate the analysis using a number of criteria. The calculation of the mean, median, or mode is sufficiently simple that the consumer can readily check for accuracy. Conclusions drawn from each measure of central tendency are different in nature, so the appropriateness of interpretation should be examined. Similarly, when assisting with the development of a research project, if measures of central tendency are proposed as a method of statistical analysis, the researcher needs to address these concerns.

CRITICAL APPRAISAL

Measures of Central Tendency

- Are the mean, median, and mode calculated correctly?

- If the mean, median, and mode are calculated correctly, are the findings expressed accurately or are conclusions drawn that are not warranted?

- Are the measures used—mean, median, and mode-appropriate to the purpose of the study?

Another descriptive measure of quantitative data is the measurement of the variation or dispersion among the results. How scores differ one from another is an important consideration when analyzing data. Although the mean, median, and mode describe something about the middle of a set of numbers, the variation among the numbers shows whether the scores cluster around the middle with few scores at either extreme. Three indices are used to measure the variation or dispersion among scores: (1) range, (2) variance, and (3) standard deviation (Cozby, 2000).

The **range** is the simplest method for examining variation among scores and simply refers to the difference between the highest and lowest values produced. The distance between the lowest score and the highest score in a distribution constitutes the range. Using the pain scores as an example, the total range would be 17 minus 3, or 14 (scores are 3, 5, 12, 12, 14, 17). Another method for examining the dispersion of scores when ordinal, interval, and ratio variables are used is to look at the data in terms of percentiles or quartiles-those scores that make up 25% of the results, 50%, 75%, and so on. For example, if an investigator assessed the weight of eight anorectic teenagers as 95, 88, 78, 91, 85, 83, 79, 81, the quartiles would be:

78 79 | 81 83 | 85 88 | 91 95

The **interquartile range** is the area between the lowest quartile and the highest quartile, or the middle 50% of the scores. In this case the interquartile range would be 81 to 88.

The concepts of variance and standard deviation are based on the difference or deviation of each score in a distribution from the mean. One method for calculating the variance is to first calculate the deviation scores. For example, given that six women breast-feed their infants for periods of 3 months, 2 months, 5 months, 1 month, 6 months, and 7 months, the mean of this distribution is 4. The deviation scores in relation to months of breast-feeding are $3 - 4 = -1$, $2 - 4 = -2$, $5 - 4 = +1$, $1 - 4 = -3$, $6 - 4 = +2$, $7 - 4 = +3$. The $\pm$ sign of the deviation score identifies whether the score is above (+) or below (−) the mean. The sum of a set of deviation scores equals zero:

$$(-1) + (-2) + (1) + (-3) + (2) + (3) = 0$$

The deviations of a distribution of scores can then be used to calculate the variance. The following formula can be used to calculate the variance, using deviation scores:

$$\tilde{\sigma}^2 = \frac{SS_x}{n}$$

where

$\tilde{\sigma}^2$ = variance of the distribution of scores
SS_x = sum of the squared deviation scores
n = number of scores in the distribution

For the above example, where six mothers breast-fed infants for 3 months, 2 months, 5 months, 1 month, 6 months, and 7 months, the variance would be calculated as follows:

$SS_x = (3-4)^2 + (2-4)^2 + (5-4)^2 + (1-4)^2 + (6-4)^2 + (7-4)^2$

$\quad = (-1)^2 + (-2)^2 + (1)^2 + (-3)^2 + (2)^2 + (3)^2$

$\quad = 1 + 4 + 1 + 9 + 4 + 9$

$\quad = 28$

$\quad = \dfrac{28}{6} = 4.66$

The variance of 4.66 is therefore the average of the sum of the squared deviation scores.

The standard deviation of a distribution of scores is the square root of the variance. For the example above the standard deviation would be calculated as follows: If we let

$$\tilde{\sigma}^2 = \text{standard deviation}$$

$$\hat{\sigma}^2 = \text{variance}$$

then

$$\tilde{\sigma} = \sqrt{4.66}$$

therefore,

$$\tilde{\sigma} = 2.16$$

Large standard deviations suggest that scores do not cluster around the mean; they are probably widely scattered. Similarly, small standard deviations suggest that there is very little difference among the scores. The calculation of the standard deviation is relatively simple if there are only a few values;

however, if there are many values, this calculation can be extremely time consuming and is generally calculated on a computer.

WORKING DEFINITION

Measures of Variance

The range, variance, and standard deviation are measures of the variation or dispersion among data. The range describes the difference between the largest and the smallest observations made; the variance and standard deviation are based on the average difference or deviation of observations from the mean.

EXAMPLE

Measures of Variance

A group of nurse investigators conduct a pilot test on the attitudes toward breast-feeding of a group of four primiparas two months before their due dates. An attitude scale is used that provides a score that ranges from 0 to 15. The following data are collected, and the range, standard deviation, and variance are calculated (hypothetical data).

Scores: 5, 7, 9, 11

Range: 11 − 5 = 6

Interquartile range: 7–9

Variance: 5

Standard deviation: 2.24

The value of the information provided by the measures of variance is an important consideration. The total range in the case of the attitudes of the primiparas toward breast-feeding is of little value if the purpose of the assessment is to try to develop an intervention that will enhance positive values toward breast-feeding. A range of scores of 5 to 11 does not convey how many are close to the negative end of the scale or, conversely, how many are close to the positive end of the scale.

The interquartile range does present information regarding the middle portion of the observations that can be helpful in designing an intervention; however, it still does not describe the extent to which scores appear at the extremes. The standard deviation does provide a description of the spread of scores and therefore could give the investigator an idea of the kind of diversity of opinion that may be present in the group studied. In addition, the calculation of the standard deviation uses each observation, thereby reflecting all of the information collected.

 PRACTICE

Measures of Variance

A nurse investigator pilot-tests the level of helplessness among ten elderly patients in a skilled nursing home. The investigator collects the following data using a paper-and-pencil questionnaire.

Scores: 23 13 14 18 15 14 23 16 21 20

Calculate: The range, the interquartile range, the variance, and the standard deviation.

Describe: The value of the information derived from these calculations given that the nurse wishes eventually to design an intervention to reduce the helplessness of these individuals.

 CRITICAL APPRAISAL

Measures of Variance

- Are the range, interquartile range, variance, and standard deviation calculated correctly?

- Are the findings expressed accurately, or are conclusions drawn that are not warranted?

- Is the measure that is used appropriate to the kind of variables being examined?

The Normal Distribution

The construct of the **normal distribution** is important to the development of an understanding of the statistical analysis of data. Although the construct of the normal distribution comes from the observation that the natural variance among variables tends to form a bell-shaped distribution, it is a theoretical concept and is not based on concrete data. This bell-shaped distribution or curve reflects the tendency of the observations concerning a specific variable to cluster in a particular manner. Most of the observations are thought to cluster at about the same scale value, while a few observations group together at either extreme (see Figure 9.3). For example, if 2000 university nursing students were assessed on their level of intelligence, results would probably show a large proportion of the 2000 at a score of 110–120 and a few at the levels of 100 and 130.

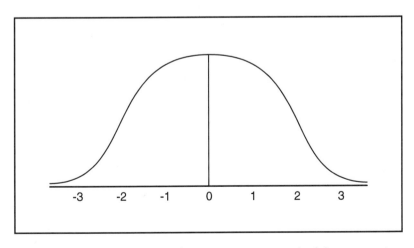

FIGURE 9.3 The unit normal curve (mean = 0, standard deviation = 1)

289

The *normal curve* can be described for any set of data given the mean and standard deviation of the data and the assumption that the characteristic under study would be normally distributed within the population. A normal distribution of data suggests that 68% of observations fall within one standard deviation of the mean, 95% fall within two standard deviations of the mean, and 99.87% fall within three standard deviations of the mean. The curve moves continually closer to the baseline but does not actually make contact. Theoretically, the range of the curve is unlimited.

Distributions of scores (weights, months, etc.) can vary in relation to the degree to which they approximate the normal curve. For example, if two groups of mothers were assessed regarding the number of months they breast-fed their children, the mean for Group A could be 4 months with a standard deviation of 4.66, and the mean of Group B might be 8 with a standard deviation of 6. A mother in Group A who breast-fed 5 months would be above average, whereas a mother in Group B who breastfed 5 months would be below average.

To make comparisons between groups, standard scores rather than raw scores can be used. When a norm-referenced measure has been used—for example, a norm has been established for the number of months women breast-feed their children—raw scores can be translated into standard scores. *Standard scores* enable the investigator to examine the position of a given score by measuring its deviation from the mean of all scores. By calculating standard scores the set of scores then has a mean of 0 and a standard deviation of 1. The unit normal curve reflects the distribution of standard scores.

To calculate standard scores (z scores), the distance between the score (x) and the mean ($\bar{x}$) is divided by the standard deviation ($\tilde{\sigma}$) . For example, where the mean equals 4 and the standard deviation equals 4.66, what is the z score equivalent of a raw score of 7?

$$z = \frac{x - \bar{x}}{\tilde{\sigma}}$$

where
z = standard score

x = individual raw score
x = mean score
$\tilde{\sigma}$ = standard deviation

$$z = \frac{(7-4)}{4.66}$$

$$= \frac{3}{4.66}$$

$$= .64$$

WORKING DEFINITION

The Normal Distribution

The normal distribution is a mathematical construct which suggests that naturally occurring observations follow a given pattern. The pattern is the normal curve, which places most observations at the mean and a lesser number of observations at either extreme.

Because the normal curve is symmetrical, the mean, median, and mode are at the same point. If the mean and standard deviation of the data observed are known, and the assumption can be made that the characteristic under investigation is normally distributed in the population, the shape of the particular curve can be calculated by plugging these numbers into the formula for the normal curve. The value in studying characteristics that can be considered normally distributed within the population is that generalizations to a larger population from a limited sample are facilitated.

EXAMPLE

The Normal Distribution

A group of nurse investigators are interested in studying obesity among female adults of average height (5 feet, 3 inches to 5 feet, 6 inches). The investigators decide that weight across this population is a characteristic that would have a normal distribution. There would probably be a large number of individuals who weigh between 110 and 160 pounds, a few individuals who would weigh less than 110 pounds, and a few individuals who would weigh more than 160 pounds.

When reading a research report or assisting in the development of a research project, it is important to examine the various judgments made regarding the statistical analysis. The logic of assuming that the characteristics under study are normally distributed should be assessed.

CRITICAL APPRAISAL

The Normal Distribution

Is it logical to assume that the characteristic under study is normally distributed within the population?

Correlation

The concept of **correlation** suggests that variation in a given variable may be related to variation in another variable. An increase in stress, for example, may be related to an increase in specific somatic symptoms.

Correlational research examines relationships among variables of interest without any active intervention on the part of the investigator. A correlation coefficient is a number ranging from -1 to $+1$ that denotes the degree and kind (positive or negative) of relationship that exists between two variables.

WORKING DEFINITION

Correlation

Correlation as it applies to research refers to the tendency of a variation in one variable to be related to a variation in another variable. Correlational research examines these relationships. A correlation coefficient describes the relationship.

292

◈ TABLE 9.1 Hypothetical Data on Weight Gain over a Six-Month Period and Average Calorie Intake/Day for Eight Diabetic Adult Females

Diabetic females	Weight gain (lbs.)	Calorie intake/day
A	3	2000
B	5	1900
C	1	1600
D	4	2100
E	6	2400
F	2	1800
G	3	1800
H	1	1500

The concept of correlation is used when an investigator wants to determine the nature and extent of the relationship among variables. For example, a group of nurse investigators studying the relationship between weight gain over a six-month period and average daily calorie intake among a group of diabetics might gather the data shown in Table 9.1. The pictorial display in Figure 9.4 reflects the data collected on weight gain and calorie intake.

From scanning the points on the scatterplot in Figure 9.4, it is apparent that some relationship exists between weight gain and average caloric intake. As caloric intake increases, to some extent weight gain also increases. A perfect positive relationship would be depicted as shown in Figure 9.5. As caloric intake increases, weight gain also increases. A perfect negative relationship would be depicted as shown in Figure 9.6. As weight

293

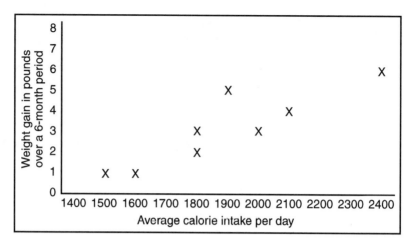

FIGURE 9.4 Scatterplot of scores presented in Table 9.1

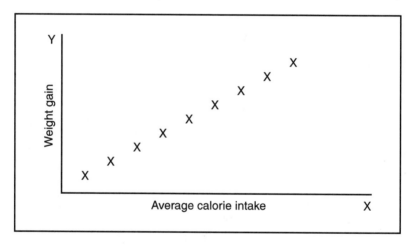

FIGURE 9.5 Perfect positive relationship of weight gain and average caloric intake

gain increases, caloric intake decreases. In most instances, relationships arc not perfect but to varying degrees approximate the perfect positive or perfect negative linear relationship.

In addition to scanning the points on a scatterplot to assess the relationship between variables, researchers can calculate a numerical index. The statistic often used to calculate a numerical index is the Pearson product-moment correlation coefficient (r_{xy}). This coefficient measures the extent to which the

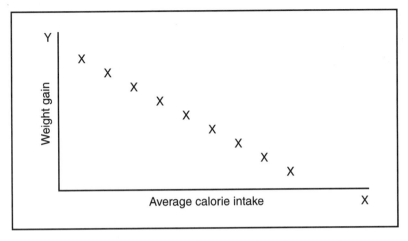

FIGURE 9.6 Perfect negative relationship of weight gain and average caloric intake

points on the scatterplot follow a straight line. In order to compute r_{xy}, two measures are needed for each participant. The formula for calculating r_{xy} from raw scores is relatively simple:

$$\text{Pearson } r = \frac{n\Sigma XY - (\Sigma X)(\Sigma Y)}{[n\Sigma X^2 - (\Sigma X)^2][n\Sigma Y^2 - (\Sigma Y)^2]}$$

where

ΣXY = the sum of the products of each participant's scores
ΣX = the sum of all X scores
ΣY = the sum of all Y scores
n = the number of participants
ΣX^2 = the sum of all squared X scores
$(\Sigma X)^2$ = the square of the sum of all X scores
ΣY^2 = the sum of all squared Y scores
$(\Sigma Y)^2$ = the square of the sum of all Y scores

 EXAMPLE

Pearson Product-Moment Correlation Coefficient

A group of nurse investigators designed a pilot study to examine the relationship between weight gain (X) and depression (Y)

295

among five inpatients at a private psychiatric hospital over a six-month period. They collected the following data (hypothetical).

Inpatient	X (lbs.)	Y (range 0–10)	X^2	Y^2	XY
A	2	4	4	16	8
B	7	9	49	81	63
C	3	6	9	36	18
D	5	7	25	49	35
E	1	3	1	9	3
	$\Sigma X = 18$	$\Sigma Y = 29$	$\Sigma X^2 = 88$	$\Sigma Y^2 = 191$	$\Sigma XY = 127$

The Pearson r was calculated as follows:

$$r = \frac{\Sigma XY - (\Sigma X)(\Sigma Y)}{\sqrt{[\Sigma X^2 - (\Sigma X)^2][\Sigma Y^2 - (\Sigma Y)^2]}}$$

$$= \frac{5(127) - (18)(29)}{\sqrt{[5(88) - 324][5(191) - 841]}}$$

$$= \frac{113}{114.9}$$

$$= .98$$

When the resulting r is squared, the value that results is the percentage of explained variance between two sets of scores. For example, if participants in a nursing research study complete a scale measuring depression and collect data related to the amount of caffeine ingested over a period of time, a possible correlation might be .40. Squaring .40 equals 0.16, suggesting that the percent of the variance shared by the variable of depression and caffeine ingestion is 16%.

The Pearson product-moment formula is a **parametric** statistical test in that an estimation of at least one parameter is involved, measurement is at an interval level, and it is assumed that the variable under study is normally distributed within the population. Spearman rho and Kendall's tau are nonparametric tests that produce a coefficient that is interpreted similarly to the Pearson r.

 PRACTICE

Pearson Product-Moment Correlation Coefficient

In the following hypothetical study, a group of nurse investigators examine the relationship between anxiety and performance on a graduate-level competency examination. Five participants received the following scores:

Participant	Anxiety score	Competency examination score
A	35	40
B	31	42
C	27	41
D	24	49
E	36	39

Calculate r and the percentage of the variance shared by the two variables.

The accurate interpretation of correlations is frequently a difficult task. Causation must not be inferred, and care must be taken neither to inflate nor underrepresent the relationship described by the coefficient. For example, if nurse investigators discover that the correlation between patient satisfaction with care and a positive attitude toward health status is high (r = .80), it means that as patients' attitudes toward their health status increase in a positive direction, their satisfaction with care tends to increase.

CRITICAL APPRAISAL

Correlation

- Does the interpretation of the correlation seem to under- or overrepresent the relationship?

- Might other variables (not identified) be affecting the outcome?

- Is causation erroneously implied?

Basic Concepts in Inferential Statistics

Probability

Although there are many inferential statistical techniques that vary considerably in their complexity, the goal of each technique is the same, namely, to determine as precisely as possible the probability of an occurrence. The probability or likelihood that something will occur is an idea that is used by clinicians at all levels of inquiry. Nurses frequently consider the likelihood of success for particular nursing interventions and, through the process of evaluation, check the accuracy of their predictions.

When working with inferential statistics, investigators analyze their data to establish the likelihood that differences in the groups under study are the result of chance as opposed to the manipulation of variables. Because errors occur whenever an attempt is made to infer characteristics from a small group to the larger population, there is always some likelihood that the differences between groups could be the result of chance (Cozby, 2000).

WORKING DEFINITION

Probability

In inferential statistics, probability refers to the likelihood that the differences between the groups under study are the result of chance.

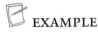

EXAMPLE

Probability

A group of nurse investigators select a sample of 100 patients who have experienced a laminectomy in order to examine the effects of preoperative teaching on pain reduction. Participants are randomly assigned to a control group and an experimental group. The purpose of the statistical analysis of the data is to determine to what degree the results were due to chance rather than intervention (preoperative teaching).

The idea of probability is basic to inferential statistics. Each researcher makes a probability statement about the likelihood that certain results are due to chance rather than the manipulation of variables. The probability that specific results are accurate (that there is little likelihood that they are the result of chance) is influenced by the degree of error that occurs when investigators attempt to measure and sample events. The question "What is the certainty that a given occurrence is due to specified factors?" is an integral component of inferential statistics.

PRACTICE

Probability

Formulate a research question such as, "How do relaxation techniques plus analgesics compare with analgesics only in reducing cancer pain?" Discuss how the concept of probability is related to the testing of the intervention.

Given that it is not possible to exclude errors completely from either the sampling or measurement processes when conducting research, there is always some probability that a given finding is a chance result. The discussion of the results of research projects should not therefore claim to have proved anything. An appropriate discussion of results includes statements about the probability that the findings are the result of chance. Acceptable levels of chance (see the section "Statistical Significance") must be specified in order to keep within the framework of the inferential process.

CRITICAL APPRAISAL

Probability

- Are the results of the study expressed in terms of probability?
- Is the level of probability specified?

Sampling Error (Standard Error)

A basic idea underlying the use of inferential statistics is that a sample of events or observations is selected to represent a larger population of those same events or observations. The sample is intended to reflect as closely as possible the characteristics of the larger population. For example, nurse investigators might collect data on every patient diagnosed with breast cancer throughout the country to try to understand the effects of a particular intervention on self-esteem following a mastectomy. This process would be costly and time consuming and would probably not be feasible given various financial constraints. Another approach would be to select a sample of patients diagnosed with breast cancer and infer the results of the investigation to the larger population.

Whenever a sample is drawn from a larger population (even if random selection is used), that sample cannot exactly duplicate all the characteristics of the larger group. The means and standard deviations calculated from the data collected on a given sample would not be the same as those calculations derived from data collected from the entire population. It is the discrepancy between the characteristics of the sample and the population that constitutes **sampling error**.

Rather than assess every individual, a researcher could select many samples from the same population and describe a range of possible means. The mean of these many means could then be calculated to give a more accurate estimate of the population mean. If 100 such samples were selected, the means would represent a normal curve. Because this normal distribution occurs, the calculation of the mean and standard deviation from one sample can be used to generate the means that would result if many samples were selected. An investigator can, therefore, state that a population mean is likely to fall within one or more standard deviations from the sample mean.

WORKING DEFINITION

Sampling Error

Sampling error refers to the discrepancies that inevitably occur when a small group (sample) is selected to represent the characteristics of a larger group (population).

In some instances, population means such as IQ have been calculated. Researchers can then identify a specific group and compare their IQs with a known population mean. In most instances, however, investigators do not have a known population mean available to them and must therefore specify the probability that the population mean will fall within a range of scores.

Null Hypothesis

Many researchers are interested in comparing population means as opposed to estimating a population mean from a sample mean. The nurse investigators interested in the attitudes toward parenting of women who have been abused as children may want to compare the attitudes of these women with a group of women who are similar in many ways but have never experienced physical abuse. To do so, the investigators assess the attitudes of all participants using an appropriate measuring device and then estimate the population means of each group.

The population means of the groups are compared by testing what is called the null hypothesis. The **null hypothesis** is a statistical statement that there is no difference between the groups under study. A statistical test is used to determine the probability that the null hypothesis is not true (rejected). The idea of the null hypothesis is congruent with the concept of probability that forms the basis for inferential statistics in that nothing is ever proven; investigators simply fail to disprove. When there is insufficient evidence to claim that groups of events or observations are different, they are considered to be the same.

 WORKING DEFINITION

Null Hypothesis

The null hypothesis is a statistical statement that predicts no difference between the groups of events or observations under study. Inferential statistics are used in an effort to reject the null, thereby showing that a difference does exist.

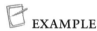 EXAMPLE

Null Hypothesis

A group of nurse investigators decide to compare the anxiety levels of children exposed to two different kinds of pretonsillectomy hospital orientation protocols. Their research hypothesis states that there is a difference in anxiety levels between children exposed to protocol A and those exposed to protocol B. The null hypothesis states that there is no difference in anxiety levels between children exposed to protocol A and those exposed to protocol B. Inferential statistical tests are used to attempt to reject the null hypothesis.

In designing a research project, or in reading research reports, the research hypothesis is clearly more important than the null. The null hypothesis is a technical necessity when using inferential statistics.

302

PRACTICE

Null Hypothesis

For the following research hypotheses, state the appropriate null hypotheses:

- Preoperative teaching designed to reduce anxiety is more effective with adults than with children.

- The combination of biofeedback and pain medication in reducing chronic back pain is more effective than pain medication alone.

- Hypnosis is an effective technique for reducing nausea among patients treated with *cis*-platinum.

Statistical Significance

The concept of **statistical significance** involves substituting a statistical value for an observed relationship and comparing the statistical value to a distribution of other statistical values to determine how likely the value of interest could have occurred by chance. If it is more likely that the observed relationship did not occur by chance alone, the null hypothesis is rejected. If it is likely that the observed relationship did occur by chance, the null hypothesis is accepted (Cozby, 2000).

The decision of whether the null hypothesis should be rejected depends on the level of error that can be tolerated. The tolerable level of error is expressed as a *level of significance* or *alpha level*. The usual (arbitrarily set) level of significance or alpha level is .05, although at times levels of .01 or .001 may be used.

A level of significance is identified to indicate the probability that the null has been incorrectly rejected and there is in fact no difference between the groups under study. The level of significance is expressed as a decimal and may be called a *p* level or an alpha level. The level of significance conveys how many times out of 100 or 1,000 the null hypothesis might have been incorrectly rejected. For example, if the null hypothesis is rejected using an alpha level of .05, there is a 5% chance, or 1 chance in 20, that the null has been incorrectly rejected and that the observed difference between groups occurred only by chance. An alpha level of .01 suggests that a difference could occur by chance 1 time out of 100. The lower the alpha level, the greater the confidence that the differences between groups did not occur by chance.

WORKING DEFINITION

Level of Significance

The level of significance (or alpha level) is determined to identify the probability that the differences between groups have occurred by chance rather than in response to the manipulation of variables.

EXAMPLE

Level of Significance

Two nurse investigators randomly assign 50 teenagers diagnosed with eating disorders to a control group and an experimental group. They evaluate the effect of a behavior modification approach on a number of destructive behaviors related to their diagnosis. They analyze the data and reject the null, which states that there will be no difference between the experimental and control groups at the .05 level of significance. The results of the data analysis suggest that only 5 times out of 100 would the differences found between the control and experimental groups be the result of chance.

If a null hypothesis has been rejected and in actuality the null is true, a **Type I error** has been made. For example, if the difference observed between the two groups in the eating disorder study was in fact the result of chance and yet statistically the null was rejected, a Type I error occurred. The more stringent the level of significance, the less likely it is that a Type I error will occur. At a level of .01 there is only 1 chance in 100 that a Type I error can occur. Similarly, at a level of .001 there is only 1 chance in 1,000 that a Type I error can occur.

A **Type II error** occurs when the null is not rejected and yet there are differences between the groups under study. In the eating disorder study, if the null was not rejected and yet there were differences between the experimental and control groups, then a Type II error was made.

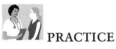 PRACTICE

Level of Significance

Explain the meaning of the following remarks.

- In a study designed to determine the effects of primary care nursing as compared with functional team nursing on patient satisfaction, a significant difference was found between the two approaches to patient care. Higher rates of satisfaction were found among patients exposed to primary care nursing ($t = 12.23$, $p < .05$).

- A literature review of the effects of one specific relaxation protocol on diminishing phantom limb pain identified two studies that reported conflicting results. The results of one study showed the relaxation intervention to be more effective than pain medication ($t = 9.48$, $p < .01$), and the results of the second study showed pain medication to be more effective than the relaxation intervention ($t = 11.42$, $p < .001$).

Levels of significance (alpha levels, p values) are not generally set beyond .05; that is, if there is more than 1 chance in 20 that the outcome of interest has occurred by chance rather than because of the manipulation of variables, the results are not considered to be of value. In studies designed to make inferences to the larger population, the level of significance is established before data are analyzed. It is important to keep in mind that even though the null hypothesis may not be rejected, important information about the topic under study can be discovered. The fact that there is no difference between groups may suggest a different methodological approach or a new way of looking at the topic of interest.

CRITICAL APPRAISAL

Level of Significance

- Is the level of significance reported?

- Are findings reported that are not significant?

- Are appropriate conclusions drawn given the significant differences found?

Inferential Statistical Tests

There are two kinds of inferential statistical tests: **parametric** and **nonparametric**. Parametric tests require the estimation of at least one variable; measurement must be at the interval or ratio level; and the variable of concern must be normally distributed within the population. The *t*-test is used when investigators wish to compare the means of two groups. The *t*-value or *t*-statistic is calculated using a formula that incorporates the means of both groups and the standard error of the difference between the means. The calculated *t*-value is used to determine the probability that the difference occurred by chance. If the *p* value is less than .05, we say that there is a significant difference.

Whether a significant difference occurs can be established through analyzing data via a computer program or analyzing data by hand and using a *t*-table. When data are analyzed by computer, the *p* value is automatically reported on the computer printout. Degrees of freedom (*df*) is a mathematical concept that describes the number of events or observations that are free to vary; for each statistical test there is a formula for calculating the appropriate *df*.

Both the *t*-value and the *df* are used to find the significance level from the t distribution table. Enter the table at the appropriate *df*; if the *t*-value is larger than the tabled value, the result is significant.

A *t*-test can be one-tailed or two-tailed. If the hypothesis of the study is directional, a one-tailed test is generally used. If the hypothesis is nondirectional, a two-tailed test is used.

WORKING DEFINITION

t-Test

A *t*-test is an inferential statistical technique used to compare the means of two groups. The reporting of the results of a *t*-test generally includes the *df*, *t*-value, and probability level.

The formula used to calculate a *t*-test can differ depending on whether the samples involved are dependent or independent. Samples are independent when there are two separate groups such as an experimental group and a control group. Samples are dependent when the participants from the two groups are paired in some manner. For example, when the same participants are assessed on a given characteristic before and after an intervention, the sample is considered dependent. Different participants may be involved in the dependent *t*-test, but there is a relationship between the participants in the groups. The form of the *t*-test that is used with a dependent sample may be termed paired, dependent, matched, or correlated.

Whether the dependent *t*-test or the independent *t*-test is used, the reporting of the results remains the same. The formulas are different for computing both the *t*-statistic and the *df*, but the manner in which the level of significance is derived and reported is identical.

EXAMPLE

t-Test

A group of nurse investigators hypothesized that women who choose midwives to provide patient care would have higher

307

patient satisfaction levels than women who choose obstetricians. They designed a study to examine this issue, collected their data, and analyzed the findings using an independent one-tailed *t*-test. They report their results as follows: A significant difference was found in the satisfaction levels of women who chose midwives to provide prenatal care as compared with women who chose obstetricians, $t(12) = 2.12$, $p < .05$.

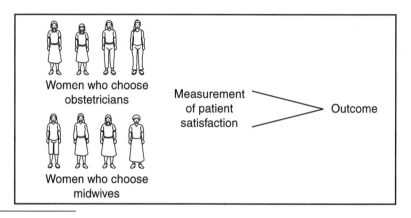

 PRACTICE

t-Test

Formulate two research questions relevant to nursing practice in which an independent *t*-test could be used to analyze the data and two questions in which a dependent t-test would be appropriate.

In reading a research report or in assisting with the design of a study it is important to be able to assess whether the appropriate kind of analysis was used and whether appropriate conclusions are drawn from the analysis conducted. In the case of the *t*-test, a knowledge of the differences between the independent and dependent *t*-tests is important. In addition, the consumer can determine whether the data collected warrant a comparison of two means and therefore the use of a *t*-test.

CRITICAL APPRAISAL

t-Test

- Is the correct form of the *t*-test—dependent versus independent—being used?

- Is the use of a comparison between means (*t*-test) appropriate considering the data that have been collected?

Whereas the *t*-test is used to test the null hypothesis that there is no difference in means between the two groups, another statistical procedure—regression analysis—is often used to predict the value of one variable given information about another variable. This procedure can describe how two continuous variables are related. For example, level of health status might be predicted from measures of height, weight, activity level, cholesterol count, and so on (Cozby, 2000).

The systematic investigation of the relationship among a number of variables is possible using regression analysis. For example, a nurse investigator can examine the relationship of a variety of personality characteristics to the uncertainty experienced in the face of a life-threatening event.

Regression analysis is generally used to examine relationships among continuous variables and is most appropriate for data that can be plotted on a graph. Data are usually plotted so that the independent variable is seen on the horizontal (*x*) axis and the dependent variable is shown on the vertical (*y*) axis. The statistical procedure of regression analysis includes a test for the significance of the relationship between two variables. Given a significant relationship between two variables, knowledge of the value of the independent variable permits a prediction of the value of the dependent variable. For example, knowledge of individuals' ages might permit prediction of their cardiac function.

One-Way Analysis of Variance (ANOVA)

Frequently in the study of nursing practice, more than two means are of interest when assessing an independent variable.

For example, nurse investigators may want to compare three different patient groups—critical care patients, ambulatory inpatients, and outpatients—in terms of their level of satisfaction with patient care. The use of several *t*-tests to make such comparisons is generally considered inappropriate in that this process distorts the probability of making a Type I error, that is, incorrectly rejecting the null hypothesis (Norman & Streiner, 1996). One-way analysis of variance (ANOVA) is an extension of the *t*-test that permits the investigator to simultaneously compare more than two means.

ANOVA, unlike the *t*-test, uses variances to calculate a value that reflects the differences among three or more means. When using ANOVA, an *F* statistic or ratio is calculated. The *F* statistic is a three- or four-digit number that is used in conjunction with degrees of freedom to establish the level of significance from an *F* distribution. The degrees of freedom are identified along with the *F* statistic when reporting the results of an ANOVA [$F(3, 54) = 8.22, p < .05$].

WORKING DEFINITION

One-Way Analysis of Variance (ANOVA)

One-way analysis of variance is a parametric inferential statistical test that enables investigators to compare two or more group means. The reporting of the results includes the *df*, *F* value, and probability level.

Researchers studying two or more groups can use ANOVA to determine whether there are differences among the groups. For example, nurse investigators who want to assess the levels of helplessness among three groups of patients—long-term, acute-care, and outpatient—can administer an instrument designed to measure levels of helplessness and then calculate an *F* ratio. The null hypothesis is that there is no difference between any two of these means. If the *F* ratio is sufficiently large, then the conclusion that there is a difference between at least two of the means can be drawn. Other tests, called post hoc comparisons, can then be used to determine which of the means differ significantly.

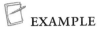 EXAMPLE

One-Way Analysis of Variance (ANOVA)

A group of nurse investigators designed a study to examine the differences in five forms of relaxation therapy used with patients suffering from chronic back pain. Pain scales were administered following each intervention, and the means and variances of each group were calculated. An analysis of variance was performed on the data, and a significant difference was found: $F(4, 26) = 8.04$, $p < .01$. A post hoc comparison test was used to determine which of the therapies was significantly different.

Fisher's LSD, Duncan's new multiple range test, the Newman-Keuls, Tukey's HSD, and Scheffé's test are the post hoc comparison tests that are most frequently used following ANOVA. The use of these tests and other similar post hoc techniques is only appropriate given that a statistically significant difference has been found using ANOVA. In some instances a post hoc comparison is not necessary because the means of the groups under consideration readily convey the differences between the groups. For example, if three groups with means of 34, 54, and 75 are being compared, and a significant difference is found using ANOVA, it is obvious where the differences lie.

 PRACTICE

One-Way Analysis of Variance (ANOVA)

Formulate four research questions relevant to nursing practice in which ANOVA would be an appropriate statistical test.

 CRITICAL APPRAISAL

One-Way Analysis of Variance (ANOVA)

- Is ANOVA used rather than multiple *t*-tests when a comparison of more than two means is required?

311

- Are post hoc comparisons used only if a significant difference has been found using ANOVA?

Factorial Analysis of Variance

Factorial analysis of variance permits the investigator to analyze the effects of two or more independent variables on the dependent variable. (One-way ANOVA is used with one independent variable and one dependent variable.) For example, in the study in which various delivery modes of nursing care were assessed in relation to patient satisfaction, the investigators might want to know whether patient satisfaction differed between males and females. If there were three modes of delivering care—primary nursing, functional team nursing, and modified primary nursing—and both males and females were to be assessed, there would be two independent variables (modes of delivering care, sex) and one dependent variable (patient satisfaction). The statistical procedure used is called a two-way (two independent variables) or factorial ANOVA.

The term *factor* is interchangeable with *independent variable* and factorial ANOVA therefore refers to the idea that data having two or more independent variables can be analyzed using this technique. Usually there are two, three, or four factors (independent variables) and a number of levels within each variable (usually no more than ten). For example, in the study on patient satisfaction, there are three levels of care delivery and two levels associated with gender:

Modes of delivery

	X_1	X_2	X_3
Sex Y_1			
Y_2			

Independent variables: Modes of delivering care, sex
Dependent variable: Patient satisfaction

WORKING DEFINITION

Factorial Analysis of Variance

Factorial analysis of variance is an inferential statistical test that enables investigators to analyze the effects of several factors or independent variables on the dependent variable.

EXAMPLE

Factorial Analysis of Variance

Staff nurses working in a community mental health center conduct a study to examine the effects of three interventions designed to resolve school phobia among boys and girls ages 7 to 10. Their design for purposes of data analysis is a 2×3 ANOVA (two independent variables, three groups within the independent variable).

	Intervention		
	A	B	C
Males			
Females			

Sex

Independent variables: Approaches to resolve school phobia, sex

Dependent variables: School phobia

Factorial ANOVA permits the investigator to make the usual null hypotheses plus an additional null hypothesis based on the interaction of the independent variables. In the example related to school phobia, the three null hypotheses would be as follows: There is no difference between male and female phobics; there is no difference between the treatment groups; and there is no difference between the two factors.

The first two null hypotheses could be tested using two one-way ANOVAs. These hypotheses could also be tested using factorial ANOVA. Two *F* ratios with corresponding levels of significance would be calculated, and they would show whether any differences occurred for each factor independent of one another. The results of these calculations are called the main or simple effects. An advantage of using factorial ANOVA is that the test is more powerful in detecting differences, and it permits the investigator to test the null hypotheses relating to interaction.

Interaction refers to the collective effect of the independent variables on the dependent variable. An *F* ratio is calculated for the interaction effect along with a corresponding level of significance. For example, there may be no significant difference between males and females relative to school phobia, and there may be no significant difference relative to the treatments used. There may, however, be a significant difference across the interventions in relation to gender. Males may respond better to treatment A than to B and C. Females may respond better to treatment B than to A and C. This interaction effect might be statistically significant even though the main effects were not significant.

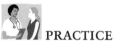 PRACTICE

Factorial Analysis of Variance

Identify a research area of interest relevant to nursing practice, and outline a study that would have two independent variables with three groups or categories and one dependent variable. The following example relates to treating chronic back pain:

Relaxation method

	A	B	C
Age 35–50			
Age 51–65			

Independent variables: Relaxation methods, age

Dependent variable: Pain

In order to make sense out of the results section of a study when factorial ANOVA has been used, the reader needs to clearly identify the variables under consideration and to have an understanding of the different implications of main effects and interaction effects. The consumer of research can then fully appreciate the findings of the study and their value to nursing practice.

CRITICAL APPRAISAL

Factorial Analysis of Variance

- Are the independent and dependent variables readily identifiable?

- Is the difference between the findings with regard to main effects versus interaction effects adequately explained?

Analysis of Covariance (ANCOVA)

Analysis of covariance (ANCOVA) is a statistical test that is similar in use to one-way or factorial ANOVA. The use of ANCOVA assists the investigator in examining possible group differences that are not controlled in the design of the study but could affect the dependent variable.

For example, nurse investigators may choose to examine compliance to a weight loss diet among three different age groups of children (male and female). They may believe that parental attitudes toward food have an effect on compliance. They therefore assess the parents of all participants regarding their attitudes toward food and determine by using ANCOVA what part of the differences in the compliance rates was the result of parental attitudes.

The variable that could confound the scores—in this case, parental attitudes toward food—is called the covariate. More than one covariate can be identified when using ANCOVA. The results are reported in a manner similar to one-way or factorial analysis.

315

WORKING DEFINITION

Analysis of Covariance (ANCOVA)

ANCOVA is an inferential statistical test that enables investigators to adjust statistically for group differences that may interfere with obtaining results that relate specifically to the effects of the independent variable(s) on the dependent variable(s).

EXAMPLE

Analysis of Covariance (ANCOVA)

A group of nurse investigators designed a study to examine the effects of institutional care versus home care on terminally ill male and female patients' levels of satisfaction. The team of investigators agreed that patients' attitudes toward health care institutions might affect their level of satisfaction. Three null hypotheses were formulated: There is no difference in patient satisfaction between institutional care and home care; there is no difference in patient satisfaction between males and females; and there is no interaction between treatment and gender. ANCOVA was computed with patients' attitudes toward institutions as the covariate. A significant difference was found between treatments ($F = 4.75$, $df = 2, 84$, $p < .05$), with a post hoc comparison showing patient satisfaction levels higher in the home care group. The gender/satisfaction interaction was not significant.

ANCOVA is often used to study groups that have not been randomly assigned but exist naturally, such as residents of a nursing home or inpatients in an acute care hospital. Although the use of ANCOVA with the identification of a covariate (or covariates) assists in diminishing the effects of variables that are not controlled in the study, it cannot take the place of randomization. Even when several covariates are identified, such as age, attitudes, or various environmental factors, the groups are not considered to be as equal as they would be had their members been randomly assigned.

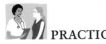

PRACTICE

Analysis of Covariance (ANCOVA)

Identify possible covariates from the following descriptions of research projects:

- The effect of patient teaching regarding mouth care on adult cancer patients receiving highly toxic chemotherapy.

- A comparison of verbal and written instructions on adult schizophrenic patients' compliance with their medication regimens.

- The effect of mother and infant bonding on the marital relationship.

In interpreting the results of a study in which ANCOVA has been used, the consumer, as well as the individual who is assisting with the design of a research project, needs to examine the usefulness in identifying the particular covariate. For example, is age, if it is identified, likely to affect the dependent variable, and are there additional covariates that should be identified?

CRITICAL APPRAISAL

Analysis of Covariance (ANCOVA)

- Is the covariate clearly identified?

- Might additional covariates be examined?

- If randomization is not used, are results interpreted with that factor in mind?

Multivariate Analysis

Before the advent of computers, simple techniques were used because the analysis had to be carried out by hand with the assistance of a calculator. The use of multivariate analysis has

317

increased as computers have become more accessible to investigators and statisticians. This statistical test enables researchers to examine multiple factors at the same time. Statistical tests described thus far have involved one dependent variable; multivariate analysis permits the examination of more than one dependent or independent variable. For example, in the studies that examine patients' satisfaction with their care, another dependent variable that might be of interest would be the patients' fears relative to survival.

It is not as appropriate to use separate univariate analyses to examine patient satisfaction and fears related to survival because, as long as these two dependent variables are related, separate analyses increase the chances of finding a difference resulting simply from the number of tests used. The computing of multivariate analysis is complex; however, the underlying principle is the same as for other inferential statistical tests—that is, there is an attempt to reject the null hypothesis at a given level of significance. Examples of specific multivariate tests include Hotelling's T^2, MANOVA, and MANCOVA.

WORKING DEFINITION

Multivariate Analysis

Multivariate analysis refers to a group of inferential statistical tests that enable the investigator to examine multiple variables simultaneously. Unlike other inferential statistical techniques, these tests permit the investigator to examine several dependent or independent variables simultaneously.

EXAMPLE

Multivariate Analysis

A group of nurse investigators designed a study to examine the effect of two forms of relaxation therapy on levels of depression and anxiety among male and female spinal-cord-injured young adults (paraplegics). Data collected in relation to the two independent variables—relaxation therapy (two groups) and gender—and the dependent variables—level of depression and level of anxiety—were analyzed using a multivariate test.

Multiple regression is another frequently used approach to analyzing data in which there are multiple variables. This statistical technique enables the investigator to examine relationships among several variables. For example, nurse investigators might want to use several criteria, such as level of depression, degree of anxiety, and concerns about survival, to predict patient satisfaction with their in-hospital experience. Using multiple regression, the three variables—level of depression, degree of anxiety, and concerns about survival—can be combined to predict the degree of patient satisfaction.

 PRACTICE

Multivariate Analysis

From a topic of interest relevant to nursing, formulate a research question identifying two independent variables and two or more dependent variables. Explain (using basic principles) how the data would be analyzed.

 CRITICAL APPRAISAL

Multivariate Analysis

Are more than one independent and more than one dependent variable used?

Correlation

Although correlation was described in the section on descriptive statistics, relationships can also be described in terms of probability. The results of a study may show that a relationship was significant; i.e., if 100 samples were drawn, it would occur by chance in only 5 samples.

Inferential Statistical Tests

Chi-Square Tests (Nonparametric)

Nonparametric statistical tests are generally used when the data analyzed are not assumed to reflect a normal distribution and when they are measured at either a nominal or ordinal level. Chi-square (X^2) is a nonparametric test that is used by nurse researchers who are interested in the number of participants or events that fall within specified categories (Munro, 2000).

For example, psychiatric clients may be categorized in relation to their compliance with a psychotropic medication regimen. The investigator may predict that clients with particular diagnoses or personality characteristics will comply more often than others.

The chi-square statistic does not give any information regarding the strength of a relationship; it only conveys the existence or nonexistence of the relationship between the variables investigated. To establish the extent and nature of the relationship, additional statistics such as phi, Cramer's V, or contingency coefficient can be used.

Critical Overview of Data Analysis

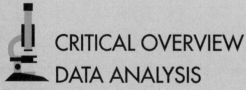

CRITICAL OVERVIEW
DATA ANALYSIS
Excerpt A

A group of nurse researchers want to investigate the psychological needs of patients newly diagnosed with acquired immunodeficiency syndrome (AIDS). No prior investigations are reported in the literature. They design a descriptive study to assess the needs of 75 male patients and use an Emotional Need Inventory that describes need for emotional support, information, and physical contact. A total score reflects the degree of "neediness."

Activity 1

- How might the team convey the results?

- Given a mean score on the "neediness" portion of the scale of 17 (possible range 1–22) and a standard deviation of 3.4, how would you interpret the findings?

- What is the value of the results of this study?

Excerpt B

The same team of nurse researchers, following their study on the psychological needs of newly diagnosed AIDS patients, design an educational intervention for these patients. They randomly assign 50 new participants to experimental and control groups and provide the experimental group with an educational package consisting of three two-hour group sessions and a collection of written materials. They want to see whether the patients' level of anxiety decreases following the intervention.

Activity 2

- What statistical test might be appropriate in analyzing the data?

- What covariate might be identified?

- What additional information might be needed to make an accurate interpretation of the results?

References

Cozby, P. C. (2000). *Methods in Behavioral Research* (7th Edition). Toronto: Mayfield Publishing Co.

Munro, B. (2000). *Statistical Methods for Health Care Research*. Philadelphia: Lippincott.

Norman, G. & Streiner, D. (1996). *PDQ Epidemiology*. St. Louis: Mosby.

Unit 4

Answering the Research Question: Qualitative Designs

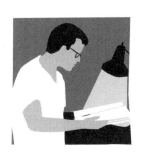

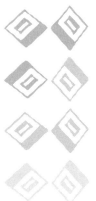

10

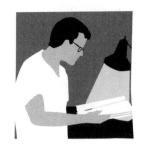

Qualitative Designs in Research

Goals

- *Describe the importance of qualitative research methods for nursing science.*
- *Examine the key elements common to various qualitative research designs.*
- *Describe strategies for implementing different types of qualitative designs.*

Introduction

Qualitative research methods are a group of approaches to conducting research that are considered increasingly important in building a body of nursing knowledge (Sandelowski, 1986). Over the past decade, a growing interest in examining qualitative methods and issues related to nursing research has appeared in the literature. Interest in research approaches that differ from the dominant scientific or quantitative methods has grown out of a concern for the need to clarify a research tradition in nursing science. Understanding qualitative research methods as an alternative form of inquiry is important in grasping the relative contribution to be made to nursing as well as the importance of adhering to guidelines that assist in maintaining scientific adequacy in the use of these research methods.

This chapter examines the issue of qualitative research: how it has evolved, how it is defined, and the purpose and concerns that the practitioner of nursing should consider when reviewing and utilizing the findings of this method. Also explored are types of qualitative approaches and ways of implementing select methodologies.

Development of Qualitative Research Designs

Research design is a term used to identify how the researcher will structure a plan to obtain the data needed to answer the research question. In traditional scientific methods, as described in Chapter 7 regarding quantitative research designs, a somewhat rigid set of rules or guidelines have been identified as important to the process. After decades of serving as the preferred mode of inquiry, traditional scientific methodology has come to be regarded as the dominant research paradigm. Qualitative research approaches have a somewhat shorter and less well-defined history.

As members of a relatively new science, nurse researchers and theoreticians have only recently sought to justify the research tradition or the manner in which knowledge is discovered or expanded (Gortner, 1983). In the process of clarifying how nursing science should be developed, nurse scientists have suggested the use of a variety of research approaches and have noted the contribution and value that qualitative methodologies can have in a discipline that is building a knowledge base. In fact, Munhall (1982) has suggested that quantitative research, or the traditional scientific method, be reconsidered in favor of methods that are more consistent with the humanistic, holistic philosophy of nursing. Nursing has historically been concerned with the wholeness of human beings. Because qualitative research is based on assumptions consistent with a belief in human wholeness, it is of value in the generation of knowledge unique to nursing.

Which method is used—qualitative or quantitative—depends on the research question because there are different assumptions with each approach. These assumptions assist the nurse researcher to select a framework most appropriate to the stated problem. For example, if the nurse researcher were interested in the accuracy of thermometers in assessing fever, a quantitative perspective would be most appropriate. However, if the nurse researcher is interested in the experience of fever from the patient's perspective, then a qualitative perspective is more appropriate. If the interest is in both phenomena, then a combined approach is most relevant.

Both qualitative and quantitative research methodologies have value for developing a unique body of nursing knowledge (Tinkle & Beaton, 1983; Phillips, 1991). It is important to remember that the differentiation between qualitative and quantitative approaches is sometimes less than clear-cut (Polit & Hungler, 1999). Philosophers of science have noted that some features typically associated with quantitative methods may also apply to qualitative research methods (Sandelowski, 1986).

Qualitative Research: Definition and Purpose

Qualitative research is a broad term referring to several research methods. Researchers conducting research using grounded theory, historical, ethnographic, philosophical, and phenomenological approaches are utilizing a few of the methods considered under the qualitative research title. Qualitative research is largely considered an inductive method that seeks to build knowledge about the meaning or relevance of a particular phenomenon or concept when little is known (Morse, 1986). Unlike quantitative methods of conducting research, qualitative strategies are useful for developing facts and concepts about an area of interest that has received little research attention, or for exploring an area that has not yet been explored from a qualitative perspective. Collectively, qualitative research strategies are often referred to as **naturalistic** investigations. The term *naturalistic* refers to the fact that this type of research often considers the study of phenomena within the everyday world.

 WORKING DEFINITION

Qualitative Research

Qualitative research is an inductive approach to discovering or expanding knowledge. It requires the involvement of the researcher in the identification of the meaning or relevance of a particular phenomenon to the individual. Analysis and interpretation of findings in this method are not generally dependent upon the quantification of observations.

It is important to remember that neither the quantitative nor the qualitative research method is better. Each research tradition is useful in a different sort of way. It is most important that the researcher choose a method that is *appropriate* for the kind of information being sought or theory being tested. For example, a nurse researcher may wish to discover what being a grandparent really means to individuals first experiencing this phase of the life process. Relatively little is known about the *meaning* of grandparenting, so the use of qualitative research methods would be a valuable and fruitful way to glean new knowledge about this concept.

328

On the other hand, some concepts or phenomena have been relatively well-researched and written about. A nurse researcher might be concerned with positioning of patients to prevent atelectasis and pulmonary infection in the postoperative phase. A significant amount of knowledge has been generated about physiological processes during the postoperative recovery phase, so it would be important to build on existing knowledge and theory in this area in an effort to expand what is already known. In this particular research instance, a quantitative approach would be most appropriate to the type of knowledge being sought.

 EXAMPLE

Qualitative Research

Following is a listing of qualitative nursing research studies:

- "The Lived Pregnancy Experience of Women in Prison" (Wismont, 2000).

- "Relinquishing Infertility: The Work of Pregnancy for Infertile Couples" (Sandelowski, Harris, & Black, 1992).

- "Mothers' Suffering: Sons Who Died of AIDS" (Gregory & Longman, 1992).

- "The Experience of Laughing at Oneself in Older Couples" (Malinski, 1991).

- "Men's Views about Hysterectomies and Women Who Have Them' (Bernhard, 1992).

The purpose of using qualitative research methodology can vary. It can be a useful, informative means of generating knowledge about an area that has received relatively little research effort. It also can be useful when bias is suspected in present knowledge or theories, or when the research question relates to understanding and describing a phenomenon (Field & Morse, 1985; Morse, 1991; Patton, 2001). Often, it is the most appropriate and efficient way of obtaining the needed

329

information. It is a misconception that qualitative research only has value as a method for obtaining preliminary, exploratory data to be used in later quantitative research efforts (Glaser & Strauss, 1966). Although that approach may be one way to use the findings, qualitative research is a legitimate activity that generates credible data for analyses through exploration, description, or expansion of existing knowledge and theory (Knafl & Howard, 1984).

Quantitative research is based on the fundamental assumptions of prediction, manipulation, and control. Qualitative research is based on gaining insight and understanding about individuals' experience and sense of reality in a fashion that does not generally involve quantification or the attachment of a number to observations in the process of recording and analyzing data. Quantitative research seeks to verify hypotheses that have been formulated to direct the research activities. Qualitative research approaches seek to examine the richness of data by determining patterns or the quality of the experience. These data are generated through the sustained interaction of the researcher with people in their own language and in their own environment (Kirk & Miller, 1986). Regardless of the research approach selected, there will be advantages and limitations that need to be considered in the context of the research question that is raised.

WORKING DEFINITION

Purpose of Qualitative Research

Qualitative research seeks to explore, describe, or expand knowledge about how reality is experienced.

The ultimate goal of nursing research is to solve scientific problems in an effort to expand knowledge in a particular area (see Figure 10.1). Research traditions, whether a qualitative or quantitative method is chosen, need not be viewed as competitive or undermining activities. Rather, research traditions

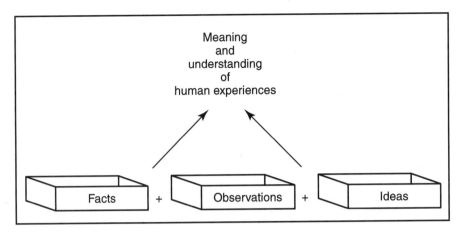

FIGURE 10.1 Knowledge generated through qualitative research

should complement one another, collaborating toward the goal of developing nursing science (Silva & Rothbart, 1984).

 PRACTICE

Purpose of Qualitative Research

Locate a research investigation that examines phenomena from a qualitative research approach. Determine the purpose for the study.

 CRITICAL APPRAISAL

Purpose of Qualitative Research

- Does the researcher identify a research question that seeks to explore, describe, or expand knowledge about how reality is experienced?

- Is the research question one that has received relatively little research attention?

331

- Has the topic only been addressed in a quantitative fashion although valuable information could be gained by conducting a qualitative investigation?

- Does the researcher clearly state the purpose for the qualitative study?

Qualitative Research Methods

Qualitative inquiry can occur in one of several forms. These forms include philosophical, historical, and grounded theory methodology; feminist methods; and phenomenology, among others. Although each method has a specific focus and goal for discovering knowledge, commonalities bind these methods together. The diversity noted between these different methods is not insignificant, however, and requires additional study of sources relevant to the method in question.

Types of Qualitative Inquiry

Developing a full understanding of the human experience requires a variety of methods for uncovering the range of experiences and intervening factors. The credibility of any given method must be evaluated within the context of the purpose, aim, goal, and "rules" governing the method. Following is a discussion of three major methods of conducting qualitative inquiry, phenomenological research, ethnographic research, and grounded theory methodology. The information presented attempts to highlight major critical guidelines for collecting and evaluating a given methodological format.

Phenomenological Research Phenomenology is a branch of philosophy that emphasizes the *meaning* that social behavior has for the individual. Thus, for any given act performed by the individual, meaning is developed that helps create a unique reality for that person. This philosophical movement was heavily influenced by the philosophers Lambert, Kant, Hegel, and Husserl, who held unique beliefs about the nature of human beings (Schmitt, 1972).

The phenomenological approach to conducting research is a relatively new emphasis for nursing science. Although there are a limited number of literature sources based on a phenomenological perspective, the popularity of the method is growing, in recognition of its value in generating knowledge.

WORKING DEFINITION

Phenomenological Research Approach

Phenomenology is a branch of philosophy that emphasizes the subjectivity of human experience. When used as the philosophical basis in research, phenomenology mandates that scientific data be generated by studying the desired information from the perspective of the research participant.

The nurse researcher who uses a phenomenological approach is concerned with the totality of the human experience. This includes all the nuances of a given experience. Phenomenological research mandates that the investigator become very attuned to research participants and their surroundings (Davis, 1978). Thus, there can be few expectations about what will be found in studying the participant and the experience. The participant generates the reality of the experience without prior hypotheses or "hunches" being established to guide what should be found. The researcher acts as an empty slate of sorts, willing to write a new chapter on the knowledge that is being sought (Omery, 1983).

EXAMPLE

Phenomenological Research Approach

A nurse working in a sleep disorder clinic is interested in exploring the impact of this human experience. She selects 25 clients who are experiencing sleep deprivation with loss of

333

REM-stage sleep and less stage-4 sleep. Although significant research has been conducted on sleep deprivation using quantitative measure, little has been done to determine the lived experience of sleep loss. The nurse interviews each client in his or her own home and at a time mutually agreed upon by the researcher and participant.

While conducting research utilizing the phenomenological method, the investigator must enter into the experience of the research participant. An effort must be made to understand the meaning of an event by participating in the process. It is through active involvement in the participant's reality that the researcher tries to make sense of and understand the meaning of the experience in question (Oiler, 1982). In this way, the researcher seeks to fully comprehend the lived experience of the phenomenon under study.

In attempting to describe the lived experience, the researcher focuses on what is happening in the life of the individual, what is important about the experience, and what alterations can be noted. Suggested steps that can be taken to guide the researcher in explicating the lived experience have been outlined by several authors (Munhall & Oiler, 1986; Oiler, 1982; Omery, 1983; Parse, Coyne, & Smith, 1985; Moustakas, 2000). It should be noted that these steps are not fixed and, in fact, vary from one philosophical perspective to another within the phenomenological movement itself.

The nurse researcher attempts to first identify the *research question*. This identification involves the determination of what specific experience is being studied. The nurse seeks to find out about that lived experience from the perspective of the participant. An example of an appropriate phenomenological research question might be "What is the experience of being a divorced, unemployed mother?"

Participants are selected that are appropriate to the research question. Of primary concern would be the selection of individuals who have recently had the experience under investigation (Omery, 1983)—for example, women who have had a stillbirth within the past three months, fathers who have lost custody of their children within the past year, or parents who have had an adult child recently diagnosed as HIV positive. The number of research participants required is highly variable in phenomenological research, as it is in other types of qualitative inquiry. Because voluminous data are frequently generated, a small number of participants are often selected. It is not unusual for the researcher to report a sample size of 10 to 20 participants or as many as 400, depending on participant availability, type of data to be collected, and time constraints. Sample size should be adequate to allow for full explanation of the phenomenon under study. The researcher needs to describe or justify the sample size but may not be able to predict the required number beforehand (Field & Morse, 1985).

The *setting* of the study is also an important consideration. To elicit the participant's feelings about a particular experience, it is beneficial to be in a relaxed environment, such as the home, community, or work environment of the participant. If a nurse were studying the experience of labor pain, however, a labor and delivery suite may be a more appropriate setting to use.

Clarifying what the experience under study means to the participant is crucial to the phenomenological method. *Bracketing* is a technique used to assist the participant in describing the lived experience by setting aside one's personal feelings so that all available perspectives can be considered in studying a phenomenon (Parse, Coyne, & Smith, 1985). Statements that would be helpful in eliciting the individual's description might be "Talk to me about what 'dying to get away from the kids' means to you" or "Tell me about your experience being a single mother."

Once participants have had an opportunity to describe their experiences fully, the researcher seeks to digest the data by systematically listing and classifying the collected information. The researcher must use *intuiting* to try to develop an awareness of the lived experience without forcing prior expectations or knowledge into the process (Oiler, 1982).

When data have been classified, the researcher seeks to reduce the number of categories to include the smallest number necessary to organize the experience. This process may mean reducing the data several times until overlap, vagueness, and irrelevancy are eliminated. The final listing of categories should reflect the lived experience captured in a coherent, meaningful manner.

The process of *analyzing* involves the difficult task of contrasting and comparing the final data to determine what patterns, themes, or threads emerge (Knaack, 1984). In the final analysis, the nurse researcher is seeking to further knowledge about some phenomenon and is trying to capture that lived experience in a concise fashion. If the knowledge is to be of relevance to other researchers, it must be understandable and clear, detailing the relationships that exist.

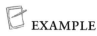 EXAMPLE

Phenomenological Research Method

A nurse working on a closed psychiatric unit was interested in investigating the experience of electroconvulsive therapy (ECT) for clients with a medical diagnosis of endogenomorphic depression. After receiving approval from the appropriate review committees, the nurse invited nine clients to participate in the study. Seven clients agreed to share their experiences with the researcher through the informal interview process.

The nurse met twice with each participant to ascertain his or her experience with the ECT process. Meetings lasted from 20 to 45 minutes, with a maximum of three weeks between interviews. The discussions took place in a comfortable lounge on the unit with no other clients present.

Participants were encouraged to share all feelings and thoughts about the ECT process. The nurse researcher refrained from commenting on the content and tried to facilitate disclosure by head nods, saying "umm-humm," and other affirmative gestures. The dialogue was tape-recorded to decrease the distraction of taking notes.

From the first interview until all interviews were completed, the nurse undertook continual analysis of the data. Attempts were made to understand the meaning of the data by pondering the content, then categorizing and recategorizing. Four patterns or themes finally emerged, and these were prioritized by determining how frequently the themes were discussed by the participant. The research process yielded knowledge valuable in generating other research questions, as well as providing a basic understanding of this lived experience.

PRACTICE

Phenomenological Research Method

Identify one research question from the practice setting that is amenable to the phenomenological approach. Discuss the number of participants that might participate, the setting for data collection, and how data collection might be accomplished.

CRITICAL APPRAISAL

Phenomenological Research Method

- Does the nurse researcher study the phenomenon from the perspective of the participant?
- Does the researcher discuss a willingness to study the experience from the participant's viewpoint?
- Does the nurse investigator engage in the research process as an active participant?

Ethnographic research Ethnographic research is generally considered to include both anthropological and historical research strategies (Shelley, 1984). Ethnographic methods involve a study of individuals, artifacts, or documents in the natural setting. The researcher is intimately involved in the data collection process and seeks to fully understand how life unfolds for the individual or group under study. The ultimate goal is to grasp the participant's point of view and understand

337

how the phenomena of health and illness are envisioned (Ragucci, 1972; Lecompte & Schensul, 1999).

WORKING DEFINITION

Ethnographic Research

Ethnographic research is a method of conducting inquiry into the life process by studying individuals, artifacts, or documents in the natural setting. It includes both anthropological and historical forms of inquiry.

Anthropology is the study of human beings under natural conditions. This type of field research seeks to understand how individuals or groups function behaviorally either by directly observing individuals or groups or by tracing former civilizations to gain insight into how they have influenced cultural groups today (Leininger, 1985).

In anthropological inquiry, the investigator collects and analyzes the data in the natural setting. The emphasis is on discovering what relationships exist under differing conditions. For example, a nurse working at a juvenile detention center is interested in studying repeat offenders. Study of these individuals would mean intensive participation with the adolescent to gather and analyze data that would provide insight into why these participants are repeat offenders. Documents that might be used to gain understanding could include diaries, observation, and interviews.

WORKING DEFINITION

Anthropological Research

Anthropological study involves the collection and analysis of data about an individual or a group under natural conditions. The investigator is immersed in the study process in an effort to fully understand the behavior and the subsequent impact on society.

338

PRACTICE

Anthropological Research

Review a newspaper for health-related articles. Identify at least one that would be appropriate for study in the natural setting. Suggest how the researcher might function to obtain the desired data.

Historical research strategies involve careful study and analysis of data from the past. Detailed analysis of what has been written or done is used to describe, explain, or interpret those events. It generally involves the review of written materials but may include oral documentation as well. The purpose of historical research is to provide meaning and understanding (Ashley, 1978). The results contribute to a clearer understanding of present or future events as they relate to nursing, health care, and the life process. For example, a nurse investigator may be interested in studying the professional nurse's role as advocate for pregnant women since World War II. Knowledge of how the advocate role has been fulfilled in the past may provide nurses with helpful information regarding how that role might best be carried out today.

WORKING DEFINITION

Historical Research

Historical research involves the careful study and analysis of data about past events. The purpose is to gain a clearer understanding of the impact of the past on present and future events related to the life process.

Use of the historical research approach is highlighted by discrete steps. First, a comprehensive *gathering of data* is undertaken. Diaries, letters, manuscripts, maps, and books are but a few of the possible documents that may be considered. The documents should be original, or primary sources, whenever

339

possible. Using primary sources may mean traveling to obtain the necessary data.

The second step is *criticism of the data*, which necessitates a comprehensive review of gathered materials. This is an arduous task requiring a sense of skepticism about the accuracy of the documents in question. Christy (1975) describes the analytic process of document review as a two-pronged activity: **external criticism**, or the establishment of validity by determining the authenticity of the source, and **internal criticism**, or the determination of reliability by correctly interpreting the contents of the document. Use of original, authentic sources, awareness of one's own biases, and the substantiation of the document in question by another collaborating source are a few of the safeguards used to ensure that interpretations are correct. It is never safe to assume that facts are accurate merely because they are in print.

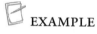 EXAMPLE

Reliability and Validity of Historical Research Sources

A nurse had read accounts of the "kinship" shared between nurse and family members during a time when health care occurred largely in the community. Curious about the impact that death in the hospital setting has for family members in the resolution of grief, the nurse conducted a historical investigation. The nurse's role in the grief process following death of a family member from 1900 to 1940 was the focus of the study. Oral accounts, family biblical records, letters, personal diaries, photographs, health records, and nursing textbooks were all used to grasp an understanding of this process.

External Criticism

The nurse ascertained that all documents were original. First-hand oral and written accounts were accepted as valid. Signatures and dates on materials were carefully reviewed. When each document selected for review clearly met the criteria for authenticity, it was then accepted as appropriate for further analysis and interpretation.

Internal Criticism

To ensure reliability, the nurse examined each document to make sure that the meaning of facts and statements was clearly understood. This process entailed seeking collaboration from individuals who may have witnessed the events in question, as well as determining the meaning of words, phrases, and colloquialisms unique to that time period.

Determining the interrelationship among facts and the meaning of the data gathered, reviewed, and recorded is the final step in historical research (Matejski, 1979). This activity is undoubtedly the most difficult and requires synthesis and resynthesis of the material to arrive at an appropriate interpretation. The nurse historian needs to sift through the data and ultimately relate the content to a larger theory or model.

The three steps identified are central to discovering the truth about the past and how it can relate to nursing and health care provided today. For example, if a nurse investigator were interested in examining the influence of early black nurse leaders in American nursing from 1870 to 1915, a historical research approach would be appropriate in generating the evidence. The historical nurse researcher could interview descendents, review professional documents, read diaries and letters, and examine photographs, among other sources (see Figure 10.2). Scrutiny of these materials should assist in the construction of the "story" of facts regarding these leaders. Ultimately, the nurse historian would synthesize the material and make a determination regarding the contribution of these leaders to nursing and health care, as well as suggestions for future change.

A more familiar example of the use of historical research methodology can be found in the work of Kalisch and Kalisch (1987). These researchers have done extensive analysis of the image of professional nurses through the examination of various documents. Documents examined have included film clips, novels, newspaper clippings, and magazine articles, among others. Intensive examination of these historical materials has

341

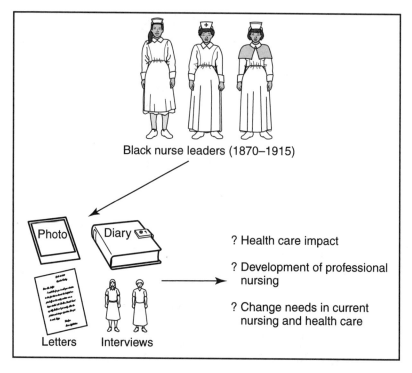

Black nurse leaders (1870–1915)

Photo Diary

Letters Interviews

? Health care impact

? Development of professional nursing

? Change needs in current nursing and health care

FIGURE 10.2 Historical research: Generating the evidence

allowed the nurse historians to identify varying images during different time periods. The result of their analyses has been a systematic evaluation of image problems currently existing within the profession.

 PRACTICE

Historical Research

Identify a topic that would be of interest for historical study. Discuss the purpose of the study, time period to be studied, and possible documents to support the focus of the investigation.

In summary, nurse historians "try to feel in body, mind, and soul what the people they are studying might have felt in their lifetime" (Ashley, 1978, p. 31). It is difficult to review documents, digest facts, and synthesize a comprehensive meaning. Contrary to what many nurses believe, historical research is the foundation of science and is a consuming task requiring scholarly insight and ability (Christy, 1975; Notter, 1972).

CRITICAL APPRAISAL

Ethnographic Research

- Does the researcher conduct the study in the natural setting?
- Is the researcher intimately involved in the data collection process?
- Does the researcher attempt to establish validity and reliability of sources?
- Does the researcher relate the study to current or future events?

Grounded Theory Methodology   Grounded theory methodology, developed by the sociologists Glaser and Strauss (1966), is an interesting means of developing theory in a manner that draws heavily on detailed social data to shape the theoretical beliefs. Although this method is frequently considered to be an inductive means of developing theory, in actuality a combined inductive and deductive process is utilized.

The investigator who selects grounded theory methodology is interested in generating a theory to explain the detailed findings gathered in the "real world." After collecting data about some area of research interest, the researcher would attempt to detail a theory to explain the data gathered and the interrelationships found therein. This is not a pure process, and the activities do not occur in isolation. The researcher gathers data, ponders relationships, suggests a theoretical explanation to capture the data found, and then repeats the process until the theory is believed to reflect the data accurately.

343

WORKING DEFINITION

Grounded Theory Methodology

Grounded theory methodology is a means of studying social data for the purpose of explaining some phenomenon. A theory is ultimately generated through inductive and deductive activity.

The nurse researcher who uses a grounded theory approach selects a single social situation or event for study. Data are then collected from as many diverse sources as possible to fully understand the experience, variations, and factors. For example, a nurse may be interested in researching the engagement behaviors of two-year-old children who are entering day care for the first time. The researcher might observe the day-care environment as well as the home environment. A combination of observation and a literature review should contribute to the development and testing of hypotheses. The nurse may manipulate the day-care environment to see if the hypotheses are accurate. These hypotheses serve to guide the researcher in observing and analyzing the data. This cyclical process of confirming what is *expected* to be found in the social situation (deductive) and what data are *actually* gathered (inductive) is a key feature of grounded theory (Stern, 1980) (see Figure 10.3).

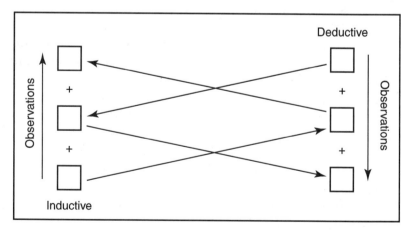

FIGURE 10.3 Building knowledge in grounded theory methodology

The ultimate purpose is to generate credible theory for further testing and study (Schreiber & Stern, 2001).

The researcher using grounded theory approach does not intend to study social situations with a totally "blank" view of the experience. Rather, throughout the research process the investigator compares and contrasts what is found in the real world of direct observation with what the literature suggests should be found. The result is the development of theory that may or may not incorporate prevailing knowledge. The natural setting and what is found by the researcher verify what will be included (Glaser & Strauss, 1966). The researcher tries to increase the credibility of the suggested theory by studying comparison groups. For example, a nurse who is studying affiliative behaviors of the homeless might also study elderly single women, childrearing families, deinstitutionalized mentally handicapped individuals, and so forth. Data that support the proposed theory would add credibility to the theory or, conversely, allow for appropriate change to accommodate the behaviors noted.

 EXAMPLE

Grounded Theory Methodology

A community health nurse is using grounded theory methodology to study scapegoating in dysfunctional families. The nurse limits the study to those families that have children (10 and under). Observation for the purpose of collecting data occurs primarily in the home. Family interaction and communication patterns are assessed through observation and interview, as well as through role-playing situations (manipulation) and observation of family members in their work or school environment. As data collection proceeds, the nurse begins to form some hypotheses regarding scapegoating activity. The literature is also reviewed to guide the researcher in asking questions and in deciding which behaviors to note.

During the process of data collection the nurse begins to categorize and code the data. Coding, or labeling the categories, assists the nurse in thinking conceptually about the data. The result of the nurse's analysis is a theory of scapegoating in dysfunctional families. To verify the theory that is generated, the nurse plans to study other dysfunctional families who use scapegoating.

PRACTICE

Grounded Theory Methodology

Identify a research project that uses grounded theory methodology. Suggest at least two comparison groups that could be used for additional study.

CRITICAL APPRAISAL

Grounded Theory Methodology

- Is the social situation or event under study clearly identified by the researcher?

- Does the researcher attempt to develop a theory about the social situation that is based on a combination of observation and literature review?

- Are comparison groups utilized to maximize credibility of the theory?

Sources of Data

Data to be used in qualitative nursing research emerge from subject and investigator participation in attempting to describe a particular experience. Because experiences of human beings unfold from everyday life, the format for collecting data may vary (Figure 10.4). For example, a nurse researcher studying the experience of being hospitalized during the preschool years may collect the data through the combined use of participant observation, therapeutic play, and art expression. Because children frequently have difficulty verbalizing the full range of their feelings, alternative methods of teasing out the meaning

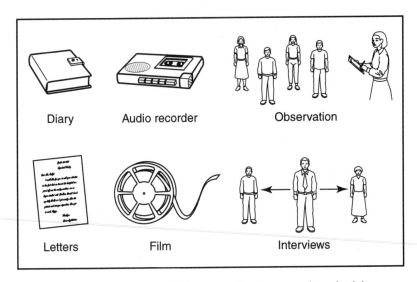

FIGURE 10.4 Sources of data in qualitative research methodology

of the experience need to be utilized by the investigator. Another nurse researcher might be investigating the impact of impotence on middle-aged men. The format selected for collecting data here might more appropriately be informal interviews or a written account of personal feelings. Still another researcher may choose to investigate weaning practices of breast-feeding mothers from 1930 to 1950. The format might be historical documents, oral histories, and interviews. Whatever the focus of inquiry, the method of collecting data should be sensitive to the needs of the research participant and the researcher as well as of the phenomenon under investigation.

A technique often used in qualitative research investigations is *triangulation*. This technique combines more than one data source or methodological technique. For example, a researcher might be interested in studying postpartum depression and might interview women during the early course of the illness. To further understand the experience, the researcher might have the patient's healthcare provider complete a survey of intensity of illness, as well as having the patient's spouse complete a checklist regarding marital relationships. Careful analysis of the data from several sources and the use of differing

347

methodologies allows for a richer, fuller description of the phenomenon than one source or approach (Thurmond, 2001).

WORKING DEFINITION

Sources of Data

Sources of data in qualitative research are the individuals, documents, or artifacts utilized to collect data about a particular phenomenon. Sources vary with the focus of inquiry, the purpose of the investigation, and guidelines suggested by the research approach being utilized.

EXAMPLE

Sources of Data

The following is a list of possible sources that could be used in collecting data relevant to the life process:

- Diaries
- Case studies
- Artwork
- Therapeutic play
- Participant observation
- Documents (historical, etc.)
- Interviews (formal and informal)
- Audio/videotape recordings

Participant observation and **semistructured interviews** are probably the two most common types of data collection in qualitative research. Both of these data collection means have the advantage of allowing flexibility in pursuing divergent topical areas that may be of concern to the participant or of interest to the researcher. Thus, new leads or relationships can be incorporated into the study.

PRACTICE

Sources of Data

Identify two possible data sources, and identify the individuals with which each one might be most appropriate for use.

CRITICAL APPRAISAL

Sources of Data

• Does the researcher discuss preparation for gathering data, including how research participants and study sites were determined?

• Are the sources of data utilized in the study appropriate to the method?

Participant Observation

Participant observation is a technique of involvement with the research participant. It evolved from sociological and anthropological field research. Participant observation has developed as a method where the observer (researcher) deliberately seeks to become involved in the experiences of the participant under study. Understanding and acknowledging the experience of the participant is purposefully and deliberately utilized (Leininger, 1985; Ragucci, 1972).

WORKING DEFINITION

Participant Observation

Participant observation is a method of researcher interaction with the participant. The researcher deliberately strives to become involved in the experience under study to facilitate fuller understanding.

There are a variety of levels of interacting with research participants during the process of data collection. These could include peripheral membership, active membership, or complete membership (Adler & Adler, 1987). Participant observation, a means of actively engaging as a member of group activity, has been identified as a particularly valuable and well-suited technique for collecting data in qualitative research study (Oiler, 1982).

It is important for the nurse researcher to decide on the level of involvement prior to the initiation of the research project. The level of participation should vary with the skills of the nurse (both personally and scientifically), the focus of the research investigation, and the needs of the participant.

A decision to participate through *peripheral* membership would mean minimal involvement with the activities of the individual or group. This may be necessary while conducting historical research, or desirable when participation may alter the data desired. The disadvantage of this role is that the nurse researcher does not feel an active part of the process and is not able to direct the data to be collected. It is less threatening than other roles, however, and may be easier for the neophyte qualitative researcher.

The *active* membership role in research involves the participation of the researcher in activities in the participant setting. The participant is largely aware of the research process and related activities. The researcher is usually able to elicit meaningful data because involvement facilitates understanding. This role may be difficult, however, because both the researcher and the participant may fail to remain cognizant of the researcher's role outside the process under study.

Acting in the *complete* membership role, a researcher is generally functioning as a full affiliative member of the group. The researcher may or may not choose to reveal his or her identity. Full acceptance as a group member yields valuable information. However, ethical concerns must be raised when full disclosure is not carried out by the investigator (Field & Morse, 1985; Orb, Eisenhauer, & Wynaden, 2001).

 EXAMPLE

Participant Observation Roles

Peripheral Membership Role

A nurse researcher is examining the development of spiritual behaviors in school-aged children. The nurse chooses to largely observe the interactions between parent and child to preserve the quality of the interactions.

Active Membership Role

Studying concerns of fathers for safety of their spouses in pregnancy after age 40, a nurse researcher elects an active membership research role. The investigator explains the nature of the study, then proceeds to interview and observe these individuals.

Complete Membership Role

A nurse is interested in investigating mental health concerns of working mothers. The researcher informs the participants of her identity and purpose but quickly moves to become a group member, sharing personal experiences as a working mother while also making observations in the data collection process.

 PRACTICE

Participant Observation Roles

Select a qualitative research report from a nursing research journal. Determine the research role utilized by the investigator: peripheral, active, or complete membership.

CRITICAL APPRAISAL

Participant Observation Roles

- Is the level of participant observation clearly identified by the researcher?

- Is the level of research participation appropriate to the focus of the study and the needs of the research participants?

Recording the Data

All forms of qualitative investigation require that the researcher, as a participant in the process, largely suspend expectations of how the data should be recorded. This requirement means that the researcher should record all aspects of data relevant to the experience under study without categorizing the data prematurely (Leininger, 1985). The purpose of conducting qualitative analysis is to discover or expand knowledge, so it is imperative that the researcher become immersed in the participants' experiences *without* deciding in advance how those individuals would feel, think, or act in those circumstances.

WORKING DEFINITION

Recording Data

Recording data in qualitative inquiry involves the full documentation of data from all sources identified for inclusion in the study. It requires a willingness to totally experience the data prior to making a decision about the meaning of the information.

Capturing the fullness of the experience involves the comprehensive documentation of data. The researcher must be careful to evaluate personal feelings prior to, during, and after data collection. Acute awareness of one's feelings and expectations helps to clarify how and why certain data might have been recorded and why these were selected over other kinds of data. For example, a nurse researcher is studying the experience of widowhood through use of the phenomenological method. If the nurse had herself been recently widowed or if she had strong feelings about the dependency of widows, it would be important to address these feelings and structure the study accordingly. Such restructuring might include asking different types of questions or using different sources of data.

This example clearly illustrates how past experience can shape the questions that are asked, the data that are recorded, and the interpretation that is rendered. In qualitative analysis the key is to *increase awareness of these expectations*, then address them as an inherent part of the investigator—participant process. When the researcher is clear about his or her own opinions, feelings, thoughts, and the like, as well as the impact they may have on the study being conducted, the study can be structured to accommodate these influences. This process is important in establishing validity in qualitative research analysis (Wilson, 1985).

 PRACTICE

Recording Data

Use the peripheral research role while sitting on a bus, train, or airplane. Record data from the conversation occurring around you (maintaining anonymity and confidentiality). Identify your feelings and thoughts about the data.

The actual recording of data is guided by the phenomenon under study and what may or may not be known about that participant. Questions such as "What factors are significant in the experience?", "What is going on in a given situation?", and "What factors alter the experience?" are all important in focusing the data needed to answer the study question. In any event, the length of time spent in gathering and recording data, as well as the way it is recorded, needs to be carefully thought out prior to study. The final research report must detail these

353

activities if the study is to be of maximum use to others (Knafl & Howard, 1984).

CRITICAL APPRAISAL

Recording Data

- Does the researcher express a willingness to fully record data about the phenomenon under study?

- Are the opinions, feelings, and thoughts of the researcher about the research topic and process addressed?

- Does the researcher discuss how much time the data collection took and how the data were recorded?

Recording for Bias

Bias is an inherent problem in both quantitative and qualitative research methodologies (Sandelowski, 1986). Bias is a feeling or influence that tends to strongly favor one side or another in an argument. This slanting of data results in research that is highly suspect. When bias is allowed to filter unchecked into the researcher's work, it can result in scientific findings that are questionable. The responsible nurse researcher attempts to identify and correct possible sources of bias in an effort to improve the reliability of the findings.

WORKING DEFINITION

Bias

Bias is a feeling or influence that strongly favors the outcome of a particular finding in a research project. When the chance of bias in a project is not addressed, the reliability of the scientific findings is considered to be highly questionable.

A practitioner of nursing would want to be sure that the findings of a particular research project were reasonably reliable before putting the findings of a study into practice. Bias is a problem in all types of research, but it has been considered a significant problem in qualitative approaches. What is probably more accurate to say is that bias is a part of all research. In qualitative approaches, the researcher bases the method and procedure on an implicit understanding that bias is present. Bias is recog*nized and incorporated* into the structure of the study, rather than making attempts to eliminate it, as is the case in quantitative methodologies (Omery, 1983).

Means of checking for unnecessary bias in conducting qualitative research have been suggested. For example, the researcher should consider the advantage of selecting unfamiliar participants, clearly state her or his own feelings and opinions about the area under study, and select a research topic that is not overly meaningful or difficult to deal with on a personal level.

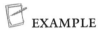 EXAMPLE

Bias

A nurse researcher is using a qualitative research approach to investigate the meaning of incorporating a cognitively impaired parent into a household. The nurse has recently had to incorporate her own in-laws into the household, both suffering from severe cognitive impairment. The nurse admits emotional strain and hostility over changes related to the move. This is probably a research topic that is too close to the researcher emotionally. Allowing a significant amount of time to pass before conducting the study or selecting a different research question would help to eliminate unnecessary bias in the study.

In qualitative research, the researcher is not considered a separate and removed observer of the research participant. Absolute objectivity is considered impossible. Each individual understands the world from his or her own bank of experiences. Instead, the observer (or researcher) is regarded as an implicit part of the scientific process. Viewing the researcher as an integral part of the individual's reality, or the reality of the investigation, is a basic assumption in qualitative designs. Accepting this position allows the researcher to build in safeguards that will permit the discovery of knowledge that is not a product of wishful thinking or bias on the part of the nurse investigator.

PRACTICE

Bias

Reflect on your own nursing practice and identify one area for study that would be difficult for you to research. Identify another study that you could initiate, and discuss ways you might incorporate sources of bias.

CRITICAL APPRAISAL

Bias

Does the researcher discuss feelings, thoughts, and attitudes about the study and subsequent means of structuring the study to incorporate those biases?

Critical Overview of Qualitative Research Designs

Qualitative research methods are an exciting means of conducting research when the problem under investigation relates to how a particular phenomenon is experienced. These methodologies are particularly useful when looking at areas that have not been well understood or studied, or when the existing theories or knowledge are suspected of being biased.

The qualitative researcher selects participants or data sources that are appropriate to the question under study. Every effort is made to understand the richness of the experience

356

from the participant's point of view and that may require varying levels of participation. Understanding the experience requires that the phenomenon is clearly identified prior to initiation of the project.

A careful recording of the data allows the researcher to gain a clearer understanding of what the experience means to the participants. Awareness and recognition of inherent bias on the part of any researcher assists in accurate data collection and subsequent analysis.

CRITICAL OVERVIEW
QUALITATIVE RESEARCH DESIGNS

Excerpt A

A nurse works in a center for the hearing impaired. Curious about this experience, the nurse structures an investigation to determine the meaning of this condition to the individual.

Excerpt B

Working in a community health center where many of the clients are Polish-speaking immigrants, a staff nurse wants to investigate cultural beliefs and customs that influence health behaviors. To facilitate an understanding, the nurse moves into an apartment in a Polish neighborhood for nine months.

Excerpt C

A nurse works on a medical-surgical unit in a large inner-city hospital. Many of the patients hospitalized on the unit express a preference for selecting their own nurse to provide health care. The nurse collaborates with a nurse colleague who has made the same observation. Together, they decide to research how the trend of nurse–patient assignment originated and what impact it has had on nursing effectiveness and patient participation in the health care system.

Select one excerpt and complete the following activities:

- Identify the type of qualitative research approach that would be most appropriate to use in the excerpt (i.e., phenomenological, anthropological, historical, or grounded theory methodology).

- Identify sources of data for the method. If human participants are utilized, how many would be desirable or feasible? How might the data sources be obtained?

- Discuss the researcher's role. If participant observation is selected, identify the level of researcher interaction.

References

Adler, P. A. & Adler, P. (1987). *Membership roles in field research*, vol. 6. Newbury Park, CA: Sage.

Ashley, J. A. (1978). Foundations for scholarship: Historical research in nursing. *Advances in Nursing Science*, 1(1): 25–36.

Bernhard, L. A. (1992). Men's views about hysterectomies and women who have them. *Image: The Journal of Nursing Scholarship*, 24(3): 177–181.

Christy, T. E. (1975). The methodology of historical research. *Nursing Research*, 24(3): 189–192.

Davis, A. J. (1978). The phenomenological approach in nursing research. In Norma L. Chaska (Ed.), *The nursing profession: Views through the mist* (pp. 186–196). New York: McGraw-Hill.

Field, P. A. & Morse, J. M. (1985). *Nursing research: The application of qualitative approaches*. Rockville, MD: Aspen Systems Corporation.

Glaser, B. G. & Strauss, A. L. (1966). The purpose and credibility of qualitative research. *Nursing Research, 15*(1): 56–61.

Gortner, S. R. (1983). The history and philosophy of nursing science and research. *Advances in Nursing Science, 5*(2): 1–7.

Gregory, D. & Longman, A. (1992). Mothers' suffering: Sons who died of AIDS. *Qualitative Health Research, 2*(3): 334–357.

Kalisch, B. J. & Kalisch, P. A. (1987). *The changing image of the nurse.* Menlo Park, CA: Addison-Wesley.

Kirk, J. & Miller, M. L. (1986). *Reliability and validity in qualitative research,* vol. 1. Newbury Park, CA: Sage.

Knaack, P. (1984). Phenomenological research, *Western Journal of Nursing Research, 6*(1): 107–114.

Knafl, K. A. & Howard, M. J. (1984). Interpreting and reporting qualitative research. *Research in Nursing and Health, 7*(1): 17–24.

Lecompte, M. D. & Schensul, J. J. (1999). *Designing and conducting ethnographic research (volume 1).* Walnut Creek, CA: Altamira Press.

Leininger, M. M. (1985). *Qualitative research methods in nursing.* New York: Grune and Stratton.

Leininger, M. M. (1992). Current issues, problems, and trends to advance qualitative paradigmatic research methods for the future. *Qualitative Health Research, 2*(4): 392–415.

Lincoln, Y. & Guba, G. (1985). *Naturalistic inquiry.* Beverly Hills, CA: Sage.

Malinski, V. M. (1991). The experience of laughing at oneself in older couples. *Nursing Science Quarterly, 4*(2): 69–75.

Matejski, M. P. (1979). Humanities: The nurse and historical research, *Image, 11*(3): 80–85.

Morse, J. M. (1986). Quantitative and qualitative research: Issues in sampling. In Peggy L. Chinn (Ed.), *Nursing research methodology* (pp. 181–193). Rockville, MD: Aspen.

Morse, J. M. (1991). Evaluating qualitative research (editorial). *Qualitative Health Research, 1*(3): 283–286.

Moustakas, C. E. (2000). *Phenomenological Research Methods.* Thousand Oaks, CA: Sage Publications.

Munhall, P. L. (1982). Nursing philosophy and nursing research: In apposition or opposition? *Nursing Research, 31*(3): 176–177, 181.

Munhall, P. L. & Oiler, C. J. (1986). *Nursing research: A qualitative perspective.* Norwalk, CT: Appleton-Century-Crofts.

Notter, L. E. (1972). The case for historical research in nursing (editorial), *Nursing Research, 21*(6): 483.

Oiler, C. (1982). The phenomenological approach in nursing research. *Nursing Research, 31*(3): 178–181.

Omery, A. (1983). Phenomenology: A method for nursing research. *Advances in Nursing Science, 5*(2): 49–63.

Orb, A., Eisenhauer, L., & Wynaden, D. (2001). Ethics in qualitative research. *Journal of Nursing Scholarship, 33*(1): 93–96.

Oxford American Dictionary. (1980). New York: Oxford University Press.

Parse, R. R., Coyne, A. B., & Smith, M. J. (1985). *Nursing research: Qualitative methods.* Bowie, MD: Brady Communications.

Patton, M. Q. (2001). *Qualitative Research & Evaluation Methods* (3rd Edition). Thousand Oaks, CA: Sage Publications.

Phillips, J. R. (1991). Different ways to skin a cat. *Nursing Science Quarterly, 4*(2): 50–51.

Polit, D. F. & Hungler, B. P. (1999). *Nursing research: Principles and methods* (6th Edition). Philadelphia: Lippincott Williams & Wilkins.

Ragucci, A. T. (1972). The ethnographic approach and nursing research. *Nursing Research, 21*(6): 485–490.

Sandelowski, M. (1986). The problem of rigor in qualitative research. *Advances in Nursing Science, 8*(3): 27–37.

Sandelowski, M., Harris, B. G., & Black B. P. (1992). Relinquishing infertility: The work of pregnancy for infertile couples. *Qualitative Health Research, 2*(3): 282–301.

Schmitt, R. (1972[1967]). Phenomenology. In Paul Edwards (Ed.), *The Encyclopedia of Philosophy*, vol. 6, (pp. 135–151). New York: Macmillan/Free Press.

Schreiber, R. & Stern, P. (2001). *Using grounded theory in nursing.* NY: Springer Publishing.

Seidel, J. V. & Clark, J. (1983). *The ethnograph: A user's guide.* Boulder: University of Colorado Computer Center.

360

Shelley, S. I. (1984). *Research methods in nursing and health*. Boston: Little, Brown.

Silva, M. C. & Rothbart, D. (1984). Philosophies of science on nursing theory development and testing. *Advances in Nursing Science*, 6(2): 1–13.

Stern, P. N. (1980). Grounded theory methodology: Its uses and processes. *Image*, 12(1): 20–23.

Swanson-Kauffman, K. M. (1986). A combined qualitative methodology for nursing research. *Advances in Nursing Science*, 8(3): 58–69.

Tesch, R. (1991). Computer programs that assist in the analysis of qualitative data: An overview. *Qualitative Health Research*, 1(3): 309–325.

Thurmond, V. A. (2001). The point of triangulation. *Journal of Nursing Scholarship*, 33(3): 253–258.

Tinkle, M. B. & Beaton, J. L. (1983). Toward a new view of science: Implications for nursing research. *Advances in Nursing Science*, 5(2): 27–36.

Wilson, H. S. (1985). *Research in nursing*. Menlo Park, CA: Addison-Wesley.

Wismont, J. M. (2000). The lived pregnancy experience of women in prison. *Journal of Midwifery & Women's Health*, 45(4): 292–300.

Bibliography

Morse, J. M. (Ed.). (1991). *Qualitative nursing research: A contemporary dialogue*, rev. ed. Newbury Park, CA: Sage.

11

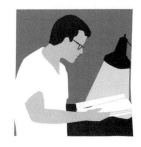

Analyzing the Data in Qualitative Research

Goals

- *Describe strategies for appropriately analyzing qualitative research data.*
- *Understand linking the qualitative research process to the review of the literature.*
- *Examine approaches to ensure scientific adequacy in qualitative designs.*

Introduction

Qualitative research designs are based on entirely different assumptions from quantitative designs. Because of differences in sample selection and methodology, data analysis is necessarily different. Large amounts of data are typically collected, and the challenge of making sense of that data can be overwhelming. The goal is to organize the data so that the reader can understand what the experience under study is like for the research participants. Analysis of the qualitative research report also requires that the researcher initiate strategies to make sure that the proposed findings and interpretation are credible or trustworthy.

Analyzing the Data

Analysis of the data that are recorded in the qualitative approach involves a careful mulling over of the possible meanings and relationships (Miles & Huberman, 1994). The researcher seeks to determine patterns, qualities, or unifying threads in the data that have been recorded. To do so requires a willingness to examine all possible meanings systematically and to let the way the research participants have experienced reality emerge without a preconceived conclusion.

WORKING DEFINITION

Analyzing the Data

Data analysis in qualitative inquiry involves the careful mulling over of recorded data to discover apparent patterns, themes, or relationships.

Analysis of qualitative data can be time-consuming. Relationships are often subtle and may require an intuitive awareness to identify. Also, the data are usually voluminous, and a quick review rarely reveals the richness of the information gleaned. Researchers using qualitative approaches frequently spend hours pondering the underlying themes and meanings of what has been recorded.

Most researchers who discuss data analysis in qualitative methodologies suggest several common steps in the process (Field & Morse, 1985; Leininger, 1985; Parse, Coyne, & Smith, 1985; Streubert & Carpenter, 1999). These include identification of themes, verifying the selected themes through reflection on the data and discussion with other researchers or experts in the area, categorizing the themes (using existing or novel categories), recording of support data for categories, and identification of propositions.

Data analysis is not a discrete step in qualitative methodology. From the beginning of the research project, the investigator has started to interpret the possible meanings of the data presented. The final conclusion about meanings of the recorded data is not made until all data have been collected, analysis has been systematically undertaken, and interrelationships have been made apparent.

For most qualitative researchers, the process of analyzing the data is a significant challenge. Part of the reason for this is that there are no set criteria for analysis. Each qualitative researcher must decide the most accurate and efficient means of summarizing the voluminous data that are generally produced during qualitative study. Most qualitative research reports generate large amounts of data that must be reviewed and put into a meaningful summary. Some researchers elect to do very little reduction of the data and instead present highlights, or excerpts, from the collected material. The challenge for the researcher is to manage the data in such a way that it can be meaningfully presented and understood while best representing the experience of the phenomenon by the research participants.

EXAMPLE

Analyzing the Data

A nurse works on a unit that provides care for patients who have debilitating orthopedic conditions. The nurse is interested in conducting historical research to determine comfort measures provided to these types of clients in the 1930s. The nurse uses a variety of historical nursing documents to determine the prevailing nursing care at the time, and also conducts interviews with individuals who had experience in this area. Data analysis here would mean spending time to look at how nursing care was provided, the basis for specific comfort measures, and how clients perceived the comfort measures and the delivery of those methods.

 PRACTICE

Analyzing the Data

Select a qualitative research study from a nursing journal and discuss how the researcher conducted preliminary data analysis: identification, verification and categorizing of themes, recording of support data, and identification of propositions.

 CRITICAL APPRAISAL

Analyzing the Data

Does the researcher discuss how the data were initially reviewed?

Literature Review

Although a limited literature review is necessary to justify the need for study, a full literature review is generally withheld in qualitative studies until the data have been collected and analyzed. (The exception is grounded theory methodology, which

366

employs an inductive-deductive process of generating theory. Continuous literature review during data collection and analysis supports this process.) This delay is considered one means of assisting the researcher in withholding preconceived ideas about what data should be found. By reviewing the literature after the data have been collected, the researcher can contrast and compare the patterns found in the study with what might have been expected from a literature standpoint.

Researchers will do a limited perusal of the literature to gain some insight into the phenomenon they are attempting to study prior to the actual investigation as well as to provide study justification. This cursory review of available literature also serves to highlight some of the areas that need to be addressed in the process of gathering data. Review of the literature prior to the actual collection of data can alert the investigator to the paucity of knowledge available or, conversely, the wealth of scientific data already generated.

At any rate, when data collection has been completed, it is wise for the researcher to review the literature carefully to ascertain relationships, the accuracy of selected categories, and areas in need of additional study.

WORKING DEFINITION

Literature Review

The literature review is a systematic review of the available literature sources about the phenomenon under study. In qualitative research methods, an intensive literature review is generally withheld until after the data have been collected.

PRACTICE

Literature Review

Select a qualitative nursing research report from a journal. Determine how the researcher conducted the literature review.

CRITICAL APPRAISAL

Literature Review

- Has a systematic literature review been conducted after the data were collected (where appropriate)?

- Is the literature review appropriate to the research question?

Analyzing the Findings

Analyzing the meaning of the data collected and how it relates to current literature sources about the phenomenon so that it can be communicated to other scientists is a major goal of qualitative methods. The researcher must decide how the findings can best be summarized: Is an existing theory from the literature best suited to highlight the data found, or does a new schema need to be developed and proposed? It is also important to realize that in qualitative methodologies, data analysis is an ongoing process. The researcher makes a final determination regarding the meaning of the data when the analytic process is completed.

Coding and categorizing of the data are generally initiated as soon as data collection begins. These categories are then refined as the data demand. Developing categories is facilitated through the use of either manual or computer activity.

Manual Analysis Manual analysis involves a thorough review of all recorded information that the researcher has documented during the course of data collection. Generally, the researcher reviews data collected from each participant. While anonymity is maintained, the participant's responses are dissected line by line (see Table 11.1). If sufficient space is left on one margin, the coding of data can take place on the data page itself. In analyzing data, the researcher looks for themes or patterns, then gives them a code name for easy referral and assimilation. For example, if a participant talked of feelings of depression and hopelessness on several occasions, the researcher might code that theme "suicide." There may be sev-

TABLE 11.1 Data Analysis: Identifying Themes from Participant Statements

Themes	Select Participant Statements: Experience of Job Loss
loss of control betrayal unpreparedness financial stress loss of self-esteem devastation	"I felt as though I was about to <u>explode!</u> I couldn't believe that <u>after 28 years of service to the company</u>—of being loyal, honest, hardworking—<u>that this could be the thanks I got. Nothing in my life prepared me for an event like this.</u> I always figured I would be the guy who got the gold watch and that I could retire with a <u>pretty good pension and a nice nest egg to fall back on.</u> Now, I have to <u>face the prospect of trying to get a job at my age and of</u> trying to tell my friends, neighbors, and colleagues. It's embarrassing and demeaning. I will <u>never get over this . . . it has ruined my life.</u>"

eral categories and codes identified within the data recorded for any given participant. The researcher works with these categories to identify those that are most prevalent or of greater priority for the individual. Constant comparison of data collected from all participants assists in the determination of the final themes, as does collaborative evidence from the literature.

Computer Analysis   Analysis of qualitative research data can be a laborious and time-consuming activity. The researcher utilizing qualitative methodology can spend hours sorting through, coding, and analyzing voluminous data recorded in the process of exploring, describing, or discovering knowledge. As in quantitative approaches, use of computer programs can be invaluable to the investigator in cutting down the hours required for manual analysis.

Several software programs are available for qualitative data analysis, though these should be selected carefully (St. John & Johnson, 2000). One available program that is particularly helpful in qualitative analyses is referred to as *Ethnograph*

369

(Seidel & Clark, 1983). These programs replace the bulk of manual work involved in sorting, coding, and storing collected data. In essence, software programs facilitate the management and reorganization of the data in preparation for interpretation. Tesch (1991) provides an excellent overview of available computer programs. Finally, it is always worthwhile to consult a computer analyst to determine which software is available to the researcher and is most useful for the project under study.

 PRACTICE

Analyzing the Findings

Following is a listing of the final categories or themes found in a qualitative inquiry about the experience of drug dependence ($n = 9$). Discuss the clarity of these categories and their relative importance.

70%	self-esteem
34%	hopelessness
83%	affiliative relationships
52%	conformity to social pressure

 CRITICAL APPRAISAL

Analyzing the Findings

- Are the importance of patterns and the interrelationships made clear?

- Does the researcher discuss the overall implications of the research findings?

Scientific Adequacy in Qualitative Designs

Scientific adequacy refers to the credibility of the findings in a qualitative investigation. In qualitative research methodology, the credibility of findings and the scientific rigor used to answer the research question is addressed by strategies designed to enhance validity and reliability. Lincoln and Guba (1985) refer to concerns regarding scientific rigor in qualitative research designs as issues of trustworthiness. They suggest specific measures in four areas: *credibility* (internal validity); *transferability* (external validity); *dependability* (reliability); and *confirmability* (neutrality).

The qualitative researcher carefully develops strategies to address possible threats to credibility of the research (Guba & Lincoln, 1992). As the researcher seeks to obtain a thick, rich construction of the meaning of an experience for the research participant(s), care is taken to ensure that scientific rigor is maintained throughout. The following example of scientific adequacy details how one researcher addressed issues of scientific adequacy in a phenomenologic investigation. This process should be evident in every qualitative study.

In evaluating a qualitative research report, the consumer needs to question whether the design used was logical and appropriate for answering the stated research question. The design should fit the nature of the phenomenon under study. In addition, the consumer needs to question the scientific rigor of the investigation and make a determination regarding how threats to credibility of findings were addressed during the course of the study.

WORKING DEFINITION

Scientific Adequacy in Qualitative Designs

Scientific adequacy refers to the trustworthiness of research findings from qualitative methods. Attention to issues of credibility, transferability, dependability, and confirmability are necessary to avoid threats and ensure scientific rigor.

371

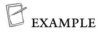
EXAMPLE

Scientific Adequacy in Qualitative Designs

Haylor (1992) used phenomenology in examining caring in families of children diagnosed with autism. Detailed narrative accounts of family members understanding of autism, caring episodes, family history, and daily family life provided the basis for developing a description for analysis. Scientific adequacy was addressed in the study as follows:

Credibility

Data were collected from several members of the family using a variety of methods. The researcher also analyzed the data in a variety of ways. Consultants were asked to examine the data, and family members were invited to provide feedback regarding the researcher's initial interpretation of the data as the study was in progress. In addition, regular debriefing sessions about the researcher's involvement with the study families were held with a mental health clinician.

Transferability

Purposive sampling was used to collect data from various family members who lived with a child with autism. The researcher commented that a limitation of the study is that the ratio of boys to girls affected by autism is 4:1. Failure to include females is an issue in transferability of findings from this investigation. In all other ways (economic, educational, religious, etc.), study families were diverse, increasing the generalizability of the findings.

Dependability

The researcher carefully logged all sessions dealing with interpretation of data and kept track of how coding strategies evolved during the course of the study. All notes were saved for future reference and further reflection. Should other researchers examine this work, a comparable logical analysis should be apparent.

Confirmability

In an effort to minimize inappropriate bias, the researcher met regularly with a mental health clinician and kept track of all interpretive work relating to data analysis. These strategies for reflective thought were important in addressing the confirmability of the findings as the researcher immersed herself in the world of the family caring for an autistic child.

 PRACTICE

Scientific Adequacy in Qualitative Designs

Obtain a qualitative research report from a research journal or arrange to meet with a nurse researcher who has conducted a research investigation using a qualitative methodology. Make a determination regarding how the issues of credibility, transferability, dependability, and confirmability were addressed throughout the study.

 CRITICAL APPRAISAL

Scientific Adequacy in Qualitative Designs

- Is the stated qualitative design a logical selection and appropriate to answer the stated research question?

- Does the design fit the nature of the phenomenon under study?

- Does the researcher address issues related to scientific rigor: credibility, transferability, dependability, and confirmability?

Critical Overview of Analyzing the Data in Qualitative Research

Following the collection of data that is generally voluminous, the qualitative researcher must decide how to analyze the information so that it both represents what the participants

373

reported and is meaningful. Data analysis can be a daunting task, and the qualitative researcher often relies on software to get a handle on the data and to help make sense of the categories, patterns, and themes that are present. Efforts should also be made to ensure that the data is credible.

CRITICAL OVERVIEW
ANALYZING THE DATA IN
QUALITATIVE RESEARCH

Select three qualitative research reports from the literature. Complete the following activities for each study:

- Describe when the literature review was conducted. What major topical areas were reviewed in the literature?

- Detail the process used to review the literature for each study. What were the major topical areas that were reviewed?

- Describe how the researcher ensured credibility of the findings.

References

Field, P. A. & Morse, J. M. (1985). *Nursing research: The application of qualitative approaches.* Rockville, MD: Aspen Systems Corporation.

Guba, E. G. & Lincoln, Y. S. (1992). *Effective evaluation: Improving the usefulness of evaluation results through responsive and naturalistic approaches.* San Francisco: Jossey-Bass.

Haylor, M. J. (1992). Caring in families of children with autism. Unpublished Ph.D. dissertation, Oregon Health Sciences University, Portland.

Leininger, M. M. (1985). *Qualitative research methods in nursing.* New York: Grune and Stratton.

Leininger, M. M. (1992). Current issues, problems, and trends to advance qualitative paradigmatic research methods for the future. *Qualitative Health Research*, 2(4): 392–415.

Lincoln, Y. & Guba, G. (1985). *Naturalistic inquiry.* Beverly Hills, CA: Sage.

Miles, M. B. & Huberman, M. (1994). *Qualitative data analysis: An expanded sourcebook* (2nd Edition). Thousand Oaks, CA: Sage Publications.

Parse, R. R., Coyne, A. B. & Smith, M. J. (1985). *Nursing research: Qualitative methods.* Bowie, MD: Brady Communications.

Seidel, J. V. & Clark, J. (1983). *The ethnograph: A user's guide.* Boulder: University of Colorado Computer Center.

St. John, W. & Johnson, P. (2000). The pros and cons of data analysis software for qualitative research. *Journal of Nursing Scholarship*, 32(4): 393–397.

Streubert, H. J. & Carpenter, D. R. (1999). *Qualitative research in nursing: Advancing the humanistic imperative* (2nd Edition). Philadelphia: Lippincott Williams & Wilkins.

Swanson-Kauffman, K. M. (1986). A combined qualitative methodology for nursing research. *Advances in Nursing Science*, 8(3): 58–69.

Tesch, R. (1991). Computer programs that assist in the analysis of qualitative data: An overview. *Qualitative Health Research*, 1(3): 309–325.

Unit 5

Promoting Evidence-Based Practice: Nurse as Researcher

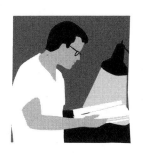

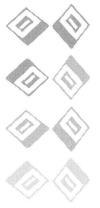

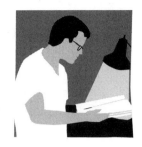

12

Reviewing the Research Findings

Goals

- *Describe various methods of conveying the results of a study.*
- *Analyze differences in methods of communicating the results of a study.*
- *Describe the process of drawing conclusions from the results of a study.*

Introduction

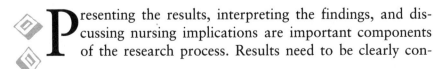

Presenting the results, interpreting the findings, and discussing nursing implications are important components of the research process. Results need to be clearly conveyed, interpretations must be accurate, and the implications for nursing should provide nurses with suggestions for practice that emanate from the study.

Presenting the Findings

The results of a study can be presented through the written word or through various kinds of **pictorial displays.** In general, both approaches are incorporated in the report of a given study. In using either the written word or pictorial displays, several factors are important to the effective communication of results. For the sake of the consumer of a study, the results must be conveyed in a clear, appropriately concise, and readily understandable fashion.

Several factors are crucial to the consumer's understanding of the outcome of the study, including the presence of a title for each pictorial display, evidence that the results presented are related to the data obtained, agreement between the written word and the pictorial display, the presentation of the actual findings in the results section (a discussion of the results is usually found in a later section), the inclusion of limitations within the study that may have influenced the results, and a generally unbiased presentation of findings (Polit & Hungler, 1999). The importance of understanding the presentation of results cannot be overemphasized; consumers who understand the results section will not be tempted to accept outcomes of research simply because they have been published.

The two major methods for communicating the results of a study using a visual or pictorial approach are the construction of graphs and tables. *Graphs* are generally used to describe the data in question, and tables are constructed to summarize the results. Criteria for evaluating the effectiveness of both graphs and tables include the clarity of the presentation, its conciseness, and its adequacy in conveying appropriate information (Wilson, 1987, p. 295).

Graphs can effectively convey information related to the data collected in a study and can be constructed in varying ways. There are bar graphs, histograms, pie diagrams, and pictorial charts, as well as graphs that depict relationships among two or more continuous variables. From looking at a well-constructed graph, the consumer of research can readily detect trends and relationships.

 WORKING DEFINITION

Graphs

A graph in the context of research is a visual display that conveys information about the topic of study. Graphs are generally used to describe the data collected in a given research project.

A *bar graph* is a visual display consisting of a number of distinct rectangular bars. The height of the bars denotes the frequency of a specified category. The categories represented are discrete and noncontinuous, reflecting the use of a nominal level of measurement. The x-axis, or abscissa (horizontal), is used to record categories of data. The y-axis, or ordinate (vertical), reflects the frequency of the event of interest.

 EXAMPLE

A Bar Graph

A group of nurse investigators display the data they have collected reflecting the number of mastectomy patients who have chosen reconstructive surgery over a period of five years in four cancer research centers.

381

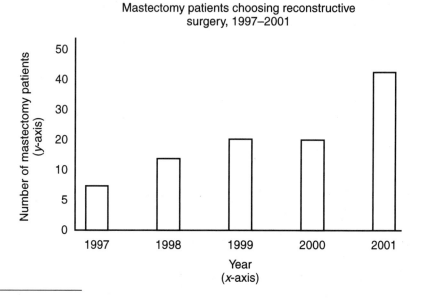

Mastectomy patients choosing reconstructive
surgery, 1997–2001

As with all pictorial displays, the consumer should be readily able to interpret the information conveyed. From this example, the consumer would conclude that the number of mastectomy patients choosing reconstructive surgery at the four specified cancer centers had increased from 1997 to 2001 and that the number making that choice was the same in 1999 and 2000.

 PRACTICE

Bar Graph

Given the following data, construct a bar graph: In order to examine the effects of a specific diet on obesity, 50 women are weighed and categorized as to the degree of their problem. The categories identified are moderately obese, very obese, and dangerously obese. Eight, thirty-seven, and five women, respectively, fall within these categories.

A **histogram** also consists of a number of rectangular bars, but unlike the bar graph it represents continuous data reflecting ordinal and interval levels of measurement. The height of the bars represents the frequency of the event. Information found on the horizontal axis describes the categories or class intervals of interest. The bars in a histogram, unlike those in a bar graph, touch one another. A space is left between the *y*-axis and the first bar, and the frequency data start at zero.

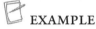

EXAMPLE

A Histogram

A group of nurse investigators display the data they have collected on the age of clients attending a series of seminars on drug abuse.

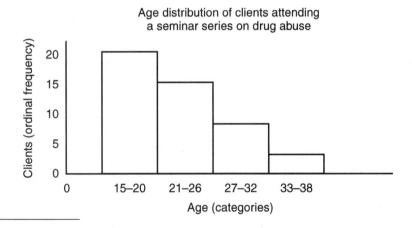

A graph called a **frequency polygon** can be constructed from a histogram by joining points in the center at the top of each column, as shown in Figure 12.1. The purpose of a frequency polygon is similar to the histogram. Once constructed, a frequency polygon allows the researcher to easily see the shape or form of the distribution of the numerical values.

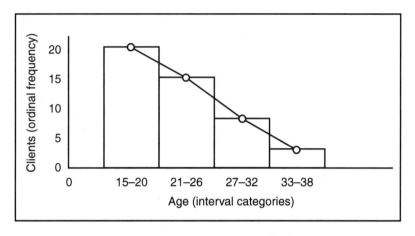

FIGURE 12.1 Frequency polygon

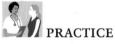 PRACTICE

A Histogram

Given the following data construct a histogram: In the process of studying breast-feeding habits among women in a rural setting, data are collected reflecting the number of months women breast-feed their first child. The time periods for breast-feeding are 0–5, 6–10, 11–15, and 16–20 months, with 24, 13, 4, and 2 women falling within those categories, respectively.

A **pie diagram** or **pie chart** is a circle that is used to compare the different components of a particular area of interest. Proportions or percentages of a given sample or population are generally shown.

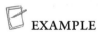 EXAMPLE

A Pie Diagram

Two nurse investigators collect data on the age range of women seeking pregnancy counseling at an urban health care center over a six-month period. Sixty-five women seek that particular service over that period of time. The investigators communicate the data collected by drawing a pie diagram that shows the percentage of women seeking pregnancy counseling.

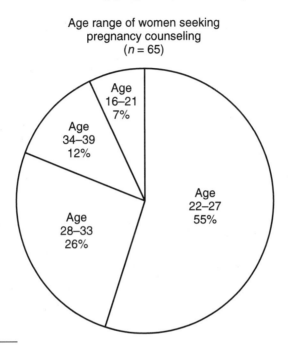

Age range of women seeking
pregnancy counseling
($n = 65$)

Age 16–21 7%

Age 34–39 12%

Age 22–27 55%

Age 28–33 26%

 PRACTICE

A Pie Diagram

For purposes of examining the relationship between two treatments for skin breakdown among adult quadriplegics, two nurse investigators collected data on the number of patients (quadriplegics) in three age ranges that suffered from skin breakdown in a given rehabilitation center. They found that 35% of patients age 21–30, 40% of patients age 31–40, and 25% of patients age 41–50 experienced skin breakdown. Construct a pie diagram using these data.

385

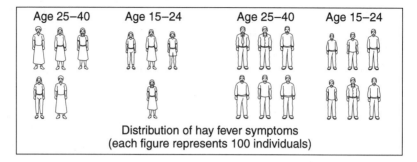

FIGURE 12.2 Pictorial chart

A **pictorial chart** uses a picture of the topic of concern to convey the data collected. For example, to communicate the distribution of hay fever symptoms among males and females of various ages, the pictorial chart in Figure 12.2 could be used.

Graphs used to describe the relationship between two or more continuous variables use the *x*-axis (horizontal line) and *y*-axis (vertical line) to plot the variables of interest. For example, the incidence of leukemia among young adults in a given area over a period of years might be conveyed as shown in Figure 12.3.

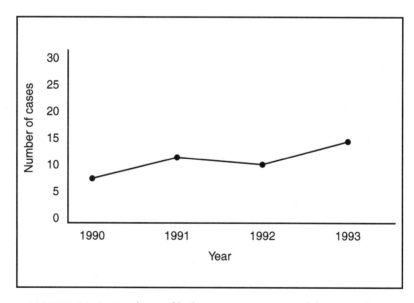

FIGURE 12.3 Incidence of leukemia among young adults in Academic County, 1990–1993

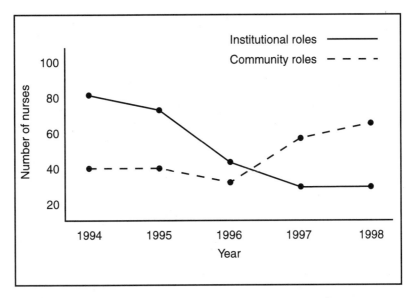

FIGURE 12.4 New graduate nurses choosing community roles versus institutional roles in Academic County, 1994–1998

Several lines may be used within a graph to describe data depending on the categories involved. Nurse investigators who want to communicate to the consumer the change in the number of nurses in a specific location who are choosing roles in the community versus roles in institutions might construct the graph shown in Figure 12.4.

The broken line communicates information about community roles from 1994 to 1998; the solid line does the same for institutional roles. The x-axis depicts the years, and the y-axis shows the number of nurses involved in each role.

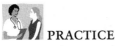 PRACTICE

Graph Showing the Relationship between Two or More Variables

Construct a graph using the following data: The x-axis represents the years 1995–1999; the y-axis represents the number of patients, male and female, who attend a self-help group focusing on alcoholism in the County of Academic. The data on males read: 1995, 27; 1996, 21; 1997, 23; 1998, 30; and

1999, 35; on females: 1995, 16; 1996, 18; 1997, 17; 1998, 19; and 1999, 24.

The inclusion of graphs in a research presentation permits the consumer to digest a considerable amount of information in a very short period of time. Graphs must, however, be clear and readily understood by the consumer to be of value. They must also fit the type of data collected; for example, bar charts and pie diagrams are generally used for nominal data, and horizontal and vertical lines drawn from points plotted against the x- and y-axes are used to represent relationships between two or more continuous variables (Lobiondo-Wood & Haber, 2002).

CRITICAL APPRAISAL

Graphs

- Is the title clear?

- If axes are used, are they labeled?

- Do the data collected fit the graph selected?

Tables are generally used to summarize the meaningful results of a study. Tables within a research presentation, whether written or oral, are numbered in sequence and are referenced within the text. The tables assist the reader to better understand the meaning of the text, thereby simplifying the consumer's task (Oyster et al., 1987, pp. 196–197).

In order to assist the reader to better understand the results of a study, tables need to be clearly labeled and have titles that accurately identify their meaning. Labels are applied to each column in the table, and the title describes what the table represents. Directly below the title, headnotes in parentheses are frequently used to provide the consumer with additional information. For example, "(numbers represent percentages)" may be used to denote that all numbers used in the table are in the form of percentages.

EXAMPLE

A Table

Percentage of Nurses from Specified Settings in Academic County Desiring Additional Education (*n* = 179)

Setting	Desire a Baccalaureate Degree	Desire a Masters Degree	Desire a Doctoral Degree	No Additional Education Desired
Critical care units (*n* = 58)	78	15	2	5
Cardiac care units (*n* = 60)	64	22	5	9
Neonatal intensive care units (*n* = 61)	55	8	1	36

Unlike graphs, the most effective use of tables is for the summarizing of data—that is, communicating relationships rather than describing characteristics. The table must clearly reflect the relationships in question, identifying the actual value of any statistical tests used and the significance probability.

 CRITICAL APPRAISAL

Tables

- Is the table appropriately labeled?
- Does the table convey the desired information in a clear, simple fashion?
- Are the variables under study clearly designated?
- Are the groups from which data were collected identified?

- Is adequate information presented relating to the statistical test used?

Although the tables should be able to stand alone, they must be accompanied by a factual, precise description of their meaning. The narrative that accompanies the tables identifies the characteristics of the sample and the statistical methods used (in such a way that the logic of the overall data analysis is clear), and provides a discussion of each research question or hypothesis.

For example, a written description should accompany the table describing the percentage of nurses desiring additional education. The description would specify the total number of nurses involved (e.g., 179) and the number of nurses representing each setting (e.g., critical care, 58; cardiac care, 60; and neonatal care, 61). Each category of additional education would be described, as well as the fact that percentages were calculated to show the interest in additional education reflected in each setting.

Interpreting the Results

The results section of a research report reflects the actual outcome of the data analysis. An additional section of the report usually focuses on the interpretation of the results. If hypotheses have been formed, the results section identifies the support or lack of support for the positions taken. When hypotheses have not been formed, the results section describes the outcome of the analytical techniques used.

Even though data have been collected and analyzed, producing a set of results, the consumer cannot assume that these results represent "facts" or that the study in question has demonstrated something. The results of a given study can provide descriptive information about a particular phenomenon or identify possible relationships among phenomena. The knowledge derived from the results as they are presented in the research report is meaningful within the context of the particular study. It is the task of the investigator to interpret the results as accurately as possible given the conceptual framework and research design previously selected (Trussell, Brandt, & Knapp, 1981, pp. 196–198).

When interpreting the results of a study, investigators share with the consumer their view of the outcome, given their involvement in designing and conducting the research. In this section, they need to tie the study together by clearly reflecting the original problem statement, the conceptual framework, the hypotheses to be tested, the literature reviewed, the characteristics of the population studied, and the limitations of the design. Consumers may agree with the investigators' interpretation of the results, or they may disagree. Positions taken may be based on a disagreement at either the conceptual or methodological level. For example, a critical research consumer who practices nursing within a self-help framework might not agree with the interpretations of a study based on a conceptual framework that emphasized caring for clients.

Methodological disagreement may be based on a difference of opinion in regard to the appropriateness of the methods used to conduct the study. Such disagreement may also result from actual errors committed by the investigators in designing the study. Abdellah and Levine (1979) have identified a number of errors related to the interpretation of results that are frequently made by investigators. Those errors that may be most readily apparent to the consumer include the following:

- Using an inappropriate statistical test of significance given the kind of data collected.

- Implying that statistical significance reflects "proof" or in some way conveys something about the quality of the study.

- Suggesting that because a relationship was found to be statistically significant there are meaningful practical implications.

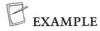 EXAMPLE

Disagreement with the Interpretation of Results

A group of beginning nurse investigators design and conduct a study to examine the patterns of family functioning among 30 teenagers who have presented themselves at a local mental

391

health center, having attempted suicide. Their conceptual framework is psychological in nature, emphasizing the effects of family dynamics on the individual family member's ability to function. They use a paper-and-pencil test (with acceptable levels of validity and reliability) that measures three levels of family functioning: healthy, problematic, and pathological. The test is based on a model of family dynamics that defines problematic and pathological behavior in terms of the quality of the interaction among family members. Each family member takes the test, and a family score is then calculated. The investigators hypothesize that each of the 30 families will score in either the problematic or pathological level of family functioning.

The results of the study show that three families score as healthy, 17 as problematic, and 10 as pathological. Among these families, 15 are of lower socioeconomic status, seven are on welfare, and eight are middle-class. Each family has more than one child, with the suicide attempter being the youngest in five families, the oldest in 11, and between the youngest and oldest in the remaining families. The investigators interpret the results to mean that unhealthy family dynamics are a major contributor to suicidal gestures among teenagers. They explain that, upon further investigation of their data, they realized that the teenagers from the three families who scored healthy made less serious attempts than did the remaining 27.

Possible Disagreements

1. Although problematic or pathological functioning as determined by the test used in this study might be a contributing factor in relation to these teenagers' suicide attempts, other important factors must be considered and analyzed, such as socioeconomic status, gender, and position in family.

2. The sample is a convenience sample, and therefore generalizations beyond the 30 teenagers studied are inappropriate.

3. The investigators hypothesize that 100% of the families will fall in the problematic or pathological level and then

excuse their result of 90% in view of new data—an inappropriate strategy.

Although other criticisms of this study could be made, the important point to note is that the interpretation of the result—90% of the families studied scored in the problematic or pathological level—is misleading. The consumer cannot take at face value the statement "Unhealthy family functioning is a major contributor to teenage suicide attempts."

Another important factor that can assist the consumer in interpreting the results of a study effectively is the investigator's handling of the limitations of the project. The investigator who clearly and accurately identifies the limitations of the study—that is, those aspects of the research that were not addressed (Nieswiadomy, 1993, p. 29)—assists the consumer to better understand the results that have been reached. For example, using Taylor's (1983) theory of cognitive adaptation, investigators may examine one of the three themes of meaning, mastery, and self-esteem. To point out in the limitations section that only meaning has been examined helps the consumer to interpret the findings within that framework alone. The interpretation can therefore be more accurate and therefore useful.

Other limitations related to the design of the study, such as small sample size, may be reported. Identification of these limitations can also help the consumer to make a better interpretation of the findings.

 PRACTICE

Evaluating the Investigator's Interpretation of Results

Select a completed study relevant to nursing practice. Summarize the investigator's interpretation of the results (usually found in the discussion section). Agree or disagree with the interpretation, providing a rationale for the position taken.

CRITICAL APPRAISAL

Interpreting the Results

- Does the interpretation of the results fit with the other components of the study (i.e., problem statement, literature review, design, and so forth)?

- Is each hypothesis (if made) addressed?

- Are the study's limitations discussed?

Drawing Conclusions

Drawing conclusions from the findings of a study requires the consumer to understand the results section of the research report and to place that understanding within the general framework of the study (conceptual framework, review of literature, research design, etc.) (Trussell et al., 1981, pp. 196–209). In order to draw conclusions that appropriately flow from the research report, the consumer has to critically evaluate the logic of the investigation as well as the methods used.

There are a number of questions a consumer can ask in relation to drawing conclusions about the findings of a research report. For example, what questions has the study answered? What questions were left unanswered? What could or should the investigator have done differently? If additional research is suggested in the area, what changes should be made? Are there reasons not to generalize the results? (Oyster et al., 1987, p. 15).

Another consideration to be addressed when attempting to draw conclusions from a research report is the risk–benefit ratio of any suggestions for practice. Research that concludes that certain nursing practices are effective but could cause harm must be investigated more extensively and with greater attention to the generalizability of results than research that suggests approaches without negative side effects.

Some research reports conclude that additional research on the topic studied should be conducted before changes in practice are considered. In deciding whether additional research should be conducted, the consumer can evaluate the reasons why the original study could not produce results that are immediately applicable. Concerns about sample selection, sample size, and the like may or may not be easily rectified in future studies.

In drawing conclusions from a research report, the consumer must remember that although some questions may be answered, nothing is proven. Application of the research process leads to the accumulation of knowledge that hopefully moves the profession toward truth; however, proof of the effectiveness of a given intervention is not an outcome. The probability that a given intervention is effective provides valuable information; however, even a high probability does not constitute proof.

Implications for Nursing

The section of the research report that focuses on nursing implications usually includes specific suggestions for practice. In order to make use of these suggestions, the consumer needs to evaluate the implications for nursing in relation to the fit between the results section and the proposed suggestions for practice. For example, if the results section shows that the hypothesis "bonding between father and infant occurs more quickly when the father is present at the time of delivery" is statistically significant, implications for revising practice must be related to that finding. It would not be appropriate to expand on that finding by suggesting that relationships between grandparents and infant could be improved by including grandparents in the delivery process.

The implications for nursing should also be evaluated in relation to the major components of the study, including such questions as the following: What are the characteristics of the population studied that permitted these implications to be suggested? Does the design used permit the generalization of findings? Are the statistical procedures used appropriate to the data collected? Does the results section assist the consumer in evaluating the proposed implications for nursing practice?

Critical Overview of Reviewing the Research Findings

CRITICAL OVERVIEW
REVIEWING THE RESEARCH
FINDINGS

Excerpt A

A research consumer has prepared the following synthesis of a research report entitled "Attribution and Chronic Illness: The Function of Meaning as It Affects the Occurrence of Depression":

Conceptual framework: Taylor's (1983) theory of cognitive adaptation, which postulates that when faced with a threatening event (such as the diagnosis of a chronic illness) individuals respond by attributing meaning to the event, regaining mastery over the event, and attempting to bolster their self-esteem.

Problem statement: What is the relationship between the attribution of meaning to the diagnosis of multiple sclerosis (MS) and the occurrence of depression?

Hypothesis: The more individuals internalize attributions regarding the diagnosis of MS, the greater will be their level of depression.

Population studied: Adults diagnosed with multiple sclerosis (MS)

Sample size: 84

Design: Correlational

Method: Participants responded to two instruments. One instrument assessed the degree to which each participant internalized the blame for the diagnosis of MS. The other instrument measured depression.

Statistical analysis: Pearson product moment correlations were calculated.

Results: $r = 0.70$

$r^2 = 0.49$ or 49%

49% of the variance in level of depression can be attributed to the degree of internalization of the cause (self-blame) of the diagnosis of MS.

Activity 1

Using the information in Excerpt A as a framework, construct a table (using fictitious data) to display the results.

Activity 2

Write a brief interpretation of the results as presented.

Activity 3

Draw conclusions from Excerpt A and the response to Activity 2.

Activity 4

Identify the implications for nursing from the information provided, the interpretation made, and the conclusions drawn.

References

Abdellah, F. G. & Levine, E. (1979). *Better patient care through nursing research.* New York: Macmillan.

Lobiondo-Wood, G. & Haber, J. (2002). *Nursing research: Methods, critical appraisal, and utilization* (5th Edition). St. Louis: Mosby—Year Book.

Nieswiadomy, R. (1993). *Foundations of nursing research* (2nd Edition). Norwalk, CT: Appleton & Lange.

Oyster, C., Hanten, W., & Liorens, L. (1987). *Introduction to research: A guide for the health science professional.* Philadelphia: Lippincott.

Polit, D. F. & Hungler, B. P. (1999). *Nursing research: Principles and methods* (6th Edition). Philadelphia: Lippincott Williams & Wilkins.

Taylor, S. (1983). Adjustment to threatening events: A theory of cognitive adaptation. *American Psychologist, 38*(11): 1161–1173.

Trussell, P., Brandt, A., & Knapp, S. (1981). *Using nursing research: Discovery, analysis and interpretation.* Wakefield, MA: Nursing Resources.

Wilson, H. (1987). *Introducing research in nursing.* Menlo Park, CA: Addison-Wesley.

13

Evaluating Research Reports

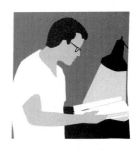

Goals

- *Describe the process of evaluating the full research report.*
- *Utilize general critique guidelines to evaluate both qualitative and quantitative research.*
- *Examine use of research findings for practice using a utilization model.*

Introduction

The primary research responsibility of the entry-level professional nurse is to critically appraise the research report. As a research consumer, the nurse makes a determination as to the merit, appropriateness, and adequacy of report findings for use in practice. Publication of a research report in no way guarantees quality, value, or relative worth. Making a determination about the overall usefulness of a research piece requires an intense, systematic review and critical appraisal of the report in toto.

Each area of the research report has been addressed in detail in the preceding chapters. This detailed analysis of each portion of the report assists in developing a formative evaluation. Completion of a formative evaluation facilitates comprehensive evaluation—a full critical overview of the report. A comprehensive evaluation includes a review of the research problem, the methodology utilized in solving the problem, the findings of the study, and the meaning of the results.

This chapter addresses the process of conducting a comprehensive evaluation of a research report. Specific attention is directed to providing general critique guidelines useful in determining the importance and usability of a report. Included are evaluation components for both quantitative and qualitative research, key considerations for applying the research findings to practice using a utilization model, and a tool for guiding the research consumer in reviewing key report elements.

Aim of Research Evaluation

The overall significance and value of a research report are determined by conducting an inventory of strengths and weaknesses. It is important to keep in mind that all research investigations have positive and negative aspects. The best research report will have flaws, and conversely, the most poorly developed and executed study will have some value for other researchers, scientists, and practitioners. The critical consumer of research is interested in weighing the strengths and weaknesses of a report and determining the overall usability of findings from an investigation.

The professional nurse is charged with developing the ability to judge a research piece in relationship to how well the research *process* was executed, as well as the product of the research findings per se (Duffy, 1985). For example, a nurse researcher has examined the effectiveness of three different methods of relieving colic in infants: motion, warmth, and secure holding. The nurse who is critically appraising the report would be most concerned with how well the investigator defined the problem, adequacy and relevance of the literature review, clarity of purpose, appropriateness of the sampling method, and so forth, as well as the study's credibility and value. The reviewer would be less concerned with the fact that there may not have been a difference in the outcomes of treatment methods. If the researcher has carried out the process well, the findings will have relevance for future research and clinical practice.

 WORKING DEFINITION

Aim of Research Evaluation

The aim of research evaluation is to determine how well the research process has been executed, as well as the credibility and value of the research findings.

 PRACTICE

Aim of Research Evaluation

Select a research textbook or journal that has published a critique of a research report. Read the report and the critique carefully. Discuss how well the components of the research were carried out, the credibility of the findings, and the overall value of the research investigation. Compare your evaluation of the report with that of the published critique, and describe the differences.

Determining the overall merit of research reports is a process that evolves over time and after repeated experiences with evaluation of research. Developing critical evaluation skill requires patience in the development of knowledge for constructive criticism of scientific work.

A variety of methodologies have been used to assist nurses in refining their ability to critique research. One common approach has been through the use of checklists that detail the elements to be considered in evaluation. A checklist is intended to be an organizational framework that assists the research consumer in making a determination of the strengths and weaknesses of each element.

It is impossible to utilize any checklist to critique a report without a basic understanding of the research process. Expertise in critiquing evolves over time and in direct relationship to knowledge of research. Thus, as the critical consumer of research conducts repeated evaluations of reports, the process will become easier, and observations about the conduct of the report will become more astute.

CRITICAL APPRAISAL

Aim of Research Evaluation

- Does the evaluation of the research report detail how well the research process was executed?

- Is the credibility of findings addressed?

- Does the reviewer discuss the overall value of the report's findings?

 # Critique Guidelines

Critique guidelines detail key elements that need to be considered in evaluating any research report. These elements, or critical appraisal components, can be very extensive and thorough, as highlighted in each of the preceding chapters. (See Appendix A for a comprehensive listing of the critical appraisal elements.) Although the critical appraiser of research synthesizes all of the many elements in making a final determination about the report, some elements generally are viewed as key in conducting an overall evaluation of the report. These abbreviated, select elements make the use of a critical appraisal checklist possible.

Table 13.1 is a listing of critical appraisal components useful in guiding the critical consumer of research in producing an evaluation of a report. Although each aspect is theoretically of equal importance in determining the worth of the report, the research consumer will consider the overall strengths and weaknesses as the ultimate determinant.

Critiquing Process

Quantitative research methodology has traditionally been the primary vehicle for generating nursing knowledge. Thus many of the available tools developed for use in critiquing the research report focus on criteria that are appropriate to quantitative research but not necessarily to qualitative research methodology. In addition to differing criteria, the sequence for evaluating the qualitative research report generally differs from the sequence for evaluating the quantitative report. Some of the elements of the research evaluation process do overlap, however, and it is difficult to identify mutually exclusive criteria. When the critical consumer is attempting to evaluate a report that utilizes a synthesis of quantitative and qualitative methodologies, criteria need to be selected to satisfy both requirements. (See Appendices B and C.)

Mapping the Research Report

Mapping the study can be a helpful part of the evaluation process. Mapping is a visual portrayal of the research project. The use of a map helps to clarify just what the investigation under review is about, as well as helping to point out gaps in the study and areas of overlap (Woods & Catanzaro, 1988). It is often easier for the reviewer to understand the problem, the proposed relationships between variables, and how each variable was measured when the study is sketched out on paper.

TABLE 13.1   Critical Evaluation Components for Research Appraisal

Research problem:

- Overview of how the problem emerged for study
- Clarity of the problem
- Significance of the problem for nursing
- Purpose and importance of the investigation
- Conceptual model
- Related literature defining the problem

Research methodology:

- Design for study
- Setting for data gathering
- Description of instruments (including validity and reliability)
- Sample utilized

Research results, findings, and interpretation:

- Data analysis strategies
- Results of data analysis
- Analysis of the research question
- Discussion of the findings and how they were interpreted
- Significance for nursing
- Recommendations for relating study findings to nursing education, practice, and additional research

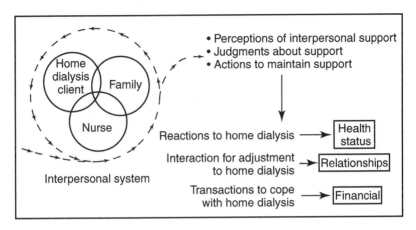

FIGURE 13.1 Mapping the research report

Mapping can be valuable in helping the consumer to synthesize what the investigation is all about and avoid a rote, piecemeal approach to evaluating the study. Figure 13.1 depicts what mapping of a research investigation might look like.

In Figure 13.1 the nurse researcher is examining relationships in home dialysis and health outcomes. Using King's (1989) theory for nursing, the researcher examines the interpersonal client-family-nurse system in connection with home dialysis. Perceptions, judgments, and actions related to support for home dialysis are studied. The researcher uses the model to examine variables related to reaction to home dialysis, interactions observed in adjusting to home dialysis, and transactions within the system for coping. The study incorporates variables related to health of family members (reaction to dialysis), family-nurse changes (support), and resource identification (interaction and transactions in adjusting and coping). Diagramming the study's concepts and the relationship between them assists in understanding how the project was developed.

Critique of the Quantitative Research Report

Evaluation of the quantitative report involves a systematic review and judgment of the adequacy of the way in which the research process was executed. The consumer conducts the appraisal with sufficient rigor to determine how much confidence can be placed in the reported findings.

Evaluation Aspects of the Quantitative Research Report   The sequence for review of the quantitative research report is straightforward and relatively inflexible. Because this method of research has been the dominant model for scientific inquiry, most textbooks address the critique process from this vantage point. The usual sequence for evaluating the quantitative report is identified in Table 13.2. Table 13.3 demonstrates how a critique of each section of a fictional quantitative research report might look.

TABLE 13.2   Evaluation Aspects of the Quantitative Research Report

Purpose of the investigation

Problem under study

   Hypothesis statement

Theoretical framework

Literature review

Research design and methods

Data collection measures

Sample

Analysis of the data

Findings/summary of study

Suggestions for use of the research findings

   Implications for education

   Implications for practice

   Implications for future research

TABLE 13.3   Evaluation of a Quantitative Research Report

Purpose

The study was designed to build on earlier studies regarding patient strategies for pain control.

Critique: The purpose is not clearly stated but is implied. It is consistent with the background data presented.

Problem under Study

The problem is, What are the self-selected methods for pain control chosen by postoperative patients?

Critique: The problem is clearly stated, important to nursing practice, and researchable. Pain and self-selected methods for control of pain are the central concepts around which the problem is formulated. The question is specific enough to provide direction for specifying the design and methodology for investigation.

Theoretical Framework

Swang (1992) has suggested that pain experiences are determined by perceived stress in conjunction with coping tactics initiated in the family of origin. The involvement of the family system in eliciting behavior effective for pain control is further outlined by Mersk (1990). Finally, Johnson (1980) asserts that properties of the relationship between the family and health care systems are crucial to a behavioral response that fosters adaptation.

Critique: Numerous references to systems, stress, and coping response suggest that systems theory, stress theory, and adaptation theory are used as a unifying framework for the study. There is no discussion regarding how the investigation is placed in a nursing framework. There is a lack of clarity regarding the relationships between variables. Finally, it is unclear how the assumed framework relates to the problem under study.

(continued)

TABLE 13.3   (continued)

Literature Review

Studies of pain and perceived control in management have demonstrated a consistent, positive relationship between feelings of control and pain level. Research by Adams (1985), Dodds (1991), Kemp (1994), Pip (1998), and Smith (1987, 1989) supports the notion that the experience of pain is closely associated with cooperation between the ill member, the family, and health care system professionals. White (1962) was a pioneer in researching the components of greatest influence in determining pain control. Differences in physiologic processing of narcotics was noted to be of greatest significance and influenced the type of medical treatment the individual sought. Finally, learned health behaviors have been found to represent a crucial aspect of controlling adverse experiences in humans (Black, 1996).

Critique: The literature review focuses on pain, perceived control, and learned health behaviors. The review fails to address the substantive area of postoperative pain as well as available strategies for self-management of pain. The review appears to be insufficient in light of the voluminous research available on the topic, and conflicting literature is not discussed. Sources are current but do not identify seminal works in the area of pain. Methodology of the studies presented was absent. Primary sources are used, and the references are complete and appropriately integrated into the development of the study.

Research Design and Methods

This descriptive study involved the use of postoperative patients to study the problem. Two forms were administered: a biographical data sheet and a survey to determine pain control methods selected by postoperative patients. Surveys were left with participants to complete within 24 hours. Participants were assured of confidentiality, anonymity, and privacy.

Critique: The research design was clearly stated and appeared appropriate to the study problem and purpose of the investigation. No hypotheses were stated or required. Neither independent nor dependent variables were specified. Unclear whether consent forms were obtained or how information on rights was provided.

(continued)

TABLE 13.3   (continued)

Data Collection Measures

The Pain Management Survey (Jones, 1996) was administered to determine methods of pain control. The survey requires the participant to identify the primary pain management method and then to rate that method using 12 scales. Alpha reliability coefficients for the scales range from 0.66 to 0.84. Content and construct validity were demonstrated.

Critique: The variables were measured using the Pain Management Survey. The instrument reflects the problem concepts as discussed in the background information. Insufficient data were presented regarding the validity and reliability, as well as the developmental aspects, of the tool. Information about the appropriateness of the instrument for use in this study was missing. Procedures for data collection were vague and would not allow for replication.

Sample

Two surgical gynecology units were selected from a large metropolitan hospital. Forty participants who met the following criteria were included: able to read and write English, free from malignancy, premenopausal, and at least 72 hours postoperative.

Critique: Insufficient detail provided about sampling procedure and available population. Significant concern centers on the nature and selection of research participants for purposes of generalizability, e.g., participant alertness, concomitant narcotic administration, whether or not surgery was emergent, etc. Sample size probably adequate.

Analysis of Data

Forty patients ranged in age from 29 to 49. Most were high school graduates and of the middle socioeconomic class (see Table 1). Median time since surgery was 5 days (see Table 2). Four strategies were utilized for management of pain: biofeedback, imagery, relaxation techniques, and self-hypnosis (see Table 3). Rating of the method

(continued)

TABLE 13.3 (continued)

by the research participant for difficulty in implementing, perceived assistance needed from others, and anticipated versus actual control of the pain suggested that imagery (35%) and relaxation techniques (28%) were least difficult, required the least assistance from others to initiate, and actually controlled the pain in closer approximation to what had been anticipated (see Table 4).

Critique: Summary of demographics was provided but was incomplete. Descriptive statistics were obviously employed, but the entire statistical program initiated was never stated. Although measures of central tendency and variability were applied, tests of correlation should have been utilized and described. Tables were accurate and easy to understand but only briefly discussed in the text of the report. Data regarding extraneous variables such as concomitant narcotic use, previous experience with pain, and so forth were not provided. The text discussion was both brief and weak. A more comprehensive discussion would facilitate reader understanding.

Findings and Summary

Interestingly, 60% of the respondents stated they had given little or no thought to self-control of pain. This finding is consistent with Doe's (1994) survey, which demonstrated that the average patient perceives having little or no control over events and experiences occurring within the health care system. Of the respondents who identified and initiated a pain-control method, a surprisingly large percentage of participants expressed success.

Critique: Conclusions were clearly stated but did not reflect the richness of the data. Those that were identified were substantiated by the data presented. The researcher failed to discuss limitations of the study methods. Unclear how the findings related to the theoretical basis of the investigation or how they contributed to the larger body of knowledge concerning the pain experience.

(continued)

TABLE 13.3   (continued)

Suggestions for Use of the Research Findings

The impact of the study is the recognition of the diverse methods of pain control selected by patients, as well as the extent to which patients fail to recognize the ability to influence their own pain experience. Patients who selected pain control methods were remarkably successful in using them. Nurses need to address their responsibility for educating patients about the importance of selecting and successfully initiating pain control methodologies. Nursing curricula need to develop courses of study related to varied pain control methodologies and strategies for teaching these innovative methods. Finally, nurse researchers need to investigate pain control more fully. This study needs to be replicated using similar as well as diverse populations and conditions.

Critique: Implications are made for nursing practice, education, and research. They are logical and relevant but are not related to a theoretical framework. No recommendations are specifically suggested. The overall worth and relevance of the study is important for nursing.

Critique of the Qualitative Research Report

The qualitative research evaluation process should be based on the researcher's stated goal (Knafl & Howard, 1986). Several authors have specified qualitative evaluation guidelines (Aamodt, 1983; Cobb & Hagemaster, 1987; Duffy, 1987; Morse, 1991; Elder & Miller, 1995). However, the qualitative research report needs to be evaluated in a fashion that is both consistent with the researcher's stated purpose and commensurate with the steps outlined in reporting the research.

Evaluation Aspects of the Qualitative Research Report   The execution of most qualitative research requires the use of a sequence of steps different from that utilized in conducting quantitative methodologies. As noted in Chapters 10 and 11, the researcher has a different purpose for each of the methodologies. Qualitative research methodology is largely an inductive approach characterized by subjectivity, description, and discovery (Reichardt & Cook, 1979). Evaluation of the qualitative report is therefore most appropriately conducted when

411

the criteria are ordered to reflect this differing purpose and methodology. Table 13.4 identifies the typical sequencing of the criteria for evaluating the qualitative research report.

 TABLE 13.4   Evaluation Aspects of the Qualitative Research Report

Researcher's stated purpose

Problem or area in need of study and related to the literature

Sample

Measures used to capture desired data

Procedure for carrying out data-gathering methods

    Method

    Time and length of study

    Nature and number of settings and participants

    How the individual became a research participant

    Researcher's feelings about the experience

    Relationship of researcher and participant

    Means of checking for biases

    Process of organizing, categorizing, and summarizing data

    Relationship of data to existing literature and theory

Scientific adequacy

    Credibility

    Transferability

    Dependability

    Confirmability

Results of the data gathered

Discussion for use of findings

Suggestions for utilizing the research findings

    Implications for education

    Implications for practice

    Implications for future research

Conducting the evaluation requires a systematic analysis of each portion of the qualitative report. Table 13.5 presents a fictitious example of each aspect of the qualitative report.

 ## TABLE 13.5   Evaluation of a Qualitative Research Report

Stated Purpose

Work with families serving as foster homes brought the investigator into close contact with children who had been relocated several times. The pervasive sense of rejection became increasingly apparent. The literature offers little about the essential structure of this lived experience.

Critique: The purpose is clearly stated. References to the literature support the need for exploratory investigation of the concept.

Identified Problem for Study

The problem in this study is: From the perspective of the foster child, what is the experience of rejection? The problem is in need of further exploration because increasing numbers of children are being placed in foster home situations. Flail (1992), Robbins (1993), and Whitter (1999) have all commented that considerable objective data exist that address numbers of children in foster care, projected numbers, and the like. What is conspicuously absent is subjective knowledge about these foster home children.

Critique: The problem is clearly stated. Justification for the problem is clear and supported by theorists and researchers involved in the study of foster children.

Sample

The sample for this study was 13 school-age children who were experiencing at least their second foster home placement. Participants needed to be able to verbalize their

(continued)

413

TABLE 13.5 (continued)

experiences. The children, their foster parents, and the placement agency were all contacted and gave written consent to be interviewed and tape-recorded.

Critique: The sample was adequately described and appropriate to the purpose of the
study. The population, however, was not described nor was the process of sampling. A
full discussion of how the participants were selected should have been detailed. Rights
of participants were appropriately addressed and discussed.

Measures for Collecting Data

A phenomenological approach was selected to gather the data in this descriptive investigation. This approach was selected as a means of exploring and coming to know
what the experience of rejection is for children placed in foster homes.

Critique: Method clearly stated. Additional information regarding the basic assumptions
of the approach would have been helpful to the reader.

Procedures for Data Collection: Method

Children were contacted and asked if they would like to participate in a nursing project
that would involve discussion about what it was like to be a child placed in foster
homes. All participants were told of the need to tape-record, and all gave permission
to do so. All participants were told the discussions could stop at any time. Discussions
with each participant were structured as follows: Describe how you felt when you were
told you were to be placed in a different foster home, and try to describe how you felt
during those first weeks in your next foster home. Participants were verbally told not
to stop talking until they felt they had been able to express their feelings fully. The
interaction with each participant was recorded and paper notations were occasionally
made by the researcher. The researcher asked questions only when the participant
seemed uncertain about sharing his or her feelings, or when the participant's feelings
needed to be clarified.

(continued)

TABLE 13.5 (continued)

Critique: The method for data gathering was clearly identified and was appropriate to the concept under study as well as to the participants. It would have been helpful if the length of the interviews had been specified. Sufficient detail was provided to allow replication of the study.

Procedures for Data Collection: Time/Length of Study

The study was conducted with children who had been relocated to a new foster home within the past six months. The length of the study was nine months.

Critique: Time framework for the study sufficiently detailed. No rationale given for the time framework.

Procedures for Data Collection: Nature/Number of Participants/Settings

The setting for the study was a rural six-county area in the western part of an eastern state in the United States. The interviews took place in the child's current foster home. The participants were 13 children who met the study criteria. They were selected from a master list of children in foster care. The researcher solicited individual participation by determining children who met the criteria and then randomly selecting a list of 13.

Critique: The participants and setting were identified in sufficient detail. The process of randomly selecting participants from a master list was unclear. The researcher did not provide a rationale for random sampling as opposed to purposive sampling. It is not clear that all children in foster care experienced "rejection." This assumption by the researcher should have been addressed.

Procedures for Data Collection: Participant Involvement

The foster children became participants after being contacted by the researcher at home. The nurse followed up the phone call with a visit to the home to talk with the foster parents and child prior to initiating the investigation.

(continued)

TABLE 13.5   (continued)

Critique: The process of involving participants in the research process was outlined. Information about what was told to the foster parents and child was not provided.

Procedures for Data Collection: Researcher's Feelings

Paterson and Zderad's (1976) humanistic nursing model describes the importance of nursing care that is directed toward holistic, intersubjective relating. Similarly, Parse's (1981, 1989) man-living–health nursing model stresses the need for coexistence in the transformation process. Providing humanistic care means that an effort is made to experience the lives of clients.

Critique: Brief but thoughtful remarks about the need for holistic care and the need for the nurse to participate actively in the process. Reference made to nursing models that are philosophically consistent with the researcher's views.

Procedures for Data Collection: Researcher-Participant Relationship

The researcher and all but one participant were not known to each other prior to the initiation of the study. The researcher knew one participant as a client in the ambulatory pediatric department three years earlier.

Critique: The relationships between the researcher and participants were clarified. The researcher was sensitive to her own knowledge about the research participants and how it might influence the sharing of the experience.

Procedures for Data Collection: Checking for Bias

In an effort to minimize unnecessary bias, the research participants and families chosen were essentially unknown to the researcher. Individual case records were not reviewed prior to the gathering of data.

(continued)

416

TABLE 13.5 (continued)

Critique: The researcher described the way in which she attempted to eliminate unnecessary bias. The researcher does not specifically address personal feelings about children placed in multiple foster homes. Doing so would be helpful in ascertaining how she had recognized and incorporated bias into the study design and methodology. Finally, the researcher did not define the terms that were used: rejection, child, experience.

Procedures for Data Collection: Organizing/Categorizing/Summarizing

The data were transcribed verbatim for each research participant within three days of the discussion. The researcher spent considerable time reading and absorbing the transcribed data to develop a feel for the child's experience. Key statements were taken from the transcription, and the meaning was explicated. This process was repeated with and between participants. Fourteen theme categories originally emerged but were reduced to four: anger, desolation, hopelessness, and shame.

Critique: The researcher included the steps taken to organize and categorize the data. However, the number of key statements and the process of collapsing the 14 theme categories into 4 was not discussed. The researcher also did not discuss how the data were summarized for ease in theme identification. The researcher failed to describe the literature, although some references were made to select aspects. Discussion of the literature would have facilitated the reader's understanding of how pattern categories were recognized and accepted.

Scientific Adequacy: Credibility/Transferability/Dependabillty/Confirmability

In an effort to maintain scientific adequacy, the researcher did not review the case records of individual research participants. In addition, consultants were solicited to review the data and the researcher met with a child mental health clinician at periodic intervals during the course of the nine-month investigation. Participants were selected from a rural eastern state and this is a limitation of the study. However, all sessions with research participants were tape recorded and carefully coded, with notations for category selections carefully documented.

(continued)

TABLE 13.5   (continued)

Critique: The researcher briefly mentioned how scientific rigor was addressed in the study. Although attention was given to eliminating bias, little attention was given to transferability (external validity) of the findings. A description of the sample, in particular, would have made it easier to determine whether the findings were generalizable. Careful notation of data during the process of interpretation, and meeting with a mental health clinician, were both strategies designed to foster scientific rigor.

Results of the Data Gathered

The meaning of rejection for children placed in multiple foster homes was represented in the data clustering around four themes: hopelessness, anger, desolation, and shame. Statements from the original text were used to validate the pattern, and this content is noted in Tables 1 through 4. Finally, the patterns were synthesized into an exhaustive description of the lived experience of rejection (see Table 5). Each participant was contacted two months after data collection had ended to confirm or assist in refinement of the final description that was synthesized.

Critique: The process of obtaining study results was clear and appropriate to phenomenological research. Although statistical analysis is not necessary using the phenomenological method, it is not stated whether any was applied. Tables were not clearly described in the text of the report. Other sources of validation for clusters and themes were not addressed.

Discussion for Use of Findings

Analysis resulted in the exhaustive description of the experience of rejection in children placed in foster home care. The four patterns suggest the overwhelmingness of the experience for these children. Consistent references to "something wrong with me" and "hating them for doing this to me" reflect the intensity of the experience. The findings suggest the need for innovative ways of being with these children and a need to rethink current care patterns.

(continued)

TABLE 13.5 (continued)

Critique: The discussion is consistent with a phenomenological method. Directions for using the study are generally addressed.

Suggestions for Use of Findings

The practitioner, educator, and researcher can use the findings to clarify how the foster child is approached through care and study.

Critique: No specific direction is given for practice, education, and research. The study has special significance for the development of theory, but this topic was not mentioned.

Basic Considerations in Evaluating Research Reports

Whether the critical consumer is evaluating a qualitative or a quantitative research report, there are several underlying evaluation elements that are important to both. These central concerns include title, author credentials, the abstract, references, style, and organization. These aspects may seem minor but, in fact, are important in disseminating the report to an appropriate audience. Additionally, when these elements are completed well they will serve to pique the reader's interest and provide a framework to support the credibility of the report. Chapter 14 describes these research elements in more detail.

Each of these underlying elements needs to be clear and appropriate to the research report. Ultimately, the consumer should get a sense that the researcher moved systematically and logically in executing the selected methodology of the investigation (Woods & Catanzaro, 1988). Table 13.6 demonstrates how a critique of the title, author credentials, and abstract might look in a fictitious example.

419

TABLE 13.6   Evaluation of Basic Elements of the Research Report

Title

Informational Needs of Adults Recently Diagnosed with Lyme Disease.

Critique: The title is informative about the contents of the study. The population (adults with Lyme Disease) is identified, as is one variable (informational needs). The title suggests that the intent of the investigator is to conduct an exploratory study, and review of the study supports this expectation.

Author Credentials

Sally Restonz, R.N., Ph.D., is a nurse researcher with the Northeast Center for Health Promotion and Disease Management in New York. The study was funded in part by a grant from the National Disease Prevention Center.

Critique: The investigator is a doctorally prepared nurse, and it can be assumed that she has basic competencies as an independent researcher. The fact that the study was funded suggests that it was reviewed by other scientists who found it meritorious. It would have been helpful if information about the researcher's professional experiences had been provided, but it is not crucial to evaluating the study.

Abstract

This study explored the informational needs of 42 adults recently diagnosed with Lyme Disease—a tick-borne bacterial infection—in relation to two parameters: physiological and psychosocial (role, interdependence, and self-concept) adaptation. Use of Roy's (1989) adaptation nursing model, as well as the findings from previous research, provided the framework for category development that would identify the informational needs supportive of an adaptive response by the participant. The Restonz Informational Needs for Adaptation Tool was used to assess participants. Par-

(continued)

TABLE 13.6 (continued)

ticipant needs for information were categorized and described in relation to physiological and psychosocial responses. Responses were further identified and categorized according to age, gender, health status, and situation-related variables. Findings from the exploratory study indicate that informational needs are most closely related to intensity of the stimuli as it impacts on perceived role and self-concept functioning.

Critique: The abstract provides baseline knowledge about the study and gives the reader enough information so that a decision can be made about whether the study merits further consideration. The article appears in *Health and Disease Management in Nursing,* which is a refereed journal and has thus been subjected to the full review process by experts. The abstract does identify the purpose, framework for studying the problem, variables under study, sample, design, and methodology. Results of statistical analysis are not provided to support the credibility of the suggested findings, but this is acceptable given the probable space limitations specified by journal guidelines.

Format and Preparation of the Research Evaluation

Conducting a research evaluation requires a systematic examination of each part of the research process (Ward & Fetler, 1979; Grove & Burns, 2001). Regardless of the purpose for evaluating the research report, it should be obvious to the reader of the critique that a systematic review has been undertaken. Development of a format to ensure this orderly process is helpful in focusing the reviewer and in maintaining a comprehensive evaluation.

Preparation of the final research critique by the research consumer generally means a two- to three-page synopsis of the strengths and weaknesses of the research report. The report is usually written in a narrative fashion and should be clearly and concisely presented. The report is relatively easy to write once the systematic evaluation of report components has been completed. The written critique is designed to communicate to others the potential value and significance of the findings. A critique is most valuable when the target audience is kept as the focus, thus fashioning the language and depth of discussion to an appropriate level.

Implementing the Research Report Findings in Practice

The professional nurse utilizes research findings in an attempt to improve, change, or support current clinical practice. Through systematic, organized review of relevant research, the nurse uses appropriate findings as the basis for practice. **Research utilization** emphasizes the transfer of specific research-based knowledge into practice (Horsley, 1987).

The manner in which research findings become an integral part of nursing practice has been an issue of concern. To date, evidence that nursing practice is based on current research findings is just beginning to grow. There have been several models proposed to facilitate the use of research by professional nurses. Some of the models that have been proposed to assist the practicing nurse in the utilization of nursing research findings are the conduct and utilization of research in nursing (CURN) model (Horsley et al., 1983); the Western Interstate Commission for Higher Education (WICHE) model (Phillips, 1986); the Stetler model for the utilization of research (Stetler & Marram, 1976); the systems model for change related to clinical research (Conway, 1978); and the Horn Video Productions model for research utilization (1991). All of the models are designed to assist nurses in establishing research-based nursing practice (Beyea & Nicoll, 1997).

Each of the research utilization models has strengths and weaknesses. However, a commonality among the models is that each stresses the need to identify the practice problem in need of scientific solution, the importance of carefully reviewing the research (quality and quantity) that has been done, and then the careful development of a plan for implementing the appropriate findings and evaluating the success of the change. The nurse who implements the research utilization process and transfers research knowledge into practice through the use of a model is helping to ensure that quality clinical nursing practice is being provided.

WORKING DEFINITION

Research Utilization

Research utilization is the process of transferring research knowledge into practice, thus facilitating an innovative change in practice or the verification of existing practice protocols.

Critical appraisal of the research report is the foundation of research utilization processes. Skill in evaluating a piece of research is important in making a determination regarding the quality of the findings. In addition to evaluating all the available relevant research, the nurse must make a decision about the strength of the research as an organized whole. Mateo and Kirchhoff (1991) have identified eight fundamental criteria that need to be considered before making the decision to adopt an innovation for nursing practice (see Table 13.7). The use of these or comparable criteria assist in an organized, systematic review of the research base that exists in relation to a particular clinical problem. When the research is carefully critiqued and criteria are used in making a determination about readiness of findings for implementation in the clinical setting, the nurse can be relatively confident that policies, protocols, and procedures will be scientifically sound.

Review of the available research that relates to a particular problem is a time-consuming task and is often most easily accomplished by a group of clinicians interested in the same nursing problem. As can be noted in the following example of

Table 13.7 Criteria for Adoption of a Research Innovation

Significance

Scientific Merit

Replication

Applicability to Practice

Utility in Directing Nursing Assessment/Observation/Intervention

Applicability of Findings

Risk-Benefit Ratio for Clients/Nurses

Feasibility

research utilization, there is often a dearth of research available on which to base the decision to implement a practice change. In such circumstances the nurse must weigh the significance of the problem with the quality of the available research.

In some areas of nursing practice, a significant amount of research has amassed about a particular problem. For example, temperature measurement, preoperative teaching, tubing feeding protocols, and pain control strategies are some of the areas where a considerable body of research exists. Findings in these and other areas should be a part of research-based practice. For the nurse who is new to research, it may also be useful to look at the *Annual Review of Nursing Research* or *Nursing Scan in Research: Application for Clinical Practice.* These publications are just two of the materials available to assist the research consumer in making a determination about practice-ready research and the significance of the research findings in developing innovative nursing practice methodologies.

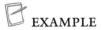

EXAMPLE

Research Utilization

Practice Problem

Many hospitalized patients receive intravenous (IV) therapy each day and IV infiltration is a significant cause of IV morbidity. The treatment of IV infiltrations is largely a nursing responsibility, yet little is known about which intervention (if any) is most effective. It is known that patients can experience considerable suffering, prolonged hospitalization, and significant cost, depending on the nature and severity of injury.

Review of the Research

Most of the literature regarding treatment of IV infiltrations is anecdotal or case reports. Three systematic investigations have been done in nursing and include treatment of the IV infiltration site in one of four ways: warm application, cold application, elevation of the affected limb, and no treatment. These therapies constitute the most common clinical interventions currently used for IV infiltration treatment.

In one investigation, Robson and Tompkins (1989) treated the caustic IV infiltrations of pediatric ICU patients ($N = 15$) with gauze soaked in ice water slush solution. They found that the immediate identification and treatment of the extravasation with ice slush resulted in 100% resolution of the tissue injury for all participants.

In a study by Hastings-Tolsma, Yucha, Tompkins, Robson, and Szeverenyi (1993), research participants ($N = 18$) were intentionally infiltrated with one of three commonly used IV solutions that varied in osmolarity (hypo-iso-hypertonic) but not in pH (all approximately 5.0). A warm or cold application was then randomly applied. At three periodic intervals postinfiltration, measurements were taken to determine differences in pain intensity, extent of surface swelling and erythema, and the volume of interstitial fluid (as determined by magnetic resonance imaging). Findings demonstrated that warmth or cold had no effect on swelling or pain intensity. However, volume remaining was always less when warmth was applied, even though the hypertonic solution doubled in size. Results indicate that the application of warmth to sites of IV infiltration produces faster resolution of a noncaustic infiltrate than does a cold application.

Finally, Yucha, Hastings-Tolsma, and Szeverenyi (1993) conducted an investigation designed to extend the work described above. The researchers intentionally infiltrated one of two solutions that were both isotonic but varied in pH (alkaline vs. acidic). Participants received one of three treatments: elevation, warmth, or no treatment (ambient temperature control). For the solutions examined, it made little difference whether the infiltrated limb received no treatment, elevation, or warmth.

Plan for Nursing Practice Change/Evaluation

For the consumer and practitioner who is struggling to make a determination regarding how best to treat IV infiltrations, the above research reports would need to be systematically evaluated to determine scientific merit and generalizability of the findings. The cited research on treatment of IV infiltrations presents results that would ideally be replicated and further investigated. Although it would not seem prudent to initiate a change in how IV infiltrations are treated when the solution is noncaustic and of a small volume, it may be important to initiate a change when the infiltrated solution is caustic (e.g., dilantin, potassium chloride) and when the infiltration occurs in children. Given the potentially costly consequence of caustic infiltrations, an innovative change in practice (the application of cold) may be warranted. Each of the criteria identified in Table 13.7 would need to be carefully attended to before a final decision could be made.

 PRACTICE

Research Utilization

Identify a problem found in clinical practice. Make a determination about the amount of research attention the topic has received, and then select and critique three or four of the research reports. Make a decision about how the problem should be addressed by nurses in the clinical setting based on a composite of research findings.

In addition to using a model and systematic approach in evaluating and critiquing the body of research available on a particular topic or problem, there are other factors that are significant in the success of implementing research-based nursing practice. These strategies have been evaluated for effectiveness in promoting nursing practice research findings (Brett, 1987).

Some facilities have a nurse researcher on staff who assists nursing personnel in using research findings appropriately, as well as assisting in the identification of problems in need of research and the implementation of research proposals. Other facilities have nurses with graduate-level preparation on staff. These individuals serve as nurse practitioners, clinical nurse specialists, educators, and clinical supervisors. Graduate preparation provides them with the skills necessary to develop, execute, evaluate, and support research relevant to clinical practice. They can serve as a valuable resource for the entry-level professional nurse who seeks to use research to improve practice.

It is important for the nurse to consider how research utilization is facilitated and implemented in clinical practice (Brooten, Youngblut, Roberts, Montgomery, Standing, Hemstrom, Suresky, & Polis, 1999). It is not unreasonable for the nurse clinician to expect resources related to research utilization to be available. These may include discussion with administrative personnel regarding the need for nurses with advanced research preparation, journal clubs, opportunities to attend conferences presenting clinically related research, and a research committee in the department of nursing or health system at large. Contact with educators, editors, and nurse researchers regarding the need for research reports that are clearly written for the practicing nurse provides impetus for change in how reports are communicated. Finally, incentives and support need to be available to encourage the utilization of relevant research findings. Such support may be demonstrated through merit pay mechanisms, promotion, or the creation of a milieu that clearly underscores a respect for creative change and empowers the nurse to act autonomously within the practice arena (Holm & Llewellyn, 1986).

427

CRITICAL APPRAISAL

Research Utilization

- Has a systematic review of the research available on a particular topic been conducted?

- Is the research-based knowledge relevant to the problem?

- Is there evidence that a practice change would be beneficial?

Critical Overview of the Research Evaluation Process

A serious gap exists between available nursing knowledge and the implementation of appropriate findings in practice. Numerous examples have been cited throughout the literature. Although most nurses have a fundamental sense of the importance of research-based practice and a desire for it, there is often a feeling of uncertainty and frustration regarding how that process might best be executed. Fear of research and inconsistent support for involvement in research activities have promulgated the gap between research and practice. As patient advocates and autonomous professionals, nurses have an obligation to become astute consumers of research. Critical appraisal of research reports becomes a primary vehicle for achieving the quality of patient care that nursing alone can provide.

CRITICAL OVERVIEW
THE RESEARCH EVALUATION
PROCESS

Find two research reports: one using a quantitative methodology and one a qualitative methodology. Using the guidelines presented in Appendices B and C, critique each and then discuss the following aspects of the reports:

• What differences exist in sequencing of the steps of the research process?

• How do the reports differ in their purpose?

• Suggest differences in implementing the findings from both reports.

References

Aamodt, A. (1983). Problems in doing nursing research: Developing criteria for evaluating qualitative research. *Western Journal of Nursing Research*, 5: 398–402.

Barnard, K. E. (1986). Research utilization: The clinician's role. *American Journal of Maternal/Child Nursing*, 11(3): 224.

Beyea, S. C. & Nicoll, L. H. (1997). Research utilization models help disseminate research findings and ultimately improve patient outcomes. *AORN Journal*, 65(3): 640–2.

Brett, J. L. L. (1987). Use of nursing practice research findings, *Nursing Research*, 36(6): 344–349.

Brooten, D., Youngblut, J. M., Roberts, B. L., Montgomery, K., Standing, T., Hemstrom, M., Suresky, J., & Polis, N. (1999). Disseminating our break-throughs: Enacting a strategic framework. *Nursing Outlook*, 47(3): 133–7.

Cobb, A. K. & Hagemaster, J. N. (1987). Ten criteria for evaluating qualitative research proposals. *Journal of Nursing Education*, 26: 138–142.

Conway, M. E. (1978). Clinical research: Instrument for change. *Journal of Nursing Administration*, 8: 27–32.

Duffy, M. E. (1985). A research appraisal checklist for evaluating nursing research reports. *Nursing and Health Care*, 6(10): 539–547.

Duffy, M. E. (1987). Methodological triangulation: A vehicle for merging quantitative and qualitative research methods. *Image: The Journal of Nursing Scholarship, 19*: 130–133.

Elder, N. C. & Miller, W. L. (1995). Reading and evaluating qualitative research studies. *Journal of Family Practice, 41*(3): 279–85.

Grove, S. K. & Burns, N. (2001). *The practice of nursing research: Conduct, critique & utilization* (4th Edition). St. Louis: W. B. Saunders.

Hastings-Tolsma, M. T., Yucha, C. B., Tompkins, J., Robson, L., & Szeverenyi, N. (1993). Effect of warm and cold applications on the resolution of IV infiltrations. *Research in Nursing and Health, 16*: 171–176.

Holm, K. & Llewellyn, J. G. (1986). *Nursing research for nursing practice.* Philadelphia: W. B. Saunders.

Horn Video Productions. (1991). *Research utilization* (video). Ida Grove, IA: Author.

Horsley, J. A. (1987, October). *The research to practice connection.* Paper presented at Research Day, Omicron, Iota/Delta Chapters of Sigma Theta Tau International, Syracuse, New York.

Horsley, J. A., Crane, J., Crabtree, M. K., & Wood, D. J. (1983). *Using research to improve nursing practice.* New York: Grime and Stratton.

King, I. M. (1989). King's general systems, framework and theory. In J. Riehl-Sisca (Ed.), *Conceptual models for nursing practice* (3rd Edition). (pp. 149–158). Norwalk, CT: Appleton and Lange.

Knafl, K. A. & Howard, M. J. (1986). Interpreting, reporting and evaluating qualitative research. In P. L. Munhall & C. J. Oiler, (Eds.), *Nursing research: A qualitative perspective.* (pp. 265–278). Norwalk, CT: Appleton-Century-Crofts.

Mateo, M. A. & Kirchhoff, K. T (1991). *Conducting and using nursing research in the clinical setting.* Baltimore, MD: Williams and Wilkins.

Morse, J. (1991). On the evaluation of qualitative proposals. *Qualitative Health Research, 1*: 147–151.

Paterson, J. G. & Zderad, L. T. (1976). *Humanistic nursing.* New York: Wiley Biomedical Publications.

Parse, R. R. (1981). *Man-living-health: A theory of nursing.* New York: Wiley.

Parse, R. R. (1989). Man–living–health: A theory of nursing. In J. Riehl-Sisca (Ed.) *Conceptual models for nursing practice* (3rd Edition). (pp. 253–257). Norwalk, CT: Appleton & Lange.

Phillips, L. R. E. (1986). *A clinician's guide to the critique and utilization of nursing research*. Norwalk, CT: Appleton-Century-Crofts.

Reichardt, C. & Cook, T., (Eds.). (1979). *Qualitative and quantitative methods in evaluation research*. Beverly Hills, CA: Sage.

Robson, L. K. & Tompkins, J. M. (1989, October). *Management of caustic intravenous infiltrations in pediatric patients: A pilot study*. Paper presented at Research Day, Omicron, Iota/Delta Chapters of Sigma Theta Tau International, Syracuse, New York.

Roy, C. & Andrews, H. A. (1991). *The Roy adaption model: The definitive statement*. Norwalk, CT: Appleton & Lange.

Stetler, C. B. & Marram, G. (1976). Evaluating research findings for applicability in practice. *Nursing Outlook, 24*(9): 559–563.

Ward, M. J. & Fetler, M. E. (1979). What guidelines should be followed in critically evaluating research reports? *Nursing Research, 27*: 120–126.

Woods, N. F. & Catanzaro, M. (1988). *Nursing research: Theory and practice*. St. Louis: C. V. Mosby.

Yucha, C., Hastings-Tolsma, M., & Szeverenyi, N. (1993, November). *Contrasts in IV extravasations made with different solutions*. Paper presented at Sigma Theta Tau International 32nd Biennial Convention, Indianapolis, IN.

14

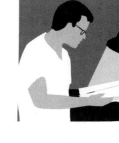

Communicating Study Results

Goals

- *Describe strategies for communicating findings from the research report.*
- *Examine key elements for effective research presentation.*

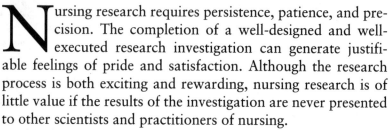

Introduction

Nursing research requires persistence, patience, and precision. The completion of a well-designed and well-executed research investigation can generate justifiable feelings of pride and satisfaction. Although the research process is both exciting and rewarding, nursing research is of little value if the results of the investigation are never presented to other scientists and practitioners of nursing.

This chapter discusses key points in developing and presenting the research report. The purpose of the nursing research report, primary areas that need to be included in the actual development of the report, and style considerations are highlighted.

The Research Report

The research report is the vehicle through which the nurse researcher disseminates crucial information about the investigation. The purpose of the research report is to give the critical consumer essential knowledge about the research question and how it was answered to allow for a full scientific evaluation. The nurse researcher needs to prepare the research report knowing that the consumer may want to evaluate the report for a variety of uses. These include possible replication, support of additional study related to the project, or clarification of a nursing practice problem.

WORKING DEFINITION

The Research Report

The research report is a means of communicating key aspects of the study to the research consumer.

If the research consumer is unable to determine how the study was conducted, comprehensive evaluation is impossible. It is important that the report be straightforward in describing the research problem, methodology, findings, and the researcher's interpretation of those findings. Access to this information allows the critical consumer the data necessary for systematic evaluation of the report's validity and utility of report findings for nursing (Haller, 1987).

Research is a costly endeavor. Considerable time, effort, money, and other resources are generally invested in the study. If the research is never reported to others, or if the report is poorly developed, the research is relatively meaningless. Research conducted in isolation will never contribute to the building of a body of nursing knowledge. Gortner (1974) suggests that one aspect of the researcher's scientific accountability is for the study findings to be published for review. Whether presented in written or oral form, a nursing research investigation should address the issue of how results will be disseminated to others prior to the inception of the study. Subsequently, the nursing investigation should be considered incomplete until the research report is prepared and presented to an appropriate nursing body.

The nursing research report needs to be shared with other nurses, regardless of the study's outcome. Nurses conducting research are often reluctant to share the results of their work if the study findings fail to answer the research question adequately because of an unclear research question, a poorly designed project, or another error in planning the project. Although there is no substitute for a well-developed and executed study, findings contrary to what the researcher expected are a valuable contribution to other researchers and consumers of research. For example, Randolph (1984) developed a study to explore the effectiveness of therapeutic touch versus physical touch in reducing anxiety levels in a healthy population. The hypotheses were not supported, possibly because of faulty assumptions on which the study was based. Despite the findings, the study makes a valuable contribution to the literature and to those who might wish to conduct an investigation using therapeutic touch. Research should be undertaken not only to support a proposed theory but also as a means of refuting a guiding theoretical conception (Batey, 1977). Negative findings can provide valuable data indicating theoretical areas in need of refinement, expansion, or change (Polit & Hungler, 1999).

EXAMPLE

The Research Report

A nurse investigator conducts an investigation to examine adaptation patterns of children with long-term health problems. Using Roy's adaptation nursing model as the framework for the study, the nurse develops a theory of child adaptation during prolonged illness. The findings do not support the proposed theory, and the nurse refines her ideas based on the data. An additional study is planned to test the revised theory for accuracy. The nurse presents the study and subsequent results to nurses attending a child rehabilitation conference. Participants provide feedback and assist in the refinement and expansion of the theoretical conceptualization.

PRACTICE

The Research Report

Select one issue of a nursing research journal or attend a research presentation. Review each research report presented. Determine whether the findings support or refute the proposed conceptual framework or stated hypotheses.

The research report is the vehicle for clearly identifying for the professional nurse how the results of the research relate to practice. The researcher has a responsibility to detail the link between research and practice. This includes spelling out significance, relevance, and benefits of the project to the practicing nurse. The title, findings, and discussion should leave little doubt regarding how the research articulates with practice (Brooten, 1982).

Elements of the Research Report

The individual who has conducted a research project has a vested interest in presenting a full picture of the investigation. Hours spent in developing and executing the research proposal make every aspect seem of great importance. However, whether reporting the study in a written or oral format, the nurse researcher must make a decision regarding what information is crucial to include and what can be omitted in the presentation. Most nurses have a limited amount of time available for literature perusal or conference attendance. The time spent in absorbing scholarly work must be maximized.

The nurse researcher should identify key elements in the research report. Those elements should be included in all forms of presentation, whether it is written or oral. The major areas include the research problem, the methodology utilized in solving the problem, and the findings of the study and what those results mean. For example, a nurse researcher prepares for an oral research presentation where 45 minutes have been allotted for discussion of each research report. The nurse decides that 10 minutes will be given to discussion of how the topic for research emerged and the formation of the research problem. Fifteen minutes are scheduled for an overview of how the research problem was solved (the methodology), and another 15 minutes are reserved for results and discussion of findings. Five minutes are reserved for questions about the project from the audience.

The elements of the research report related to the major areas of presentation are identified in Table 14.1. It should be noted that the sequence of presenting these elements may vary depending on whether the researcher is examining knowledge from a qualitative or quantitative perspective.

The elements identified in Table 14.1 are generally recognized as essential in presenting a comprehensive picture of the research report. The researcher would need to make a decision

437

TABLE 14.1   Major Elements of the Research Report for Presentation

Research problem:

- Introduction/overview of how the problem for study emerged
- Formation of the problem
- Purpose and importance of the investigation
- Conceptual model and related literature defining the problem

Research methodology:

- Design for study
- Date collection strategies and setting for data gathering (including description of instruments, and validity and reliability issues)
- Sample utilized

Research results, findings, and interpretation:

- Data analysis strategies and results
- Analysis of the research question
- Discussion of the findings and how they were interpreted
- Significance for nursing
- Recommendations for relating study findings to nursing education, practice, and additional research

about the depth to be presented in each area (based on time, audience, and format). Providing at least baseline information in each area gives the consumer of nursing research sufficient data to make an appropriate decision about the value of the investigation and the potential it holds for application and further study.

PRACTICE

The Research Report

Attend a research presentation (formal or informal) or locate a written research report. Determine if major areas of the research report were identified, as well as the relative attention directed to each area.

CRITICAL APPRAISAL

The Research Report

- Does the researcher discuss key elements of the research report: the research problem, the methodology for solving the problem, the results, and the meaning of the findings?

- Does the researcher clearly identify how the study results relate to nursing practice?

Selecting the Target Audience

The project investigator needs to consider carefully the most appropriate format for presenting the findings of the study. A decision must be made whether to present the findings in oral format (e.g., formal or informal conference presentation) or written format (e.g., journal or scientific bulletin). The researcher decides the most appropriate professional group toward which to direct the report. For example, a research investigation that examines the relationship between night wakings in toddlers and pregnancy for multiparous women would be most relevant to maternal–child health nursing professionals. Although this investigation is peripherally related to other areas of practice, the research investigator would target nurses working in settings where current childbearing and child-rearing knowledge is crucial in maintaining competency in nursing practice. The report might be presented at a maternal–child health research conference, or the study and findings could be prepared for publication in a general nursing research or maternal–child specialty journal.

The nurse may find an appropriate source for disseminating information about the research project by examining current research journals to determine whether there are plans to concentrate on themes to which the report may be especially well suited. Where journals do not plan specific thematic issues, the researcher should communicate directly with the editor to inquire about interest in the investigation.

Another way of determining how to reach the target audience is to watch for announcements of upcoming research conferences. These conferences seek research reports that are relevant to a planned theme or to the interests of a specific body of nursing professionals. Research conferences are generally announced to both the researcher and consumer through the use of the **call for abstracts**.

 WORKING DEFINITION

Call for Abstracts

A call for abstracts is a general announcement seeking research reports for presentation at a preplanned research conference.

The call for abstracts is meant to be a brief synopsis giving conference sponsors, specific theme and target audience, date and location of the conference, deadline for abstract submission, and contact person. The sponsoring organization generally places the call for abstracts in several journals and sends the announcement to individuals likely to be interested in attending. Nurses interested in being notified of upcoming research conferences can contact sponsoring organizations and ask to be placed on the mailing list, as well as closely watch the journals for information.

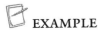 EXAMPLE

Call for Abstracts

Following is an example of a call for abstracts that might appear in a journal:

Call for Abstracts

The National Society for Promotion of Family Health Nursing is holding its fifth annual research conference on May 31 at Midwestern University. Deadline for research abstracts is March 1. The theme of the conference is "Family Health: Advocacy and Anarchy." For further information write Edith Jones, R.N., Ph.D., Conference Chair, Midwestern University College of Nursing, 5555 Beltline Boulevard, Globaline, IA 55555.

 PRACTICE

Selecting the Target Audience

Obtain a current issue of a nursing research journal that contains a "call for abstracts" section. Select one upcoming research conference that has a planned theme and one conference that has no planned theme but targets a specific group of nurse professionals. For each conference, select a research report in the journal that would be appropriate for presentation.

 CRITICAL APPRAISAL

Selecting the Target Audience

Does the researcher present the project to the most appropriate target audience?

Selecting the Mode of Presentation

There are a variety of ways to present the research project. Oral presentations at conferences, meetings, or informal gatherings; poster presentations; written reports in journals, books, or newsletters; and the thesis or dissertation are some of the major formats selected for disseminating the research project. The researcher needs to consider the nature of the project and the need for rapid circulation of the findings to interested and concerned nurses before making a decision about the mode of presentation. For example, a nurse researcher may conduct an investigation that evaluates three different nursing care strategies for children medically diagnosed with acquired immunodeficiency syndrome (AIDS). Because AIDS has been identified as a major public health problem, timely dissemination of the findings would seem crucial. The nurse researcher would make a valuable contribution to practicing nurses who work with AIDS patients by presenting the research findings in an oral format.

Regardless of the mode of presentation—that is, written or oral—the presentation should address the major elements of the research report. The research problem and its importance, the methodology used to answer the research question, and the study results and proposed impact should each be addressed in whatever form of presentation is chosen. Some methods will mandate more or less detail about the exact nature of the project. Guidelines relevant to each mode of presentation should be followed as appropriate.

Written Research Reports

Most critical consumers of research are familiar with the written report found in the research journal. Written reports, however, may be prepared several ways and for several different audiences. A written report may mean preparing a book chapter, describing the study in a more condensed format for inclusion in a scientific bulletin, preparing a detailed report for a sponsoring agency, or completing a thesis or dissertation as a requirement for an educational degree.

Written research reports usually have the advantage of allowing the researcher time and space to give in-depth detail about the investigation. The researcher is able to spend time carefully thinking how aspects of the study would best be presented in the manuscript. The written report also tends to reach a wider audience, because circulation is greater and accessibility permanent. The primary disadvantage of the written report is that many journals and books have printing delays of one year or more.

 PRACTICE

Written Research Reports

Visit a health sciences library and obtain a nursing research report published in each of the following forms: a dissertation or thesis, a scientific bulletin, a nursing journal, and a book chapter. Compare differences in presenting the research report.

Oral Research Reports

Oral presentations can be delivered at professional meetings, at informal gatherings, or through poster presentations. There are advantages to choosing an oral presentation. First, the oral presentation is generally more current and up to date. Thus, interested persons have access to scientific findings offering knowledge that has been promptly disseminated. The second advantage of the oral report is that immediate feedback is available from the participants who attend the presentation. This feedback can be invaluable in helping to interpret study results as well as helping to shape related research investigations.

Oral research reports can be anxiety-producing, however, especially for the novice nurse researcher. For the individual who has not previously had the opportunity to present at a conference, it may be helpful first to present at a more informal gathering, such as a research luncheon for colleagues, a seminar, or a clinical postconference setting. Presentation in one of these settings allows for the refinement of ideas under less pressure.

Oral reports also mandate time restrictions; therefore, fewer details about the study may be given. It is not unusual for the researcher to have a time limitation on the presentation, which may vary from 20 to 60 minutes. The researcher must make crucial decisions about deleting less important aspects of the study without dropping key elements that need to be included.

Finally, the oral research presentation is limited to a prescribed number of participants. Only those individuals who actually attend the conference have knowledge of the material. Oral presentation also prevents the detailed evaluation that the written report allows, because some data may have to be abbreviated in the presentation due to time restrictions. Some researchers presenting at a conference compensate for this disadvantage by providing participants with a written summary of the project. Some conference organizers also provide a written account of the research presentations in a booklet format referred to as **conference proceedings**. This is one way of increasing the size of the audience and encouraging utilization of the findings.

The critical consumer of nursing research can develop evaluation skills by actively seeking out research presentations. It is a worthwhile activity to ask about attending a research luncheon or to seek out a research conference presenting investigations relevant to nursing practice. Repeated exposure to nurse researchers who are sharing their findings heightens awareness of scientific and technical research language, as well as increases understanding of how to evaluate and synthesize the data.

Tips for Presenting the Research Report

Whether the research investigator selects a written or oral format, several points need to be considered in preparation of the presentation. Effective communication of the project requires attention to the level of presentation, adherence to guidelines for the presentation, and clear organization.

The audience that the researcher is addressing is a central consideration in preparing the report. It should be remembered that the purpose of the research report is to inform the audience about the project (Jackie, 1989). Regardless of the educational or professional background of the investigator of the research report, clear, direct, straightforward language should be used. A highly technical and esoteric style is difficult to follow and unnecessary. The report should also focus on presenting the essential elements of the research report without interjecting opinions.

Considerable criticism has been leveled at researchers who make little effort to prepare a project report that is understandable to the practicing professional nurse. Nevertheless, not every research project has direct applicability to the practice arena. Fawcett (1984) identifies two forms of nursing research utilization: use in a realm of nursing practice, and use of findings to develop additional study in a program of nursing research. Thus, although research can have two different utilization aims, the consumer should find that the report clearly indicates what the aim is and how it can best be achieved.

The presentation of the report should be prepared in an interesting fashion. The researcher who develops a dry, dull report falls short of stimulating an attitude of scientific inquiry in the audience. Lindeman (1984) has noted that the general state of written research reports is such that most fail to stimulate a visual image for the reader. Failure to describe the perceptions that led to the initiation of the project has resulted in a loss of the richness of the research experience. Observations and intuition are important aspects of the research process, and describing them emphasizes the uniqueness of knowledge in nursing.

Whether the research report is prepared for a journal, book, or conference, the investigator should make every effort to use aids that will enhance audience understanding and interest. These may include audiovisuals, tables, graphs, or photographs. Combined with close attention to the characteristics of the target audience, succinct organization, and clarity, the research report can be an exciting tool for communicating to others the impact of the research.

CRITICAL APPRAISAL

Mode of Presentation for the Research Report

- Does the researcher present the research report in a clear, understandable, exciting fashion?

- Does the researcher follow guidelines for presenting the report and make the presentation organized and logical?

◈ Basic Considerations in Facilitating Use of the Research Report

The research consumer can use several parameters in making a determination about the general worth of a study and whether or not to engage in an in-depth evaluation of the report. These parameters include the title of the report, abstract, references, and credentials of the investigator.

Titling the Research Report

The title of the research report is the research consumer's first exposure to the study. Ideally a title can be generated that not only is concise, but also stimulates interest in reading the full report. The title of the research project should reflect the major emphasis and nature of the investigation. Generally the title that is selected identifies the major variables as well as the population under study (Polit & Hungler, 1999).

WORKING DEFINITION

Research Report Title

The title of the research report is a brief phrase that indicates the major study variables and the population under investigation.

EXAMPLE

Research Report Title

Following is a list of titles that might be utilized in conducting different types of research investigations:

- "The Role of the Nurse in Development of Health Promotion Behaviors, 1950–1985"

- "Ingestion of Milk Products During Breast-feeding and the Incidence of Fussiness During Infancy"

- "The Experience of Being a Minority Student in a Private University"

- "Adolescent Satisfaction in Male–Female Relationships and Consistency in Using Contraceptives"

 PRACTICE

Research Report Title

Select a nursing research journal. Read a report and determine whether the title reflects the major variables under study as well as the population. If not, suggest a title that might be more appropriate.

Research Abstract

The research abstract is a brief summary of the main components of the research project. The description, which is generally 300–400 words long, is a means of briefly informing the research consumer of the project highlights. The abstract is intended to provide a synopsis of the study, thus giving the consumer enough information about the investigation to decide whether the entire report needs to be examined.

 WORKING DEFINITION

The Research Abstract

The research abstract is a 300–400-word synopsis of the research investigation. It is designed to provide the consumer with sufficient information to decide whether additional time needs to be spent on the report.

The abstract is usually placed directly under the title and precedes the actual research report. The consumer of research should utilize the abstract in determining a study's potential worth. Considerable time can be saved by using the abstract as a means of capturing the essentials of the investigation without having to pore over the entire article. For the researcher, skill and attention in developing the abstract is paramount in facilitating communication of the project and subsequent findings (Juhl & Norman, 1989).

The research consumer needs to be aware that a research abstract does not always accompany a written report. In the event that the journal does not require the inclusion of an abstract, the consumer should turn to the end of the study and review the section identified as the summary. The summary generally pulls together the major aspects of the study and can serve as a barometer regarding whether the consumer might wish to read further.

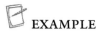 EXAMPLE

The Research Abstract

Following is an example of an abstract that might accompany a nursing research study published in a journal:

This study examined pain perception of the preschool child following attendance at the birth of a sibling. Using Neuman's (1982) systems nursing model and drawing on pain theory literature, the following research question was formulated: What is the relationship between the preschooler's attendance at a sibling birth and the perception of pain? A convenience sample of 44 preschool children who were attending their first sibling birth at a large intercommunity birthing center was selected. Parental and child consent was obtained. Data were collected using a structured questionnaire developed for use with parents, and the Pain Perception Scale for Children (PPSC) and informal interview were used with preschool participants. Data were collected over a six-month period of time by the investigators. A correlational design was utilized. Scores of the PPSC were positively correlated with parental evaluation of the difficulty of the birth. A positive but weak association was shown between length of second-stage labor and the perception of pain. Further testing of the PPSC is indicated.

 PRACTICE

The Research Abstract

Select an issue of a nursing research journal. Choose one report that does not have an abstract accompanying it, and write an abstract.

References

Review of the references accompanying the research report is one of the first considerations that the critical consumer should make. The reference list informs the potential reader whether the project was based on current literature sources and whether the sources are relevant to the project. Because the nurse must keep abreast of voluminous nursing literature, outdated or irrelevant sources should be one consideration in choosing whether to review a particular report.

Although the consumer may not be particularly knowledgeable about a given research topic, the nurse should be able to draw some general conclusions about the appropriateness of the references. For example, are the sources that are identified up to date (generally within the past five years, unless a classic)? Are the references related to the major variables for study?

The consumer should take into account the purpose of the research investigation. If the investigator is conducting a historical investigation, the references would need to be appropriate to the period of time under investigation. For example, if a nurse historian were conducting an investigation to examine the evolution of the midwife role from 1850 to 1975, the research consumer would expect to see references related to that time period. On the other hand, if a nurse researcher were conducting a comparative investigation to determine whether there was greater preparation for childbirth with each succeeding cohort group of primiparas, the consumer would be concerned if references did not reflect current sources. If the researcher identified literature dated only through the 1970s, the consumer should consider the literature review incomplete because a great deal of knowledge has been generated since that time.

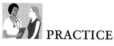 PRACTICE

References for the Research Report

Select a research report and review the references. Determine whether the sources are up to date and appropriate to the variables under study.

The Investigator's Background and Credentials

A final area to consider in attempting to determine the general worth of an investigation is the information provided about the researcher. Although some journals do not give any background data about the researcher's professional preparation and experience, many journals do provide at least basic information. This information is usually provided when researchers presenting reports at a conference are introduced, or the participants have an opportunity to inquire.

The researcher's background refers to professional experiences that have assisted in preparing the investigator for conducting the study. For example, if a nurse researcher conducts an investigation examining factors that influence self-extubation in patients after thoracic surgery, the research consumer would be cautious in reading the report if the researcher has had no professional experience in working with critically ill clients. The employment site and past work experiences related to the problem under investigation are also frequently identified.

Educational preparation of the researcher is equally important. Most reports specify the researcher's earned degrees. Knowing that the researcher is a nurse, as opposed to a social worker, psychologist, or physician, would be an overall consideration about the worth of the study. Although collaborative research is extremely valuable, the practitioner of nursing should be concerned with the credibility of research that is conducted by non-nurses without nursing input or a nurse coinvestigator. Nurses are in the best position to examine nursing care problems and develop nursing knowledge.

Past experience in conducting research is also an element to be considered. Most reports do not indicate the depth or breadth of the investigator's research preparation. The reader can draw some conclusions, however, from the information about earned degrees. For example, some master's programs in nursing require a thesis or research project. Likewise, the nurse who has earned a doctoral degree has at least some supervised experience in conducting independent nursing research.

 WORKING DEFINITION

Background and Credentials of the Researcher

The background and credentials of the researcher are the professional, educational, and research experiences that qualify the investigator to conduct the research.

Finally, the consumer should attempt to ascertain the funding sources of the research project. These are important for two reasons. First, the fact that a project has been funded means that a review process has been undertaken and some merit has been attached to the study. Second, researcher bias can exist when funding conflicts with the purpose of the study. For example, a nurse might be employed as a researcher for a large company that manufactures disposable garments for individuals with urinary incontinence. If the nurse were to conduct a comparative investigation of the efficacy of several different disposable garments utilizing funds provided by the employer, the consumer would be concerned with bias on the part of the researcher. Although this situation implies questions about the reliability of the findings, this concern would not necessarily arise in all situations. The consumer would want to know, however, that the researcher had built in adequate safeguards to prevent undue bias.

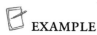 EXAMPLE

Background and Credentials of the Researcher

Following is an example of information about the researcher that might be identified in a research report:

> Sandra Anderson Jones, R.N., Ph.D., is an assistant professor in the Department of Family Nursing, School of Nursing, Western University, Noso, Idaho. The researcher has had extensive experience in counseling families experiencing the death of a child and has worked in both pediatrics and community health nursing.

 PRACTICE

Background and Credentials of the Researcher

Following is the title of a nursing research report and the background and credentials of the nurse researcher. Discuss the researcher's qualifications in conducting the study.

> *Project title:* An Analysis of Comfort Needs of Adult Patients with End-Stage Renal Disease.
>
> *About the author:* Angelina Smith, R.N., MA, is a lecturer at Central Community Hospital School of Nursing,

Touchkin, Alabama. Ms. Smith has had several years experience working on a urology service, as well as contact with patients undergoing prolonged kidney dialysis.

CRITICAL APPRAISAL

Facilitating Use of the Research Report

- Does the title of the research report identify the major study variables and the population under investigation?

- Is the research abstract clearly written, highlighting the major features of the investigation?

- Are references current, relevant, and complete?

- Does the researcher have appropriate professional, educational, and research experience to support participation in the study?

Critical Overview of Communicating Research

Communicating nursing research findings is fundamental to the development of nursing knowledge. Careful attention needs to be given to the research report. Appropriate development and delivery of the research report will contribute to an increased utilization of research findings in nursing practice.

Nursing theory, practice, and research are inextricably related. To fully develop a nursing science, however, the researcher and the consumer of nursing research must be willing to disseminate and carefully critique the value of each piece of research. Effective communication of the research report entails the search for creative, fresh ways of stimulating the reporting and use of the project and related findings.

CRITICAL OVERVIEW
COMMUNICATING RESEARCH

Ellen Varner is a nurse practicing on a surgical unit in a small rural hospital. In conducting the health history with patients, the nurse notes that several individuals report altered gastrointestinal functioning and mood changes after ingesting certain types of foods. Interested in learning more about this phenomenon and the best advice to give patients, Ellen attends a research conference entitled "Nutritional Intake, Health Promotion, and the Role of the Nurse." Several sessions focus on the well adult patient who experiences difficulty following ingestion of specific foods.

Ellen attends one session of particular interest. Following is an overview of the research presentation attended:

Research Report Title:	"Food Additives and Reported Adverse Responses"
Researcher:	Georgeann Geiorgi, R.N., M.S.N.
Overview of Problem:	The researcher works in a wellness center where many of the clients are obese and have reported adverse reactions to foods ingested while attempting weight reduction. The researcher became interested in examining the primary offending foods, additives intentionally added by the manufacturer, and reported symptoms.
Conceptual Model:	Roy's adaptation nursing model
Related Literature:	The primary areas reviewed were related to safety of food additives, nutritional needs, and physiological

	alterations during weight reduction of middle-aged women.
Problem Formation:	What adverse physiological and psychological symptoms do women attempting weight reduction and ingesting products with food additives report?
Research Methodology:	Descriptive survey
Data Collection:	A 50-item paper-and-pencil questionnaire measuring adverse symptoms
Sample:	100 women ages 40–55 who were attending a wellness center, had been on a prescribed weight reduction program for at least three weeks, and desired a weight loss of 50–75 pounds.
Data Analysis:	Descriptive analysis
Results:	Psychological symptoms were most frequently reported: feeling tired (82%), mood swings (80%), and feelings of depression (39%). Physical symptoms reported were an increase in appetite (73%), GI upset (45%), and diarrhea (30%). Women ingesting four or more diet soft drinks per day reported the highest number of symptoms.
Importance to Nursing:	Findings indicate that women who ingest foods known to have chemical additives report a higher incidence of adverse reactions, particularly psychological. Women in weight reduction programs need to be counseled about the selection of foods with chemical additives. Additional research is needed to examine

behaviors prior to the initiation of the weight reduction program, the relationship between specific types of chemical additives and reported symptoms, and specific educational programs needed for these patients.

Activity 1

- Review the research report. Identify which elements of the research report were included and which were not.
- Discuss the target audience selected and the appropriateness of the mode of presentation.

Activity 2

- Prepare a research abstract for the research report.
- Identify weaknesses in the title of the research report and suggest a more appropriate title, if necessary.
- Were the literature areas reviewed appropriate to the investigation? Were any areas deleted?
- Discuss the author's credentials and background. What strengths and weaknesses does the investigator bring to the project?

Activity 3

- Discuss strategies for facilitating the dissemination of the report findings into practice.

References

Batey, M. V. (1977). Conceptualization: Knowledge and logic guiding empirical research. *Nursing Research, 26*(5): 324–329.

Brooten, D. A. (1982). Is soft sell enough? (editorial), *Nursing Research*, *31*(4): 195.

Fawcett, J. (1984). Another look at utilization of nursing research. *Image: The Journal of Nursing Scholarship*, *16*(2): 59–62.

Gortner, S. R. (1974). Scientific accountability in nursing. *Nursing Outlook*, 22(12): 764–768.

Haller, K. B. (1987). Readying research for practice. *American Journal of Maternal/Child Nursing*, 12(3): 226.

Jackle, M. (1989). Presenting research to nurses in clinical practice. *Applied Nursing Research*, 2(4): 191–193.

Juhl, N. & Norman, V. L. (1989). Writing an effective abstract. *Applied Nursing Research*, 2(4): 189–193.

Lindeman, C. A. (1984). Dissemination of nursing research. *Image: The Journal of Nursing Scholarship*, *16*(2): 57–58.

Neuman, B. (1982). The Neuman systems model. Norwalk, CT: Appleton-Century-Crofts.

Polit, D. F. & Hungler, B. P. (1999). *Essentials of Nursing Research: Methods and Applications* (6th Edition). Philadelphia: Lippincott Williams & Wilkins.

Randolph, G. L. (1984). Therapeutic and physical touch: Physiological response to stressful stimuli. *Nursing Research*, *33*(1): 33–36.

15

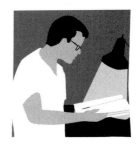

Research and the Entry-Level Professional Nurse

Goals

- *Describe professional nursing expectations for participation in research.*
- *Understand grantsmanship activities in supporting research.*
- *Identify strategies for fostering evidence-based practice in the workplace.*

Introduction

Professional nurses have the responsibility to participate in the promotion of evidence-based practice. Such expectation is both societal and professional. The mandate for research involvement and the requisite level of activity are detailed by professional organizations and provide structure for the practicing nurse. Adherence to these guidelines facilitates utilization of research findings in practice. If evidence-based practice is a major goal of nursing, then research skill and involvement become critical.

Guidelines for Participating in Research

Building a body of nursing knowledge is the ultimate goal of research. Until recently, there has been some confusion regarding who is responsible for carrying out research activities and the extent of responsibility. In the last decade, the scope of research activities for which nurses are responsible has been clearly enunciated. This research focus has evolved from within the nursing profession, from society at large, and as a result of interprofessional influences.

Expectations of the Profession

As a relatively new science, nursing has only recently come to grips with entry-level educational requirements for the professional nurse. In addition, nurses prepared at the graduate level have been a small minority of the overall number of nurses. Given the tremendous need for new knowledge, research activities have fallen largely on the nurse interested and willing to participate in research.

This confusion regarding the research role led to misplaced expectations for the entry-level nurse to design and produce research, among other activities. Research expectations have been reexamined with emphasis on the performance of activities appropriate to the educational preparation of the nurse. For the entry-level professional nurse, this reexamination has meant a thorough review of curriculum and role expectations for research.

The research role has been actively addressed by educators in professional nursing programs. Spruck (1980) reported that of 286 baccalaureate nursing programs surveyed, all accredited by the National League for Nursing (NLN) (response rate: 263, or 92%), 83% incorporated research content in the nursing curriculum in some fashion. Similarly, Thomas and Price (1980) found that 96.6% of NLN-accredited baccalaureate programs taught research as a required part of the nursing curriculum. The findings from these studies clearly indicate an early recognition of the importance of socializing professional nurses to research.

For the nurse prepared at the baccalaureate level, the mandate for participating in research is clear. Primary emphasis centers on the role of research consumer, with secondary responsibility for designing, replicating, and collecting data. For the nurse prepared at the associate degree level, emphasis is on the role of the research consumer who is able to appreciate research. Other activities for these nurses include collecting data and actively identifying problems in need of study by the researcher.

Societal Expectations

Responsibility for participating in and conducting research activities is a basic expectation of society, as well as the nursing profession. Society provides nurses with the power they hold to provide nursing care to individuals in need of health services. An implicit societal expectation is that the nursing care rendered is based on current knowledge, and that research is being conducted to improve that care.

Nursing has historically provided care to patients that was based on experience and wisdom. Soaring health care costs, highly technical health care services, and a rising number of litigations all require that nursing care be based on sound scientific findings.

Interprofessional Influences

The impact of working with other health care professionals has stimulated the development and clarification of research roles in nursing. Psychology and medicine are among those disciplines that have a more established research tradition. Professionals in those and other health-related disciplines have had an influence on nursing research. Active research endeavors related to clinical studies have helped to spark nursing participation in interdisciplinary, collaborative projects, as well as in independent nursing investigations.

461

Nurses frequently receive their first exposure to clinical research projects while functioning in a staff position within an institution. It is not uncommon for nurses to be asked to participate in clinical investigations conducted by pharmacists, physicians, or other health care professionals. Nurses sometimes feel obligated to participate in research conducted by researchers from other disciplines because of a perceived power imbalance.

Many nurses have expressed confusion about the need to assist in research activities conducted under the auspices of another researcher. Regardless of whether the researcher is a physician, pharmacist, social worker, or another nurse, the nurse is never obligated to participate. However, the nurse does have an obligation to evaluate the proposed project to ensure that the patient's rights are protected and to consider the importance of the study in generating new knowledge.

There are two major considerations that need to be addressed prior to making a decision about involvement in a proposed research project. First, the decision to participate in a given research project should be based on the merits of the project. Coercion used to obtain assistance with a research project is inappropriate. Job requirements should not imply that the nurse must participate in research activities as a condition of employment (American Nurses Association, 1985). When the decision is made to participate in research activities, the nurse needs to be considered a member of the research team. This team involvement should include a link with decision-making research approval committees, as well as input into decisions about the course of the study and its evaluation.

A second consideration crucial to a decision about participating in a research project centers on ethical considerations. The nurse needs to have sufficient knowledge about the proposed research to make an informed decision regarding how well research participants will be protected. Chapter 5 addresses specific ethical concerns that need to be considered.

Participating in a team research effort can be immensely rewarding. The nurse who has had limited contact with research activities may find that working with a team of researchers may help to refine research skills. Furthermore, an interdisciplinary involvement in research may have a significant impact on producing knowledge useful to effecting broad change within the health care system.

Research and the Entry-Level Professional Nurse

The entry-level professional nurse, with educational preparation at the baccalaureate level, has taken foundational courses that provide the basic skills for understanding the research process. For example, most baccalaureate nurses have studied statistics and research methods and taken courses related to nursing issues and leadership. These courses lay the groundwork for articulating research responsibilities as a professional nurse.

Expectations for the professional nurse's participation in research activities have been clearly enunciated by members of the chief nursing organizations, the National League for Nursing (NLN) and the American Nurses Association (ANA), as well as other nursing organizations such as the American Association of Colleges of Nursing.

NLN and ANA Guidelines for Functioning

The NLN and the ANA, both concerned with how well the nursing needs of the individual and society are met, have taken responsibility for fostering the growth of nursing research. The NLN, whose membership extends beyond nurses, is primarily concerned with nursing education and service. Since 1972, the NLN has expressed concern with the need for nurses to have an opportunity to experience the research process. Nurse educators were charged with addressing how this could best be done. This concern was further explicated in 1979, when the NLN outlined specifications for research in baccalaureate nursing programs. To date, the NLN has not specified research expectations in associate degree programs, although an increasing number of programs have identified criteria for their graduates.

The ANA, the voice of organized nursing, has likewise worked to establish guidelines for facilitating the research role. Guidelines have been established that identify the general competencies expected of nurses graduating from associate degree, baccalaureate, and graduate degree programs (American Nurses Association Commission on Nursing Research, 1981).

The baccalaureate nurse is expected to participate in research activities in practice that are related to the following guidelines:

1. Read, interpret, and evaluate research for applicability to nursing practice.

2. Identify nursing problems that need to be investigated and participate in implementation of findings.

3. Use nursing practice as a means of gathering data and refining practice.

4. Apply established research findings to nursing practice.

5. Share research findings with colleagues.

Research expectations for the associate degree nurse relate to the following guidelines:

1. Demonstrate awareness of the value and relevance of research in nursing.

2. Identify problem areas in nursing practice.

3. Participate in data collection within a structured format.

These guidelines provide the structure for the nurse to initiate research activities. They also encompass multiple research activities that can be carried out singularly or in unison. These research roles include those of consumer, collaborator in designing and producing research, replicator of research, and data collector (Mallick, 1983).

 WORKING DEFINITION

Research Expectations for the Professional Nurse

Expectations for participation in research activities by the professional nurse as detailed by professional nursing organizations.

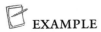

EXAMPLE

Research Expectations for the Professional Nurse

Helen is a new baccalaureate nurse graduate who has interviewed for a job in the burn unit of a large metropolitan hospital. She is told that there are many ongoing research projects being conducted, although there is no mention of what level of participation will be expected of her. She is interested in furthering her career, in promoting good patient care, and in research involvement. Before she accepts the position, she requests a second meeting to clarify what research activity she can expect and how she will be evaluated on this professional expectation.

PRACTICE

Research Expectations for the Professional Nurse

Ask the nurse manager on a unit that you are doing clinical to share with you the job description and evaluation criteria for baccalaureate-prepared, entry-level nurses. What expectations regarding research participation can be found? If research involvement is not clearly stated, ask the nurse manager what would be expected on employment.

Research Proposal

Regardless of the research role assumed by the nurse, it is important that there be a clear understanding of how to evaluate a research proposal. A proposal is a paper that details what the researcher plans to study, how the problem will be solved, how research participants will be protected, how much the project will cost, and the timetable for completion. The research proposal is submitted to appropriate institutional committees, funding agencies, and involved research personnel as a means of communicating the significance of the scientific work.

465

Nurses involved in research as consumer, data collector, or collaborator in designing and producing a research project need to develop the skills to determine the soundness of a proposal. It is the nurse's responsibility to participate in the evaluation of a research proposal when serving on institutional research committees or when acting as a member of the research team.

WORKING DEFINITION

Research Proposal

The research proposal is a formal means of presenting the scientific merits of a study to others. It details the problem under study, how it will be solved, how research participants will be protected, and cost considerations for the project.

The research proposal should be clearly written and understandable by those from other disciplines. Exact specifications for what should be included in the proposal are usually well defined by the institutional committee or funding agency reviewing the proposal. For example, federal funding sources will provide a packet of materials to be completed by the researcher when monies are sought from government agencies. These documents are very specific regarding the type of information needed before funding can be determined. Similarly, many academic and health care agencies have prepared packets appropriate to those settings. Table 15.1 presents components of the research proposal basic to any well-prepared report.

A well-written proposal helps the researcher to plan for potential problems and execute a better project. Preparing the document assists the researcher in troubleshooting prior to the actual study. It also allows other scientists, who may have greater objectivity, to make suggestions for refinement prior to the actual implementation of the investigation.

TABLE 15.1 Components of a Research Proposal

- Description of the problems to be researched
- Review of the literature with theoretical rationale
- Description of the research design
- Research methodology: research participants, instruments, research setting, and plans for data analysis
- Other relevant information: cost (financial, time, resources, etc.), qualifications of the research team

 PRACTICE

Research Proposal

Contact a member of the research review committee at an academic or health care institution and obtain a copy of the criteria for research proposal submission. Compare and contrast the requirements with the listing in Table 15.1.

 CRITICAL APPRAISAL

Research Proposal

Does the research report describe the proposal development phase of the project?

Skill in evaluating research reports allows the professional nurse to participate in decisions about research activity. Knowledge of the components that should be articulated in the proposal and skill in critiquing the strength of those components enables the nurse to be a valued participant in project development and evaluation.

Participating in Grant Applications

The entry-level professional nurse needs to have some familiarity with grant applications because support for research is often dependent on this activity. The nurse may be involved with grants in a variety of capacities. For example, the nurse may be actively involved in the design and production of a nursing research investigation or an investigation conducted by a multidisciplinary team where monies are being sought to conduct the study. The nurse might also be exposed to grant applications when asked to serve as a data collector for another investigator's research project. Prior to consenting to serve as a source of support for the proposed project, the nurse needs to understand what the project is about and what participation would mean. If asked to review a grant application as a means of obtaining information about the study, the nurse should be knowledgeable about the impact of the grant application.

Conducting research is costly even if the investigation is fairly simple. Paper, duplication of materials, salaries of support personnel, computer time, and literature searches are a few examples of the areas needing cost consideration. Most researchers do not have the personal finances available to permit costly investigations. Similarly, many academic and health care facilities lack the resources to support a research project of considerable cost.

Knowledge of how to obtain available research monies is important at a time when competition is keen and resources sometimes scarce. The ability to solicit funding for research purposes is referred to as **grantsmanship**. As nurses become more involved in research, it will be increasingly important to develop finely honed research skills and the ability to seek out funding sources to aid research efforts (Sexton, 1982; Tornquist & Funk, 1990).

468

WORKING DEFINITION

Grantsmanship

Grantsmanship is the ability to obtain funding to aid in the support of research activities.

Finding out what funds are available for research activities requires diligence. Many institutions have a grant office where diverse information about available research monies is centralized. The researcher can save a vast amount of time by contacting the chief grant officer to locate the most viable sources for support.

Sources of funding can be categorized into one of several areas. The federal government (e.g., National Institutes of Health, National Center for Health Services Research, Health Care Finances Administration, and Office of Human Developmental Services) is the largest contributor in support of research activities. Competition from federal agencies is also very keen.

Other funding sources include state and local governments, foundations (e.g., Kellogg, Robert Wood Johnson, Pew), business and industry (e.g., Exxon, Baxter), in-house (e.g., university/college and school of nursing), professional organizations (e.g., American Nurses Foundation, Sigma Theta Tau International), and philanthropic organizations and individuals.

It is difficult to keep abreast of available research monies. In addition to maintaining frequent contact with the grant officer, it is worthwhile for the researcher to regularly review publications dealing with available grants. *The Directory of Research Grants, Grants Register,* and *Foundation Grants to Individuals* are helpful directories available at most institutional libraries. Finally, there are other federal government publications (e.g., *Commerce Business Daily, NIH Guide for Grants and Contracts*) as well as journal and newsletter listings that can direct the researcher to available resources.

Preparing materials for application for grant monies involves the completion of the proposal and related materials specific to the granting agency. Most funding agencies have targeted deadlines to submit applications by, and the

469

researcher must watch these dates carefully. Tornquist and Funk (1990) describe crucial aspects of preparing a successful research grant application. *The Complete Grants Source Book for Nursing and Health* (Bauer & American Association of Colleges of Nursing, 1988) is a useful publication that addresses grant preparation as well as funding sources. For the researcher preparing a first grant application, the process may seem excessive. It is important to remember that grantsmanship requires practice to perfect. Many researchers, both experienced and inexperienced, have applications rejected. Although it may be discouraging to have an application rejected, funding agencies generally provide a summary statement (often referred to as the "pink sheet") of the review ("The Pink Sheet," 1985). This feedback can be used to revise the research proposal for resubmission to the same agency or to an alternative funding source. With each application, the researcher develops grantsmanship skill.

 EXAMPLE

Grantsmanship

A nurse who works in an inner-city community health clinic is interested in developing a research project that would promote self and clinical breast examination in homeless women. After developing a research proposal and calculating the costs of the project, she contacts a local nurse researcher for suggestions about tightening the proposal design and possible funding sources. After making changes to the proposal, she completes an application for funding to two local agencies.

 PRACTICE

Grantsmanship

Identify a topic of clinical research interest. Contact a grant officer or nurse researcher to discuss what resources might be available for supporting a research project.

CRITICAL APPRAISAL

Grantsmanship

- Does the proposal realistically detail costs of conducting the research?

- Is the topic likely to be funded?

- Is at least one category of grant funding likely to be interested in the research proposal?

Promoting Evidence-Based Practice in the Workplace

Hinshaw (2000) has stated that there is a dramatic number of opportunities and challenges for generating knowledge for nursing, but the greatest challenge is translating that knowledge into practice. Although several models have been presented to facilitate research utilization in practice, fostering the process has met with mixed success and efficiency in doing so remains a high priority.

The literature demonstrates several models that assist the nurse in changing to evidence-based practice. One model described by Rosswurm and Larrabee (1999) is particularly useful. The model guides the nurse through the process of developing and integrating an evidence-based practice change. The process involves six steps to assist nurses in the integration of evidence-based knowledge into practice. These steps include: *assess* need for practice change (involve stakeholders, collect data about current practice, compare internal and external data, identify problem), *link* the problem interventions and outcomes (identify potential interventions, select outcome indicators), *synthesize* best evidence (literature search, critique and weigh evidence, synthesize evidence, assess feasibility, determine benefits and risk), *design* practice change (define proposed change, identify needed resources, plan change based on defined outcomes), *implement and evaluate* change in practice (pilot study, evaluate process and outcome, decide to adapt/adopt/reject proposal change), and *integrate*

471

and maintain change in practice (communicate recommended change to those affected, inservice education, rewrite standards of practice to include change, monitor process and outcomes).

EXAMPLE

Promoting Evidence-Based Practice

A community health nurse is interested in promoting a change in practice based on best evidence found in the literature: early and consistent contact with breastfeeding mothers in the early postpartum period significantly increases the rate of breastfeeding at six and 10 months. She knows that fewer than 20% of their babies are breastfed at six weeks. She initiated the following steps to create the practice change:

First, she examined the need to create change. She discussed the problem with nursing colleagues and providers at the community health center. She examined the only available data regarding the current rate of breastfeeding at discharge from the hospital, at two and six weeks postpartum, and at one year of age. State data was also sought to ascertain the rates of breastfeeding at birth and at six weeks. The low rates of breastfeeding were a decided problem.

The nurse then linked the problem with potential interventions and activities by listing the current strategies that were being utilized to promote breastfeeding: discussion at a prenatal class, visits by the lactation consultant in the hospital, and a hotline that patients were told they could call if breastfeeding problems developed. The desired outcome was also identified: a minimum of 60% of mothers would be breastfeeding at six and 10 months as measured by self-report.

A review of the literature was conducted to determine the best available evidence. Five reports dealing with promotion of breastfeeding were located. Each report was critiqued and assessed for the level of evidence and the strength of the association. Also described at this point was the feasibility of the change, as well as benefits and risks.

Convinced that the evidence for change was well-detailed in the literature, the nurse decided to move forward with a planned change. She listed the activities that needed to be performed and thought out a plan for meeting the desired outcomes. She also met with all providers to allow them a chance to discuss the proposed change and what role each would have in the piloting process.

The pilot study was implemented for six months. It became immediately apparent that the plan to promote increased rates of breastfeeding was successful. Preliminary data demonstrated that 45% of mothers were now breastfeeding at six weeks. Data collection continued during the entire pilot period and at the end of that time, a decision was made to adopt the practice change with minor revisions.

The nurse wrote up new guidelines for supporting the breastfeeding mother. The guidelines were widely circulated. Several inservice sessions were planned to educate staff about the new guidelines. Finally, a plan was detailed for periodic monitoring of outcomes related to breastfeeding rates.

CRITICAL APPRAISAL

Promoting Evidence-Based Practice

Is a plan for research utilization in place?

For nurses interested in promoting the use of research findings in practice, one of the most difficult aspects is determining how to create an environment receptive to change. Implementing evidence-based practice quite literally means change and this is often difficult to incite in the institutional setting. In many systems, the rewards for maintaining the "way we always do things" is a powerful deterrent to initiating new and more efficient patient care approaches.

The nurse who is committed to promoting care that is evidence-based, however, can consider relatively simple strategies that will help create a milieu that values use of research findings. These strategies might include posting a well-done research report in the nurses' lounge or offering to review the literature on a particular patient problem and preparing a poster board that details the findings and subsequent suggestions for patient care. The nurse could suggest that the unit or facility initiate a journal club to meet on a regular basis to critique a study on a topic of common interest. Research grand rounds could be held for a variety of purposes: to allow nurses a forum to dialogue about a particular research issue, for the review of research strategies for study of a particular problem, or for the presentation of new research findings.

The nurse might also suggest careful development (or redevelopment) of the evaluation tool for nurses' performance so that it clearly identifies research involvement as a valued activity. Participation in the writing of unit protocols and standards is also an invaluable means of moving research findings into practice. Another useful strategy is to request that the administration purchase clinical journals that regularly publish research findings that would be of interest in the clinical specialty. Having some easy-to-read journals accessible for the practicing nurse can assist staff in becoming knowledgeable about innovative findings.

Finally, the nurse might consider making an appointment with the institution's nurse researcher. Many facilities have a nurse researcher on staff who is available to meet with nurses about clinical problems in need of study, to assist in the development of a proposal, or to support other research activity. If the facility does not have a nurse researcher, consider contacting faculty at a local college or university. Many faculty are interested in ways to increase their participation in clinical research and such a merger can be of enormous value for both the clinician and the faculty researcher.

Although not an exhaustive list, the strategies listed here can be relatively easy to initiate and the impact profound. However, change does not have to be on a grand scale. Offering each patient care that is based on current research findings *is* the promotion of evidence-based practice. Each nurse has the ability to create change in the practice milieu by delivering care known to be clinically significant.

Critical Overview of Research and the Entry-Level Professional Nurse

Clear societal and professional expectations exist regarding the importance of the nurse's participation in research activities. Involvement can be in a variety of ways and levels but all research should essentially work to promote evidence-based practice. The nurse needs knowledge and skill to participate in the review of proposals and to participate in research activities important in patient care. Understanding what is required to do research and develop a proposal are key elements to successfully seeking and securing research monies offered through grant programs. Use of current study findings, as well as conducting new and innovative projects to address current health care problems, are important aspects in developing evidence-based practice. The practicing professional nurse is in an excellent position to create change that demonstrates quality care that is cost-effective.

CRITICAL OVERVIEW
RESEARCH AND THE ENTRY-LEVEL
PROFESSIONAL NURSE

Excerpt A

A group of nurses working on a labor and delivery unit are concerned about staffing patterns that do not allow for staff to stay with patients during active labor. They conduct a review of the literature and find several studies supporting the use of a doula. Labor is shorter, there is less use of analgesia, and patient satisfaction is improved, among other outcomes, when a doula was present.

Activity 1

- Suggest a study for replication where the sample could be labor and delivery nurses.

- Suggest three sources of potential funding for the study.

- Ask the nurse manager of a local labor and delivery unit for a copy of the unit's staff nurse evaluation tool. Review the tool for consistency with the research findings above.

- Detail three strategies that could be used to promote the use of the findings into clinical practice on labor and delivery units.

Excerpt B

A nurse working in an extended care facility is concerned that relatively few programs are available to involve patients in physical activity. She has spoken with the nursing supervisor about how to increase opportunities for physical activity for the elderly patients, but nothing has come of the discussion.

Activity 2

- Who might the nurse talk with to assist her in developing care plans that are evidence-based?

- Suggest strategies that could be useful in introducing change based on research.

- Suggest activities that would integrate and maintain the change in practice.

Excerpt C

A nurse works with women suffering from stress urinary incontinence. She has noted an increasing number of young women coming to the clinic and is interested in primary prevention strategies that could be taught to women.

Activity 3

- Select a model for research utilization (e.g., Rosswurm and Larrabee's model). Using the steps of the model, create a table to detail your plan for creating evidence-based change in practice.

References

American Nurses Association. (1985). *Human rights guidelines for nurses in clinical and other research*. Kansas City, MO: Author.

American Nurses Association Commission on Nursing Research. (1981). *Guidelines for the investigative function of nurses*. Kansas City, MO: American Nurses Association.

Bauer, D. G. & American Association of Colleges of Nursing. (1988). *The complete grants source book for nursing and health*. New York: Macmillan.

Hinshaw, A. S. (2000). Nursing knowledge for the 21st century: Opportunities and challenges. *Journal of Nursing Scholarship, 32*(2): 117–123.

Mallick, M. J. (1983). A constant comparative method for teaching research critiquing to the baccalaureate nursing students. *Image: The Journal of Nursing Scholarship, 15*(4): 120–123.

The Pink Sheet: Review and recommendations by a special review committee of the Division of Nursing. (1985). *Western Journal of Nursing Research, 7*(2): 244–248.

Rosswurm, M. A. & Larrabee, J. H. (1999). A model for change to evidence-based practice. *Journal of Nursing Scholarship, 31*(4): 317–322.

Sexton, D. L. (1982). Developing skills in grant writing. *Nursing Outlook, 30*(1): 31–38.

Spruck, M. (1980). Teaching research at the undergraduate level. *Nursing Research*, 29(4): 257–261.

Thomas, B. & Price, M. (1980). Research preparation in baccalaureate nursing education. *Nursing Research*, 29(4): 259–261.

Tornquist, E. M. & Funk, S. G. (1990). How to write a research grant proposal. *Image: The Journal of Nursing Scholarship*, 22(4): 44–51.

Appendices

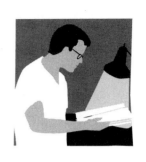

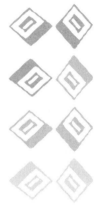

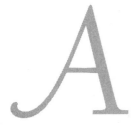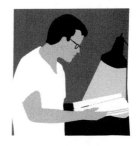

A

Elements of Critical Appraisal

Chapter 1: Evolution of a Body of Nursing Knowledge

- Does the researcher describe how the study relates to the development of the art and science of nursing?
- Does the discovered knowledge seek to contribute to understanding the patient and the health experience?
- Does the researcher answer a research question, as well as generate new questions for nursing study?
- Is the investigation consistent with the purpose and aim of nursing research?
- Does the researcher link the study to other related studies?
- Is the way the researcher discovers new knowledge appropriate to nursing concerns?
- Does the research support the development of scientific, ethical, esthetic, or personal knowledge?

- Does the researcher identify how the four major concepts for nursing study (person, environment, health, and nursing) articulate with the project under investigation?
- Does the research project focus on studying an area of concern to nursing?
- Does the research report appear in a journal that is refereed?

Chapter 2: Promoting Evidence-Based Nursing Practice

- Has a researchable problem relevant to nursing been identified?
- Does the investigation examine a problem that is related to phenomena of nursing concern?
- Can the consumer systematically appraise the research report?
- Are judgments made regarding the strengths and weaknesses of the report?
- Has a plan for studying the problem been clearly identified and executed?
- Does the researcher virtually duplicate a study that has already been completed?
- Does the replicator of the research make suggestions for improving generalizability?
- Does the researcher inform the data collector about the full nature of the project, including the impact of participation on research participants?
- Are the reports that are reviewed clearly identified?
- Are the criteria for selecting and evaluating the reports described?
- Is the level of evidence (I through III) identified and a rationale provided?
- Are the criteria specified in the guidelines clearly stated in the review of the research reports?
- Are relevant studies identified for analysis?
- At what level are the studies done?
- What is the strength of association when relevant study findings are considered altogether?

◈ Chapter 3: Initiating a Study

- If there are problems with the findings of the study, are they due to misunderstandings regarding the feasibility of the research?
- Does the purpose describe why the study was designed?
- Does the purpose reflect how results will be used?
- Is the purpose clearly specified?
- In the review of a databased article, is the area under study related to national or professional priorities?
- Is a clear benefit to nursing theoretically or practically apparent?
- Is the research designed to make predictions about phenomena under study, with no attention given to direct application?
- Is the research designed to have an immediate impact on nursing care?
- What kind of information is presented: Descriptive? Explanatory? Predictive?
- What is the knowledge base in a particular area?
- What is the proposed use for the findings of the investigation?
- Is a clear conceptual model (framework) described in the study?
- Are the major concepts of the model identified and defined?
- Are the relationships among concepts within the model described?
- Is the conceptual model relevant to nursing research?
- Does the conceptual model presented make logical sense?
- Are the concepts under study clearly identified and defined?
- Does the selected model best explain the phenomena under study?
- Is the model discussed as it relates to nursing's four key concepts (human, environment, health, and nursing)?
- Does the theory clearly describe a notion, explain an idea, or predict what might be observed?
- Is the purpose for using selected theories stated?
- Is the theory useful to nursing practice, education, and research?

- Are the propositions in the theory clearly identifiable?
- Does the researcher state the relevance of the propositions?
- Is the theorem to be tested clearly stated?
- Are the concepts defined in terms of their relationship to other concepts?
- Are the variables clearly defined?
- Are the constructs directly or indirectly observable?
- Are the variables defined in a specific manner?
- Are the variables measurable?
- Is the stated measurement of the variables logical?
- Is the researcher using inductive or deductive reasoning?
- If an inductive approach is identified, is there an appropriate theory that could be used?
- If a deductive approach is identified, is it appropriate to the task at hand?
- Are the topic and concept of interest clearly identified?
- Is the relationship between concept and topic of interest readily apparent?
- Is the focus of the study clear?
- Is the choice of focus logical?
- Is the choice of focus consistent throughout the research report?

Chapter 4: Review of the Literature

- Has an in-depth review been conducted (how many publications)?
- Has an evaluation of the prior research been presented along with the results?
- Are the criteria for evaluating each publication clearly identified?
- How recent are the identified publications?
- Have primary sources been used?
- Is the literature review comprehensive?
- Are all sides of the issue presented?

- Has the methodology of the studies been presented in the description?
- Has the evidence presented been evaluated in relation to design and method?

Chapter 5: Protecting Research Participants

- Has the researcher identified the necessity for using a population that is at increased risk (or vulnerability) for harm or injury?
- Could the researcher have used a less vulnerable population and still have gained the same knowledge?
- Does the researcher clearly describe the type of risk or harm to which the participant is particularly vulnerable?
- Have emotional, physical, spiritual, economic, social, and legal risks been assessed?
- Does the researcher indicate whether informed consent was obtained?
- Does the researcher outline how informed consent was obtained?
- Is the method used to obtain informed consent appropriate for the developmental and situational needs of the participant?
- Has the researcher informed participants of their rights to anonymity and confidentiality?
- Have steps been taken to protect the individual's privacy, anonymity, and confidentiality?
- Have data been reported so that the participants' anonymity is protected?
- Have data results been discussed only as they relate to the study's purpose?
- Has the investigator informed potential participants of their right to leave the study at any time?
- Has the investigator informed participants that withdrawal from the study will not affect them negatively?
- Does the researcher use every possible means of protecting the participant from deception?

- Does the research project seem straightforward; that is, is there no hidden agenda in the study's purpose?
- If full disclosure is not possible, is the participant so informed?
- If full disclosure is not given prior to the study, does the researcher describe plans for doing so?
- Have appropriate agencies been consulted for review of the research proposal, and have measures been taken to protect participants?
- Does the researcher identify how informed consent procedures were carried out?

Chapter 6: Measurement

- Is the level of data (nominal, ordinal, interval, ratio) appropriate given the focus of the study?
- How valid and reliable are the instruments used in the study?

Chapter 7: Quantitative Designs in Research

- Is there a comparison between or among groups?
- Is there equivalence between or among groups?
- Is there manipulation of the independent variable?
- Are extraneous variables controlled to the greatest extent possible?
- If a control group is lacking, how might that omission have affected the results?
- If participants were not randomly assigned to an experimental and control group, how might the omission of that process have affected the results?
- Are the findings inappropriately generalized to the larger population?
- Do the study findings provide information that can be useful in further examination of the particular area of interest?
- Are controls applied to the study to the greatest extent possible?

- Does the research problem and design require the formation of a hypothesis or hypotheses?
- Are hypotheses clearly and succinctly stated?
- Is the independent variable adequately specified?
- Is the dependent variable adequately specified?
- Does the operational definition specify the method for measuring the variable?
- Are the extraneous variables identified or taken into account in the design of the study?
- If a random sampling was used, has the process been described?
- Are there any factors related to the process that may have caused the sample to be biased (nonrepresentative of the larger group)?
- Are generalizations made that are not warranted given the sampling procedure used?

Chapter 8: Epidemiologic Research

- Is the study focused on a particular health care issue within a specified population?
- Are the characteristics of the population clearly described?
- Are desired health care outcomes evident?
- Are the studies that were included in the meta-analysis clearly identified?
- Is there clear discussion on why studies were included in the analysis?
- Were the individual study findings similar to the findings from the meta-analysis?
- Does the weight of the evidence from the meta-analysis lead to the conclusion that there is cause-and-effect association?
- If causation is implied in a report, have several criteria been met?
- Are multiple causes considered?
- What evidence supports the notion that a particular factor poses a risk?

- Have ratios, rates, and proportions been correctly calculated?
- Do the calculations provide useful information?
- Is the confidence interval interpreted as the frequency with which the population mean lies between the stated limits?
- Are all confounding variables taken into account?
- Is there any evidence of bias in relation to the methods used?

Chapter 9: Data Analysis

- Are the mean, median, and mode calculated correctly?
- If the mean, median, and mode are calculated correctly, are the findings expressed accurately or are conclusions drawn that are not warranted?
- Are the measures used—mean, median, and mode— appropriate to the purpose of the study?
- Are the range, interquartile range, variance, and standard deviation calculated correctly?
- Is the measure that is used appropriate to the kind of variables being examined?
- Is it logical to assume that the characteristic under study is normally distributed within the population?
- Does the interpretation of the correlation seem to under- or overrepresent the relationship?
- Might other variables (not identified) be affecting the outcome?
- Is causation erroneously implied?
- Are the results of the study expressed in terms of probability?
- Is the level of probability specified?
- Is the level of significance reported?
- Are findings reported that are not significant?
- Are appropriate conclusions drawn given the significant differences found?
- Is the correct form of the t-test—dependent versus independent—being used?
- Is the use of a comparison between means (t-test) appropriate considering the data that have been collected?

- Is ANOVA used rather than multiple *t*-tests when a comparison of more than two means is required?
- Are post hoc comparisons used only if a significant difference has been found using ANOVA?
- Are the independent and dependent variables readily identifiable?
- Is the difference between the findings with regard to main effects versus interaction effects adequately explained?
- Is the covariate clearly identified?
- Might additional covariates be examined?
- If randomization is not used, are results interpreted with that factor in mind?
- Are more than one independent and more than one dependent variable used?

Chapter 10: Qualitative Designs in Research

- Does the researcher identify a research question that seeks to explore, describe, or expand knowledge about how reality is experienced?
- Is the research question one that has received relatively little research attention?
- Has the topic only been addressed in a quantitative fashion although valuable information could be gained by conducting a qualitative investigation?
- Does the researcher clearly state the purpose for the qualitative study?
- Does the nurse researcher study the phenomenon from the perspective of the participant?
- Does the researcher discuss a willingness to study the experience form the participant's viewpoint?
- Does the nurse investigator engage in the research process as an active participant?
- Does the researcher conduct the study in the natural setting?
- Is the researcher intimately involved in the data collection process?

- Does the researcher attempt to establish validity and reliability of sources?

- Does the researcher relate the study to current or future events?

- Is the social situation or event under study clearly identified by the researcher?

- Does the researcher attempt to develop a theory about the social situation that is based on a combination of observation and literature review?

- Are comparison groups utilized to maximize credibility of the theory?

- Does the researcher discuss preparation for gathering data, including how research participants and study sites were determined?

- Are the sources of data utilized in the study appropriate to the method?

- Is the level of participant observation clearly identified by the researcher?

- Is the level of research participation appropriate to the focus of the study and the needs of the research participants?

- Does the researcher express a willingness to fully record data about the phenomenon under study?

- Are the opinions, feelings, and thoughts of the researcher about the research topic and process addressed?

- Does the researcher discuss how much time the data collection took and how the data were recorded?

- Does the researcher discuss feelings, thoughts, and attitudes about the study and subsequent means of structuring the study to incorporate those biases?

Chapter 11: Analyzing the Data in Qualitative Research

- Does the researcher discuss how the data were initially reviewed?

- Has a systematic literature review been conducted after the data were collected (where appropriate)?

- Is the literature review appropriate to the research question?

- Are the importance of patterns and the interrelationships made clear?
- Does the researcher discuss the overall implications of the research findings?
- Is the stated qualitative design a logical selection and appropriate to answer the stated research question?
- Does the design fit the nature of the phenomenon under study?
- Does the researcher address issues related to scientific rigor: credibility, transferability, dependability, and confirmability?

Chapter 12: Reviewing the Research Findings

- Is the title clear?
- If axes are used, are they labeled?
- Do the data collected fit the graph selected?
- Is the table appropriately labeled?
- Does the table convey the desired information in a clear, simple fashion?
- Are the variables under study clearly designated?
- Are the groups from which data were collected identified?
- Is adequate information presented relating to the statistical test used?
- Does the interpretation of the results fit with other components of the study, i.e., problem statement, literature review, design, etc.?
- Is each hypothesis (if made) addressed?
- Are the study's limitations discussed?

Chapter 13: Evaluating Research Reports

- Does the evaluation of the research report detail how well the research process was executed?
- Is the credibility of findings addressed?
- Does the reviewer discuss the overall value of the report's findings?

- Has a systematic review of the research available on a particular topic been conducted?
- Is the research-based knowledge relevant to the problem?
- Is there evidence that a practice change would be beneficial?

Chapter 14: Communicating Study Results

- Does the researcher discuss key elements of the research report: the research problem, the methodology for solving the problem, the results, and the meaning of the findings?
- Does the researcher clearly identify how the study results relate to nursing practice?
- Does the researcher present the project to the most appropriate target audience?
- Does the researcher present the research report in a clear, understandable, exciting fashion?
- Does the researcher follow guidelines for presenting the report and make the presentation organized and logical?
- Does the title of the research report identify the major study variables and the population under investigation?
- Is the research abstract clearly written, highlighting the major features of the investigation?
- Are references current, relevant, and complete?
- Does the researcher have appropriate professional, educational, and research experience to support participation in the study?

Chapter 15: Research and the Entry-Level Professional Nurse

- Does the research report describe the proposal development phase of the project?
- Does the proposal realistically detail costs of conducting the research?
- Is the topic likely to be funded?
- Is at least one category of grant funding likely to be interested in the research proposal?
- Is a plan for research utilization in place?

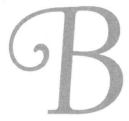

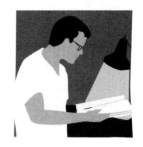

Format for Evaluation of the Quantitative Research Report

Directions: Following is a list of the key components that need to be evaluated in conducting a research critique. Rate each component based on the critical appraisal elements developed for each area. Critical appraisal elements can be found in Appendix A under the respective chapter numbers. Support your rating by making a suggestion for improvement of the component (where appropriate). Describe how the component rating might affect the reader, the conduct, the design, or the findings of the study.

Rating Key:
1 = weak or absent
2 = appropriate
3 = strong   Evaluator's Name _____

Critical Appraisal Elements	Components	Rating
13, 14	**Title:**	1 2 3
	Suggested Improvement: _____	
	Potential Impact on Reader: _____	
	_____	
	_____	
14	**Abstract:**	1 2 3
	Suggested Improvement: _____	
	Potential Impact on Reader: _____	
	_____	
	_____	
14	**Author Credentials:**	1 2 3
	Suggested Improvement: _____	
	Potential Impact on Conduct of Study: ___	
	_____	
	_____	
14	**Style/Organization:**	1 2 3
	Suggested Improvement: _____	
	Potential Impact on Reader: _____	
	_____	
	_____	

Critical Appraisal Elements	Components	Rating
3	**Purpose of Study:**	1 2 3
	Suggested Improvement: _____	
	Potential Impact on Design of Study: _____	
	_____	
	_____	
3, 7	**Problem/Hypothesis Under Study:**	1 2 3
	Suggested Improvement: _____	
	Potential Impact on Conduct of Study: ___	
	_____	
	_____	
3	**Theoretical Framework:**	1 2 3
	Suggested Improvement: _____	
	Potential Impact on Findings: _____	
	_____	
	_____	
4	**Literature Review:**	1 2 3
	Suggested Improvement: _____	
	Potential Impact on Conduct of Study: ___	
	_____	
	_____	

Critical Appraisal Elements	Components	Rating
7	**Research Design/Methods:**	1 2 3
	Suggested Improvement: _____	
	Potential Impact on Findings: _____	
	_____	
	_____	
6	**Data Collection Measures:**	1 2 3
	Suggested Improvement: _____	
	Potential Impact on Findings: _____	
	_____	
	_____	
5, 7	**Sample:**	1 2 3
	Suggested Improvement: _____	
	Potential Impact on Findings: _____	
	_____	
	_____	
8, 9, 12	**Analysis of the Data:**	1 2 3
	Suggested Improvement: _____	
	Potential Impact on Findings: _____	
	_____	
	_____	

Critical Appraisal Elements	Components	Rating
12	**Findings/Summary of Study:**	1 2 3
	Suggested Improvement: _____	
	Potential Impact on Findings: _____	
	_____	
	_____	
12, 14	**Suggestions for Use of Findings:**	1 2 3
	Suggested Improvement: _____	
	Potential Impact on Findings: _____	
	_____	
	_____	

Summative Evaluation

Strengths: _____
_____
_____
_____

Weaknesses: _____
_____
_____
_____

Overall Comments: _____
_____
_____
_____
_____

497

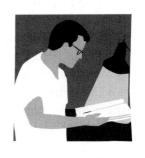

Format for Evaluation of the Qualitative Research Report

Directions: Following is a list of the key components that need to be evaluated in conducting a research critique. Rate each component based on the critical appraisal elements developed for each area. Critical appraisal elements can be found in Appendix A under the respective chapter numbers. Support your rating by making a suggestion for improvement of the component (where appropriate). Describe how the component rating might affect the reader, the conduct, the design, or the findings of the study.

Rating Key:
1 = weak or absent
2 = appropriate
3 = strong   Evaluator's Name _____

Critical Appraisal Elements	Components	Rating
12, 14	**Title:**	1 2 3
	Suggested Improvement: _____	
	Potential Impact on Reader: _____	
	_____	
	_____	
14	**Abstract:**	1 2 3
	Suggested Improvement: _____	
	Potential Impact on Reader: _____	
	_____	
	_____	

Critical Appraisal Elements	Components	Rating
14	**Author Credentials:**	1 2 3
	Suggested Improvement: _____	
	Potential Impact on Conduct of Study: ____	
	_____	
	_____	
14	**Style/Organization:**	1 2 3
	Suggested Improvement: _____	
	Potential Impact on Reader: _____	
	_____	
	_____	
3, 10	**Purpose:**	1 2 3
	Suggested Improvement: _____	
	Potential Impact on Design of Study: _____	
	_____	
	_____	
3, 10	**Problem for Study:**	1 2 3
	Suggested Improvement: _____	
	Potential Impact on Conduct of Study: ____	
	_____	
	_____	

Critical Appraisal Elements	Components	Rating
5, 7, 10	**Sample:**	1 2 3
	Suggested Improvement: _____	
	Potential Impact on Findings: _____	
	_____	
	_____	
10	**Mcasures for Collecting Data:**	1 2 3
	Suggested Improvement: _____	
	Potential Impact on Findings: _____	
	_____	
	_____	
10	**Procedures for Data Collection Method:**	1 2 3
	Suggested Improvement: _____	
	Potential Impact on Findings: _____	
	_____	
	_____	
10	**Procedures of Data Collection: Time/Length of Study:**	1 2 3
	Suggested Improvement: _____	
	Potential Impact on Findings: _____	
	_____	
	_____	

502

Critical Appraisal Elements	Components	Rating
10	**Procedures for Data Collection: Nature/Number of Participants/Settings:**	1 2 3
	Suggested Improvement: _____	
	Potential Impact on Findings: _____	
	_____	
	_____	
10	**Procedures for Data Collection: Subject Involvement:**	1 2 3
	Suggested Improvement: _____	
	Potential Impact on Findings: _____	
	_____	
	_____	
10, 11	**Procedures for Data Collection: Researcher's Feelings:**	1 2 3
	Suggested Improvement: _____	
	Potential Impact on Findings: _____	
	_____	
	_____	
3, 10	**Procedures for Data Collection: Researcher-Participant Relationship:**	1 2 3
	Suggested Improvement: _____	
	Potential Impact on Findings: _____	
	_____	
	_____	

Critical Appraisal Elements	Components	Rating
10, 11	**Procedures for Data Collection: Checking for Bias:**	1 2 3
	Suggested Improvement: _____	
	Potential Impact on Findings: _____	
	_____	
	_____	
10, 11	**Procedures for Data Collection: Organizing/Categorizing/Summarizing:**	1 2 3
	Suggested Improvement: _____	
	Potential Impact on Findings: _____	
	_____	
	_____	
10, 11	**Scientific Adequacy: Credibility/Transferability/Dependability/ Confirmability:**	1 2 3
	Suggested Improvement: _____	
	Potential Impact on Findings: _____	
	_____	
	_____	
10, 11	**Results of the Data Gathered:**	1 2 3
	Suggested Improvement: _____	
	Potential Impact on Findings: _____	
	_____	
	_____	

Critical Appraisal Elements	Components	Rating
10, 12	**Discussion for Use of Findings:**	1 2 3
	Suggested Improvement: _____	
	Potential Impact on Findings: _____	
	_____	
	_____	
12, 14	**Suggestions for Use of Findings:**	1 2 3
	Suggested Improvement: _____	
	Potential Impact on Findings: _____	
	_____	
	_____	

Summative Evaluation

Strengths: _____

_____

_____

_____

Weaknesses: _____

_____

_____

_____

Overall Comments: _____

_____

_____

_____

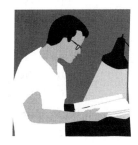

Glossary

Aim of nursing research The aim of nursing research is the identification and understanding of knowledge relevant to the patient and the experience of health.

Aim of research evaluation The aim of research evaluation is to determine how well the research process has been executed, as well as the credibility and value of the research findings.

Analysis of covariance (ANCOVA) ANCOVA is an inferential statistical test that enables investigators to adjust statistically for group differences that may interfere with obtaining results that relate specifically to the effects of the independent variable(s) on the dependent variable(s).

Analyzing the data Data analysis in qualitative inquiry involves careful examination of recorded data to discover apparent patterns, themes, or relationships.

Anonymity Anonymity refers to the act of keeping participants nameless in relation to their participation in a research project.

Anthropological research Anthropological study involves the collection and analysis of data about an individual or a group under natural conditions. The investigator is immersed in the study process in an effort to fully understand the behavior and the subsequent impact on society.

Applied research Applied research is designed to produce findings that can be used to remediate or modify a given situation.

Axiom Axioms are statements that link the concepts of a theory. The links or relationships between concepts are assumed to be true.

Background and credentials of the researcher The background and credentials of the researcher are the professional, educational, and research experiences that qualify the investigator to conduct the research.

Basic research Basic research seeks to gain knowledge for its own sake and therefore does not specify an application of the findings.

Bias Bias is a feeling or influence that strongly favors the outcome of a particular finding in a research project. When the chance of bias in a project is not addressed, the reliability of the scientific findings is considered to be highly questionable.

Borrowed models Borrowed models are conceptual models taken from scientific disciplines outside of nursing that are thought to provide a better explanation of what we see in nursing and a more relevant explanation of how the world operates.

Boundaries for nursing study Boundaries for nursing study have been identified as the body of knowledge formed by the interrelationship of the concepts of individual (person), environment, health, and nursing.

Call for abstracts A call for abstracts is a general announcement seeking research reports for presentation at a pre-planned research conference.

Causation Within the epidemiological framework, causation refers to the degree to which it can be suggested that a particular cause or set of causes leads to a particular outcome.

Cohort A cohort relates to epidemiologic research and refers to a group of individuals who share a common attribute, such as age or a specific diagnosis.

Computer search A computer search of the literature involves the use of a computer to search a prescribed number and kind of journals to provide a list of references that relate to a specific topic.

Concept Concepts are imaginary, abstract pictures or mental images formed from real-world observations of things, objects, or events that an individual has experienced.

Conceptual model A conceptual model provides organization for thinking, observing, and interpreting what is seen; gives direction to the search for identifying a question to ask about the phenomena; and points out solutions to problems.

Confidence intervals Confidence intervals are a statistical method of describing data.

Confidentiality Confidentiality refers to the researcher's responsibility to protect all data gathered within the scope of the project from being divulged to others.

Confounding variables Confounding variables are variables that can inappropriately influence the outcome of a study.

Construct A construct reflects the specific, potentially observable characteristics of a concept and thus facilitates testing of the idea.

Correlation Correlation as it applies to research refers to the tendency of a variation in one variable to be related to a variation in another variable. Correlational research examines these relationships. A correlation coefficient describes the relationship.

Data collector in research Acting as a data collector in a research project involves participation in gathering data relevant to the problem under investigation.

Debriefing Debriefing refers to the process of providing participants with information about the study that had previously been withheld to protect the validity of the research. Debriefing also refers to sharing the results of the study with all participants prior to publication or public presentation.

Deception Deception involves a failure to adequately inform potential research participants about the full nature of the research, thereby preventing them from making an informed decision on their participation.

Deductive reasoning Deductive reasoning is a method of thinking that begins with a general statement of belief and moves to obtain specific observations. Reasoning moves from the general to the specific.

Dependent variable The dependent variable represents the area of interest under investigation. It reflects the effect of or the response to the independent variable.

Descriptive research Descriptive research is present-oriented. It attempts to describe what exists. Variables are not deliberately manipulated, nor is the setting controlled. The analysis of data often leads to the formation of hypotheses that can then be tested experimentally.

Ethnographic research Ethnographic research is a method of conducting inquiry into the life process by studying individuals, artifacts, or documents in the natural setting. It includes both anthropological and historical forms of inquiry.

Extraneous variable Extraneous variables are those variables that can influence the relationship between the independent and dependent variable and must be controlled through statistical analysis or research design.

Factorial analysis of variance Factorial analysis of variance is an inferential statistical test that enables investigators to analyze data in which there is more than one independent variable and two or more groups within the independent variable.

Feasibility Feasibility refers to the ease (or conversely the difficulty) of completing a study.

Grantsmanship Grantsmanship is the ability to obtain funding to aid in the support of research activities.

Graphs A graph in the context of research is a visual display that conveys information about the topic of study. Graphs are generally used to describe the data collected in a given research project.

Grounded theory research methodology Grounded theory methodology is a means of studying social data for the purpose of explaining some phenomenon. A theory is ultimately generated through inductive and deductive activity.

Historical research Historical research involves the careful study and analysis of data about past events. The purpose is to gain a clearer understanding of the impact of the past on present and future events related to the life process.

Hypothesis formation A hypothesis is a tentative statement that suggests a relationship between two or more phenomena. The proposed relationship provides a focus for the study.

Importance of study The importance of the study to nursing is related to national priorities, local needs, and researcher interest. In terms of funding, clinical studies are more likely to receive support than educational projects.

Incidence Incidence is a mathematical reflection of the number of cases of a health problem in a given population.

Independent variable The independent variable (often referred to in an experimental or quasi-experimental study as the experimental or treatment variable) is an antecedent to other variables. In an experiment or quasi-experiment, it is the variable that is manipulated, and its effect on the dependent variable is observed.

Inductive reasoning Inductive reasoning involves the collection of observations related to a particular event. From these observations a theory or general explanation regarding the event can evolve. Reasoning moves from the specific to the general.

Informed consent Informed consent is the process of providing an individual with sufficient understandable information regarding his or her participation in a research project. It includes providing potential participants with information about their rights and responsibilities within the project and documenting the nature of the agreement.

Initial search of the literature The initial search of the literature is a cursory examination of available publications related to the major variables under study. This review is related to the area of interest and is conducted to assist the investigator in making decisions about proceeding with a given research idea.

Institutional review board (IRB) The IRB is a committee established by each agency (institution) for the express purpose of evaluating all research conducted in that facility. The IRB is concerned with the protection of human rights and evaluates research proposals in accordance with federal guidelines.

Instrument An instrument is a device used to measure the concept of interest in a research project. An instrument may be a paper-and-pencil test, a structured interview, or a piece of equipment.

Interval level of measurement Interval measurement refers to the third level of measurement in relation to the complexity of statistical techniques that can be used to analyze data. Variables within this level of measurement are assessed incrementally, and the increments are equal. A wide range of statistical techniques can be used to analyze interval variables.

Kind of investigation The kind of investigation used refers to (1) the type of information desired, (2) the present knowledge base in the topic area, and (3) the proposed use of information derived from conducting the study.

Level of significance The level of significance (or alpha level) is determined in order to identify the probability that the differences between groups have occurred by chance rather than in response to the manipulation of variables.

Literature review The literature review is a systematic review of the available literature sources about the phenomenon under study. In qualitative research methods, a full review is generally withheld until after the data have been collected.

Manual search A manual search of the literature requires the investigator to examine each of the mechanisms in the library-card catalog, indexes, abstracts, and references associated with specific articles for references relevant to the topic of interest.

Measures of central tendency Measures of central tendency—the mean, median, and mode—are calculated to identify the average, the most typical, or the most common values, respectively, among the data collected.

Measures of variance   The range, variance, and standard deviation are measures of the variation or dispersion among data. The range describes the difference between the largest and the smallest observations made; the variance and standard deviation are based on the average difference or deviation of observations from the mean.

Meta-analysis   Meta-analysis is a technique in which the findings from several small clinical trials are analyzed together. Although the findings from each study alone may not be powerful enough to allow for decisions affecting clinical practice, when analyzed together, the findings may be much more powerful.

Multivariate analysis   Multivariate analysis refers to a group of inferential statistical tests that enable the investigator to examine multiple variables simultaneously. Unlike other inferential statistical techniques, these tests permit the investigator to examine several dependent or independent variables simultaneously.

Nominal level of measurement   The nominal level of measurement is the most primitive method of classifying information. Nominal implies that categories of people, events, and other phenomena are named, are exhaustive in nature, and are mutually exclusive. These categories are discrete and noncontinuous.

Nonexperimental   Nonexperimental research is generally present-oriented. It attempts to describe what exists. Variables are not deliberately manipulated, nor is the setting controlled. The analysis of data often leads to the formation of hypotheses that can then be tested experimentally.

Nonprobability sampling   Nonprobability sampling is a selection process in which the probability that any one individual may be selected is not equal to the probability that another individual may be chosen. The probability of inclusion and the degree to which the sample represents the population are unknown.

Normal distribution   The normal distribution is a mathematical construct that suggests that naturally occurring observations follow a given pattern. The pattern is the normal curve, which places most observations at the mean and a lesser number of observations at either extreme.

Null hypothesis   The null hypothesis is a statistical statement that there is no difference between the groups of events or observations under study. Inferential statistics are used in an effort to reject the null, thereby showing that a difference does exist.

Nursing research   Nursing research is the application of scientific inquiry to the phenomena of concern to nursing: clients (individual/family/community) and their health experience.

Nursing science   Nursing science is the body of knowledge unique to the discipline of nursing. It is the discovery of information that explains, describes, and predicts relationships about the individual and his or her health experience.

One-way analysis of variance (ANOVA)   One-way analysis of variance is an inferential statistical test that enables investigators to examine differences when more than two means are involved. The reporting of the results includes the df, F value, and probability level.

Operational definition   An operational definition assigns meaning to a variable and describes the activities required to measure it.

Ordinal level of measurement   The ordinal level of measurement is another means of classifying information. Ordinal implies that the values of variables can be rank-ordered from highest to lowest.

Paradox of nursing research   The paradox of nursing research is the dual nature of research: the attempt to answer a question and the attempt to generate further questions for study.

Participant observation   Participant observation is a method of researcher interaction with the participants. The researcher deliberately strives to become involved in the experience under study to facilitate fuller understanding.

Participants at risk   Subjects at risk are individuals who may be harmed physically, emotionally, spiritually, economically, socially, or legally through participation in a research study.

Phenomenological research approach Phenomenology is a branch of philosophy that emphasizes the subjectivity of human experience. When used as the philosophical basis in research, phenomenology mandates that scientific data be generated by studying the desired information from the perspective of the research participant.

Population The population is the entire group of persons or objects that is of interest to the investigator. The population is designated by specific criteria such as age, gender, and illness state.

Population health Research in this area looks at why some people are healthy and others are not healthy. This type of study seeks to understand the determinants of health and to improve the health of populations.

Prevalence Prevalence is the population level of various diseases, risk factors, and exposures.

Probability In inferential statistics, probability refers to the likelihood that the differences between the groups under study are the result of chance.

Problem-solving process The problem-solving process is the practical determination of a solution to an immediate problem.

Problem statement The problem statement presents the topic under study, provides a rationale for the choice of topic, represents a synthesis of fact and theory, and directs the selection of the design.

Proportions Proportions, along with ratios and rates, are mathematical means for representing relationships of important variables related to population issues.

Proposition A proposition is a statement that suggests a specific relationship between two or more concepts. A proposition may take the form of an axiom or a theorem.

Purpose of nursing research The purpose of nursing research is to develop a unique body of nursing knowledge for the eventual improvement of the nursing care that patients receive.

Purpose of qualitative research Qualitative research seeks to explore, describe, or expand knowledge about how reality is experienced.

Purpose of the study The purpose of a study describes why the study has been designed. The purpose reflects the intent of the investigator and the use of the knowledge derived.

Qualitative research Qualitative research is an inductive approach to discovering or expanding knowledge. It requires the involvement of the researcher in the identification of the meaning or relevance of a particular phenomenon to the individual. Analysis and interpretation of findings in this method are not generally dependent on the quantification of observations.

Quantitative research Quantitative research is an approach to structuring knowledge by determining how much of a given behavior, characteristic, or phenomenon is present. Quantitative research methods are particularly concerned with objectivity and the ability to generalize findings to others.

Quasi-experimental design Quasi-experimental designs require the manipulation of the independent variable but may lack randomization to the control group or may not have a control group.

Random sampling Random sampling is a selection process that ensures each participant the same probability of being selected. Random sampling is the best method for ensuring that a sample is representative of the larger population.

Rates Rates are numerical representations of data collected by epidemiologists. They describe population parameters of interest and assist with the determination of risk and causation.

Ratio level of measurement The ratio level of measurement is the fourth and least primitive method of classifying information. Ratio implies that the variables reflect the characteristics of ordinal and interval measurement and can also be compared by ratios; that is, the number representing a given variable can be compared by describing it as two or three times another number or as one-third, one-quarter, and so on. The ratio level of measurement, unlike the other three levels, has an absolute zero.

Ratios Ratio is a more generic term than rate. All rates are ratios but not all ratios are necessarily rates. Ratios do not relate to a particular time. Ratios are the number of events that meet a set of criteria divided by the number of events that meet a different criterion. For example, the sex ratio is the number of liveborn males divided by the number of liveborn females.

Recording the data Recording data in qualitative inquiry involves the full documentation of data from all sources identified for inclusion in the study. It requires a willingness to totally experience the data prior to making a decision about the meaning of the information.

Refereed journal A refereed journal submits manuscripts to a review process using a panel of experts to determine the quality of the work.

Reliability Reliability is a characteristic of an instrument that reflects the degree to which the instrument provokes consistent responses. Three characteristics of reliability that are commonly evaluated are:

Stability (test-retest): Degree of consistency when individuals respond to an instrument on two separate occasions.

Internal consistency: A reflection of the degree to which all subparts of an instrument measure the same characteristic.

Equivalence: Degree of agreement when different observers are assessing the same characteristic.

Replicator of research Replicating research involves the repetition of a research investigation that has been conducted previously.

Research abstract The research abstract is a 300-400-word synopsis of the research investigation. It is designed to provide the consumer with sufficient information to decide whether additional time needs to be spent on the report.

Research consumer The research consumer determines the quality and merit of a given research report through systematic review and critique.

Research critique The research critique is the process of summarizing the key aspects of a research report, and then determining the quality and merit of the study based on predetermined criteria.

517

Research designer and producer   The process of designing and producing research involves the identification of a relevant problem for nursing study, as well as a clear plan for carrying out a relevant research design.

Research expertise   The researcher's expertise is a product of formal learning and practical experience. Qualitative in nature, the range of expertise varies from a sophisticated approach to the evaluation of specific studies, to a basic knowledge of the concepts necessary to conduct a simple investigation.

Research process   The research process is the examination and analysis of systematically gathered facts about a particular problem. The aim of the research process is the discovery or validation of knowledge.

Research proposal   The research proposal is a formal means of presenting the scientific merits of a study to others. It details the problem under study, how it will be solved, how participants will be protected, and cost considerations for the project.

Research report   The research report is a means of communicating key aspects of the study to the research consumer.

Research report title   The title of the research report is a brief phrase that indicates the major study variables and the population under investigation.

Research review   A research review is the summarization of the key points and characteristics of a research report.

Research utilization   Research utilization is the process of transferring research knowledge into practice, thus facilitating an innovative change in practice or the verification of existing practice protocols.

Review of the literature   A review of the literature is a comprehensive description as well as an evaluation of prior efforts to investigate a given topic.

Risk   Risk within the framework of epidemiology refers to the possibility of developing a health problem.

Risk-benefit ratio   A risk-benefit ratio represents the possible risk of harm in relation to possible benefits that may be incurred by an individual who participates in a given research project.

Sample   The sample is a subset of the population selected by the investigator to participate in a research project.

Sampling error   Sampling error refers to the discrepancies that inevitably occur when a small group (sample) is selected to represent the characteristics of a larger group (population).

Scholarly publications   Scholarly publications are the documents that serve to communicate to other professionals the methods and achievements produced through academic study and research investigation.

Scientific adequacy in qualitative designs   Scientific adequacy is the trustworthiness of research findings from qualitative methods. Attention to issues of credibility, transferability, dependability, and confirmability are necessary to avoid threats to the credibility of findings and ensure scientific rigor.

Scientific inquiry   Scientific inquiry is the process of critically analyzing the data that are systematically gathered about a particular phenomenon.

Secondary search of the literature   The secondary search of the literature involves an in-depth, critically evaluated search of all publications relevant to the topic of interest.

Self-determination   Self-determination is the right of the individual to decide what will happen in his or her life, as well as in which activities to become involved.

Sources of data   Sources of data in qualitative research are the individuals, documents, or artifacts used to collect data about a particular phenomenon. Sources vary with the focus of inquiry, the purpose of the investigation, and the specific approach to the research.

_t_-Test   A t-test is an inferential statistical technique used to compare the means of two groups. The reporting of the results of a _t_-test generally includes the _df, t_ value, and probability level.

Theorem   A theorem is a statement that designates a relationship between concepts that are deduced from relationships already formed by axioms.

Theory   A theory is composed of specific concepts and propositions that attempt to account for a particular notion that is observed in the real world. Theory assumes that a particular conceptual model is utilized. The purpose of using theory is to describe a notion, to explain an idea, or to predict what might be observed.

True experiment   A true experiment is a research design that is characterized by a comparison among groups that are as equal as possible, the manipulation of an independent variable, the use of inferential statistics, and stringent control of extraneous variables.

Unique body of nursing knowledge   A unique body of nursing knowledge represents the knowing, experiencing, and understanding of the phenomena related to providing nursing care to patients.

Validity of an instrument   Validity describes the usefulness of an instrument given the context in which it is applied. It reflects how well an instrument has measured what it was supposed to measure given a particular set of circumstances. The following kinds of validity are frequently assessed in trying to make a judgment about a given instrument:

Content: All important areas of concern are reflected.

Predictive: Events are accurately predicted.

Concurrent: Accurate differences are shown in the present.

Construct: The attribute of interest is actually being measured.

Variable   A variable is a concept (construct) that has been so specifically defined that precise observations, and therefore measurement, can be accomplished.

Ways of knowing   Ways of knowing are the variety of modes available through which to find new knowledge. They include intuition, problem solving, practical experience, and scientific inquiry.

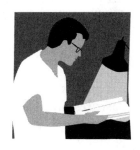

Index

Abstracts, 447-449
  call for, 440-441
  example critique of, 420-421
Abuse of participants, 161-162
Accidental sampling, 249
Accuracy of measurement, 194, 195
Adaptation model (Roy), 97, 97-98, 99, 100
Advances in Nursing Science, 26
Aim of nursing research, 15-16
Alpha level, 303-306
American Academy of Nursing, 310
American Journal of Maternal Child Nursing, 27-28
American Nurses Association (ANA), 30, 162, 462
  cabinet on nursing research, 16-17
  guidelines for research roles, 463-464
American Nurses Foundation, 30, 469

Analysis of covariance (ANCOVA), 315-317
Analysis of data. *See* Data analysis
Analysis of variance (ANOVA), 309-315
  definition, 310
  factorial, 278, 312-315
ANCOVA (analysis of covariance), 315-317
Animals used in research, 190
Annual Review of Nursing Scan in Research: Application for Clinical Practice, 424
Anonymity of research participants, 160, 171, 175, 176-181
  definition, 176
  protecting, 177-180
ANOVA. *See* Analysis of variance
Anthropology, 338-339, 349
Applied Nursing Research, 26
Applied research, 90-92
  vs. basic, 88

Art of nursing, 8-10
Attributable risk (AR), 270
Axiom, 108, 109, 110-111
    definition, 109-110

Bar graphs, 280, 281, 381-382
Basic research, 88-90
    vs. applied, 88
Baxter, 469
Bell curve, 289
Bias, 72, 263
    definition, 354
    in qualitative research, 340,
        354-356, 373, 416-417
    sampling, 272-274
    selection, 252
Biologic gradient, 72
Biologic plausibility, 72
Borrowed models, 102-105
    definition, 103
Boundaries of professional study,
    96, 96-97
Bowlby, John, 142
Bradford-Hill Criteria, 71-73,
    263, 264
Brown Report, 6

Care, evidence-based. *See* Evidence-based practice
Case-control studies, 258, 270
Causation, epidemiological, 261-262.
    See also Cause-and-effect
    relationships
Cause-and-effect relationships, 73-75, 223, 226, 233, 262-264
Center for Nursing Research, 30

Central tendency, measures of,
    280-287
    definition, 282
Children, as participants, 174.
    See also Populations, vulnerable
Chi-square tests, 278, 320
CINAHL, 146
Cluster sampling, 248
Codes, identification, 178-179
Cohort studies, 258-259
Commerce Business Daily, 469
Communicating research findings.
    See Research report
*Complete Grants Source Book for
    Nursing and Health*, 470
Computer resources for literature
    review, 145-146, 369-370
Computer-assisted data analysis,
    317-318
    and Ethnograph, 369-370
Concepts
    abstract nature of, 100-102
    choosing as research topic,
        121-125
    definition, 102
    key, in nursing, 96-97, 103,
        105
    relationships between, 125
    specifying, 112-113
    within a conceptual model,
        111-112
    within a theory, 111-112,
        114, 115, 116
Conceptual maps, 126
Conceptual models, 96-100
    definition, 96-97

in nursing, 97-100
Concurrent validity, 211, 211-212, 213, 214
Confidence intervals, 272, 273-274
Confidentiality of research participants, 160, 171, 175-176, 176-178
   definition, 175
   protecting, 177-180
Confirmability, 371, 373
Confounding variables, 72, 233, 242
Consent form, example, 171-172
Consent, informed, 160, 168-173, 187
   definition, 169
   methods of recording, 170
   obtaining, 174-175
Consistency, 72
Construct validity, 211, 212, 213, 214
Constructs, 113-114, 114, 115-116
Consumer of research, 49-52, 110, 114, 123, 130, 240
   communicating results to, 380, 388
   and credentials of investigator, 450
   definition, 50-51
   as evaluator, 52, 104-105, 399-400, 419
   and facilitating use of reports, 446
   and interpretation of results, 391

and literature review, 143
and problem statement, 120-121
and references, 449
and use of abstracts, 447, 447-448
See also Nurse; Nurse researcher, roles; Utilization of research findings
Content validity, 211, 213
Control group, 223, 226, 227, 307
   in quasi-experimental designs, 230, 231
Controlled experiments, 95
Controls
   experimental, 93-94, 94
   in nonexperimental research, 234
Convenience sampling, 249, 393
Correlation, 292-298, 319
Correlation coefficient, 215, 217
Correlational designs, 232, 234
Covariance, 278
Covariance, analysis of (ANCOVA), 315-317
Credentials, of research investigator
   example of critique of, 420
Credibility, 371, 372, 373, 374
Criterion-referenced measurement, 207, 208
Critical incident technique, 232
Critique, 64
   constructive purpose of, 54, 56

Critique *(continued)*
  definition, 54
  framework for, 56-58
  guidelines, 56, 57-58, 402-403, 404
  and mapping the report, 403, 405
  of qualitative report, example, 411-419
  of quantitative report, example, 405-411
  vs. review, 52, 53
  See also Evaluation of research reports
Cross-over designs, 258
Cross-sectional studies, 258
Cumulative Index to Nursing and Allied Health Literature (CINAHL), 146
CURN model, 422

Data analysis
  computer assisted, 317-318, 369-370
  example of critique of methods, 409-410, 418-419
  qualitative, 336, 336-337, 341-342, 345-346, 364-366
  See also Statistics, inferential; Statistics, descriptive
Data collection
  example of critique of methods, 409, 414-417
  instruments for, 206-209
  and nurse, 62-63
Data, sources of, 346-349
Debriefing of participants, 160, 184-185, 372

Deception of research participants, 160, 182-183, 182-184
Deductive reasoning, 110-111, 117-118, 120, 343, 344
Degrees of freedom (df), 306-307, 310
Delphi Survey of Clinical Research Priorities, 16
Dependability, in qualitative research, 371, 372, 373
Descartes, Rene, 13-14
Descriptive research, 93, 95, 232. *See also* Nonexperimental designs
Descriptive statistics, 280-297
Df (degrees of freedom), 310
Directory of Research Grants, 469

Ecological research designs, 258
Education, nursing, 6-7
Epidemiologists, 260
Epidemiology
  concepts in, 272-274
  definition, 274
  and health care policy, 257
Equivalence, as measure of reliability, 217
Errors
  of measurement, 209-210, 299
  sampling, 299-302
  Type I, 304-305
  Type II, 304-305
Ethical considerations, 462
  See also Participants, protecting
Ethnograph (computer program), 369-370

Ethnographic research, 327, 337-343
Evaluation of research reports
aim of, 400-402
basic considerations, 419-421
format and preparation of report, 421-422
levels of evidence in, 70-76
for use in practice, 64
See also Critique; Qualitative research, evaluation of; Quantitative research, evaluation of; Research report
Evaluation research, 91, 93
Evidence-based practice, 40, 64, 76-77
benefits of, 76
promoting, 471-474
See also Utilization of research findings
Evidence-based recommendations, making, 73-76
Evidence, categorizing, 64, 66, 69, 71
and Bradford-Hill criteria, 71-73
by level, 70-71, 73-75, 76, 77
Experiment, the, 222-227
definition, 226
Experimental designs, 222-229, 238-239
reviewing, 227
Experimental group, 226, 227, 307
in quasi-experimental designs, 230, 231
Experimental mortality, as extraneous variable, 251, 253

Experimental research, 93-94, 258
Explanatory research, 93, 94, 95, 106, 223, 232
Exploratory studies, 232
Extraneous variables, 242, 251-254
controlling for, 226, 242-243
and internal validity, 251-253
Exxon, 469

F value, 310
F.A.A.N., 30
Factorial analysis of variance, 278, 312-315
Feasibility of research, 82-83, 195
Fellow of the American Academy of Nursing, 30
Findings, presenting, 380-390
Flawed studies, value of, 435
Foundation Grants to Individuals, 469
Frameworks. *See* Conceptual models
Frequency polygons, 280, 383
Freud, Sigmund, 138-139, 142
Funding, 84-85, 86, 162-163
sources of, 469
See also grantsmanship

Generalizability, 19, 60, 61, 194, 232, 394
See also Validity, external
Goldmark Report, 6
Grants Register, 469
Grantsmanship, 468-471. *See also* Funding
Graphs, 380-388
Grounded theory, 327
methodology, 343-346

Guidelines for conducting research
  federal, 162-164
  professional, 161-162, 463

Health Care Finances Administration, 469
Hierarchy of Needs (Maslow), 142
Helsinki Declaration, 162
HIH Guide for Grants and Contracts, 469
Histograms, 280, 281, 383-384, 384
Historical research, 95, 327, 339-343, 366
  definition, 339
  reliability and validity of sources, 340-341
History, as extraneous variable, 251, 252, 254
Holism, 19, 327
Horn Video Productions model for research
  utilization, 422
Hotelling's T^2, 318
Human rights and self-determination, 168-169.
  See also Participants, rights of
Human Rights Guidelines for Nurses in Clinical Research (American Nurses Association), 162, 163
Humanism, 327
Hypotheses, 106, 231
Hypothesis formation, 235-236
Hypothesis, null, 301-303

Identification codes, 177-179

Incidence, as measure of morbidity, 268
Index Medicus, 146
Inductive reasoning, 118-120, 328, 343, 344
Inferential statistics, 298-321
Informed consent, 160, 168-173, 187
  definition, 169
  methods of recording, 170
  obtaining, 174-175
Institutional review boards (IRBs), 163-164
  role of, 185-187
Instruments of measurement, 206-209
  definition, 207
  reliability of, 215-219
  validity of, 211-215
Internal consistency, 216-217, 219
International Nursing Index, 146
Interquartile range, 285, 288
Interval level of measurement, 194, 195, 201-204, 278, 285, 306
  definition, 202
Interval sampling, 250
Intuition, use of, 12, 116, 335, 364
Investigation, kinds of, 92-95
IRBs (Institutional Review Boards), 163-164, 185-187
  composition of, 185-186
  nurses' role on, 186
  role of, 185-187

Johnson's behavioral systems model, 99

Journal of Nursing Scholarship, 31
Journals, 26-31
  in literature review, 146, 149
  refereed, 28-30
  relevance of, 139

Kellogg Foundation, 469
Kendall's tau, 297
King's open systems model, 99, 405
Knowing, ways of, 12
Knowledge, nursing, dissemination of, 27.
  See also Nursing practice, evidence-based; Utilization of research findings

Leading of respondents, 336
Level of significance, 303-306
Levels of measurement, 219, 220, 278
  interval, 194, 195, 201-204, 278
  nominal, 194, 195, 196-198, 278
  ordinal, 194, 195, 198-201, 278
  ratio, 194, 195, 204-206, 278
Literature review, 137-157, 232
  and clinical opinion, 142
  computer-assisted, 144-148
  critical overview of, 154-157
  critique of example, 408
  definition, 147
  example of, 152-153

identifying publications for, 144-149
initial search, 139-141
keeping record of, 149-151, 232
manual, 148-149, 368-369
of qualitative research, 368-370
secondary search, 141-144
writing, 152, 153-154
Literature, primary vs. secondary sources, 142
Lived experience, researching. *See* Qualitative research
Logic, 12.
  See also Inductive reasoning, Deductive reasoning

MANCOVA, 317-319
Manipulation of variables, 223, 224, 230, 237, 238-239
MANOVA (multivariate analysis of variance), 317-319
Mapping the research report, 403, 405
Maps, conceptual, 126
Maslow, Abraham, 103, 103-104
  Hierarchy of Needs, 142
Maturation, as extraneous variable, 251, 252, 254
Mean, 279, 282, 300
  and normal curve, 290.
  See also Central tendency
Measurement
  choosing strategy for, 194-195
  errors of, 209-210, 299
  levels of, 194, 219, 220, 299

Measurement *(continued)*
    methods of, 206-220
    norm-referenced, 207
    theory of, 207
Median, 279, 282.
    See also Central tendency
Medical Literature Analysis and
    Retrieval System
    (MEDLARS), 145-146, 147
MEDLINE, 146, 147
Meta-analysis, 72, 263, 265-266
Methodological studies, 258
Minors, as participants, 174
    See also Populations, vulnerable
Mode, 279, 282.
    See also Central tendency
Models
    borrowed, 102-105
    nursing, 96-100, 104, 105
Morbidity, concept in epidemiology, 268
Mortality, experimental, 251, 253, 254
Mulidisciplinary research, 461, 462-463
Multivariate analysis, 278, 317-319

National Center for Health Services Research, 469
National Center for Nursing Research, 16-17, 31, 82
National Center for Nursing Scholarship, 31
National Institute for Nursing Research, 31, 86, 87
National Institutes of Health, 469

National Laboratory of Medicine, 146
National League for Nursing, guidelines for research roles, 463
National Library of Medicine, 146
Naturalistic research, 328
Nazis, 161
Neuman's systems model, 99
Newman-Keuls test, 311
Nightingale, Florence, 6
    Notes on Nursing, 5
Nominal level of measurement, 194, 196-198, 278
    definition, 196
Nonexperimental designs, 231-234, 234
Nonparametric tests, 306, 320
Nonprobability sampling, 249-251
Normal curve, 301
Normal distribution, 289-292
    definition, 291
Normative data, 194
Notes on Nursing (Nightingale), 5
Null hypothesis, 301-303, 310
    definition, 302
Nuremberg Code, 161
Nurse
    as advocate for research participant, 62-63
    associate degree. *See* Nurse, entry-level
    baccalaureate degree. *See* Nurse, entry-level
    considerations for research participation of, 462-463
    as data collector, 62-63

as research designer, 58-59
role as consumer of research, 49-52
role in promoting utilization of research findings, 473-474
Nurse researcher
responsibilities of, 436-437
role as data collector, 62-63
role as replicator, 60-61
role as research designer, 58-60
role as research producer, 58-60
role in IRBs, 186
role in protection of participants, 187-190
role in research review committee, 186
staff, 427
Nurse, entry-level, 468
research responsibilities of, 399-400, 463-464, 475-477
Nursing
art of, 8-10
boundaries of professional study, 23-25, 96-97
conceptual models in, 96-100, 104, 105, 416
education, 6-7, 463
holistic philosophy of, 327
Nursing knowledge
body of, 10-12
development of, 18
evolution of, 33-34
structuring, 22-23
Nursing practice

evidence-based, 40, 76, 428, 459-460
implications of research for, 395-396, 453
Nursing profession
expectations for, 460-465
image of, 341-342
Nursing research
definition, 5-6, 46-48
future of, 32-33
history of, 5, 6-7
paradox of, 14-15
priorities for, 15-17
promotion of, 30-32
purpose of, 15-17
roles in, 49, 62-63
value of, 4-5
vs. research in nursing, 46-48
Nursing Research, 7, 26, 174
Nursing science, 32
definition, 5
Nursing shortage, 87
Nursing Studies Index, 7
Nursing theory, 32

Observational research, 258
Office of Human Developmental Services, 469
Oncology Nursing Forum, 27-28
Oncology Nursing Society, 87
One-way analysis of variance (ANOVA), 309-312
definition, 310
Operationalization, 240-242. *See also* Constructs; Variables, defining
Opinion, expert, 93, 137-138

Ordinal level of measurement, 194, 195, 198-201, 278, 285
definition, 200
Orem's self-care model, 97, 98

P values, 279-280, 305-306
See also Probability
Paradox of nursing research, 14-15
Parametric tests, 306
Parse's man-living-health nursing model, 416
Parsons, Talcott, 102
Participant abuse, 161-162
Participant observation, 349-352
Participants, research
abuse of, 161-162
animals as, 190
at risk, 164-168
debriefing, 63
nurse as advocate for, 62-63
protection of, 160-161, 164, 187-190
rights of, 159-160
selection of, 334-335
vulnerable, 166-168
withdrawal from study, 160, 171, 181-182
Paterson and Zderad's humanistic nursing model, 416
Pearson coefficient, 294-296, 397
Peplau, Hildegard, 7, 8
Peplau's interpersonal relations model, 99
Pew Charitable Trust, 469
Phenomenological research, 327-328, 332-337, 353

method, critique of example, 414
Philosophical research, 327
Physics, 96
Pictorial displays, 380-390
Pie diagrams, 280, 281, 384-385
Pink sheet, 470
Population
definition, 245
Population health, 258, 259, 260-261
Population under study, 129-130
Populations, vulnerable, 166-168
Positivism, 222
Posttest, 228
Predictive studies, 94, 95, 106, 223
Predictive validity, 211, 213
Pretest-posttest, 227, 228, 228-229
Prevalence, as measure of morbidity, 268, 269
Probability, 280, 298, 298-301, 302
Probability sampling, 244-245
Problem statements, 120-121, 131
critique of examples, 407, 413
and study focus, 127
Problem-solving process, 40-43
definition, 42
Proportion, 270, 271-272
Proposals for research, 465-468
Propositions, 108-109, 111, 115-116
definition, 108.
See also Axiom; Theorem
Psychology, 96

and borrowed conceptual
models, 103-104
Publications, scholarly, 25-28
definition, 25
Purpose of nursing research, 15-17
and study focus, 127, 130
Purpose statement of research
study
critique of example, 413
Purposive sampling, 249, 372
P-values, 306

Qualitative research, 19, 20-22,
46, 64, 94
analysis of data, 336, 336-
337, 341-342, 345-346,
364-366
definition, 327-329
evaluation of, 64, 67-69, 411-
419
interpreting results, 390-394
maintaining objectivity, 352,
352-353
purpose of, 327-328, 330-332
themes in, 365, 369
vs. quantitative, 326-329,
330
Qualitative research designs
anthropological, 338-339
development of, 326-327
ethnographic, 337-343
grounded theory, 343-346
historical, 338, 339-343
phenomenological, 332-337
and recording data, 352-354,
357
and recording for bias, 354-
356, 356, 357

scientific adequacy of, 371-
374
and sources of data, 346-352,
356
vs. quantitative, 222, 364
Qualitative research, critique of
framework and example,
411-419
Quantitative research, 19-21, 46,
64, 94
critique of report, 405, 411
definition, 20
evaluation of, 64, 65-66, 405-
411
vs. qualitative, 326-329, 330.
See also Statistics, inferential;
Statistics, descriptive
Quantitative research designs,
221-255
critique of example, 408-409
experimental, 222-229
and hypothesis formation,
235-236
nonexperimental, 231-234
quasi-experimental, 229-231
and sampling, 244-251
and validity, 251-255
variables in, 236-244
vs. qualitative, 222, 364
Quasi-experimental designs, 229-
231, 238-239
Quota sampling, 249

Random sampling, 245-249
Randomization, 223, 224, 226,
230, 231
purpose of, 229
Randomized controlled trials, 258

Range, of variables, 285
Rates and ratios, 269-271
Ratio level of measurement, 194,
    195, 204-206, 285, 306
    definition, 205
Ratio, risk-benefit, 164
Raw scores, 290
Ray's adaptation model, 420
Reasoning, scientific, 116-120
Refereed journals, 28-30
Regression analysis, 278, 309
Regression toward the mean, 252
Relative odds (RO), 270
Reliability, 32, 194, 392
    of historical research sources,
        340-341
    of instruments, 215-219, 219
    measures of, in qualitative
        research, 371-373
Reliability of instrument
    and equivalence, 215
    and internal consistency, 215
    and stability, 215
Replication of results, 60-61
Research
    applied, 84, 90-92
    basic, 84, 88-90
    disagreement on interpreta-
        tion of, 391-393
    elements of process, 55-56
    experimental, 258
    explanatory, 232
    exploratory, 232
    guidelines for conducting,
        160-164, 161-164
    historical, 95
    initiating a study, 130-132
    interprofessional, 461, 462-
        463

observational, 258
process of, 43-45
proposals, 465-468
purpose of, 84-86
review of, 52-54
utilization of. See Utilization
Research-based care. See Evi-
    dence-based practice
Research consumer, 49-52
    definition, 50
Research critique, 53-58
    definition, 54. See also
        Critique
Research designer
    nurse as, 58-59
Research designs, 58-60
    qualitative. See Qualitative
        research designs
    quantitative. See Quantita-
        tive research designs
Research evaluation. See Evalua-
    tion of research reports
Research findings, use of, 92-95.
    See also Utilization of
        research findings
Research in Nursing and Health,
    26
Research in nursing vs. nursing
    research, 46-48
Research journals, 26-31
Research methods, qualitative.
    See Qualitative research
        designs
Research process, 43-45
    definition, 44
    and study focus, 126-129.
    See also Problem-solving
        process
Research proposals, 465-468

definition, 466
Research report
definition, 434
elements of, 437-439
evaluation of. *See* Evaluation of research reports
implementation of findings. *See* Utilization
and investigator's credentials, 420, 450-453
and nursing practice, 436-437, 453
in oral form, 442, 443-444
presentation of, 444-445, 445-446
references, 449-450
target audience, 439-440, 441
title of, 420, 446-447
and undesirable outcomes, 435-436
in written form, 442-443. *See also* Critique
Research review committee
nurse's role in, 186
role of, 185-187
Research topic. *See* Topic, research; Topic selection
Research, nursing
definition, 46
roles in, 49
Research, qualitative. *See* Qualitative research
Research, quantitative. *See* Quantitative research
Review vs. critique, 52, 53
Review committees
role of, 160. *See also* Institutional Review Boards

Review of literature. *See* Literature review
Risk, 263, 266-267
relative, 270
Risk-benefit ratio, 164, 394
RO (relative odds), 270
Robert Wood Johnson Foundation, 469
Rogers, Martha, 12-13
Roy's adaptation model, 97, 97-98, 99, 100, 436
RR (relative risk), 265, 270

Sample selection methods, 244-251
example of critique, 409, 413-414
Sample, definition, 245
Samples, dependent and independent, 307
Sampling
accidental, 249
bias, 250-251
convenience, 393
error, 299-302
interval, 250
nonprobability, 249-251
probability, 244-245
purposive, 249, 372
quota, 249
systematic, 250
Sampling, random, 245-249
simple, 246-247
stratified, 247-248
Scales of measurement. *See* Measurement, levels of
Scheffe's test, 311
Scholarly publications, 25-27
Science of nursing, 5, 7-10, 32

Scientific adequacy, 371-374
  evaluation, in example, 417-418
Scientific inquiry, 12
  definition, 13-14
Scientific reasoning, 116-120
SD (standard deviation), 279
Selection bias, 251, 252, 254
Self-actualization, 103-104
Self-care model (Orem), 97, 98
Self-determination, and human rights, 168-169
Sick role (Parsons), 102
Sigma Theta Tau International, 31, 32, 469
Simple random sampling, 246-247
Sociology, 96, 349
Spearman rho, 297
Specificity, 72
Standard deviation (SD), 279, 300, 301
  calculation of, 285-287
  and normal curve, 290
Standard error, 300-302, 306
Standard scores, 290
Statistical analysis, 195, 397
Statistical estimates, 272
Statistical regression, 251, 252, 254
Statistical significance, 303-306
Statistics, descriptive, 279-297
  and correlation, 292-298
  and measurement of variation, 284-289
  and measures of central tendency, 280, 282-284
  and normal distribution, 289-292
  pictorial displays in, 280-281

Statistics, inferential, 224, 279, 298-321
  and analysis of covariance, 315-318
  chi square test, 320
  and factorial analysis, 312-315
  and multivariate analysis, 318-319
  null hypothesis in, 301-303, 304
  and one-way analysis, 309-312
  and probability, 298-300
  and sampling error (standard error), 300-301
  and statistical significance, 303-306
  and statistical tests, 306-321
  t-tests, 307-309
Stetler model for the utilization of research, 422
Stratified random sampling, 247-248
Strength of association, 72
Subjects, research. See Participants
Systematic sampling, 250
Systems model for change related to clinical research, 422

Tables, 380, 388-390
Temporality, 72
Testing, as extraneous variable, 251, 252, 254
Test-retest, 215, 215-216, 217
Themes, in qualitative research, 369
  example, 417, 418

Theorem, 108, 110-111
  definition, 110
Theoretical framework. *See* Concepts; Conceptual models
Theory, 105-107
  compared to conceptual model, 105-106, 111-112
  definition, 106
  and development of propositions. *See* Axioms; Theorems
  of measurement, 207
  nursing, 32
Title, of research report
  example critique of, 420
Topic selection
  and feasibility, 81-84, 92-93, 130
  and funding, 84-85, 86-88, 131
  and statement of purpose, 84-86
Topic, research
  and focus of the study, 127
  specifying, 121-125
Transferability, 371, 372, 373. *See also* Validity, external
Treatment group, 223
Treatment, withholding, 161. *See also* Abuse of participants
Triangulation, 347-348
T-test, 278, 306-309
Tukey's HSD test, 311
Type I and II errors, 304-305

Utilization of research findings, 400, 422-426, 453
  definition, 423
  example, 425-426

models for, 400

Validity, 32, 194, 392
  content, 211
  external, 19, 60, 210-211, 253, 272, 371-374. *See also* Generalizability
  of historical research sources, 340-341
  of instruments, 211-215, 219
  of instruments, assessing, 214-215
  internal, 210-211, 251-255, 272, 371-374
  measures of, in qualitative research, 371-373
  in qualitative research, 353
  and research design, 251-253
Variables
  cause-and-effect relationships between, 73-75
  confounding, 72, 233, 242, 263, 273-274, 315
  defining of, 114-116, 240-242
  dependent, 224, 236-240
  experimental, 238
  extraneous, 225, 242, 242-244
  identifying, 236
  independent, 224, 236-240
  manipulation of, 223, 224, 225, 230, 231, 237, 298
  measurement of. *See* Measurement
  operationalizing, 240-242
  treatment, 238
Variance
  analysis of, 278, 309-319

Variance *(continued)*
    calculation of, 285-286
    measures of, 285-289

Webster's II New College Dictionary, 8
Western Interstate Commission for Higher Education (WICHE), 422

Western Journal of Nursing Research, 26
Wholism, 19, 327
WICHE (Western Interstate Commission for Higher Education), 422
Withdrawal of participants, 181-182